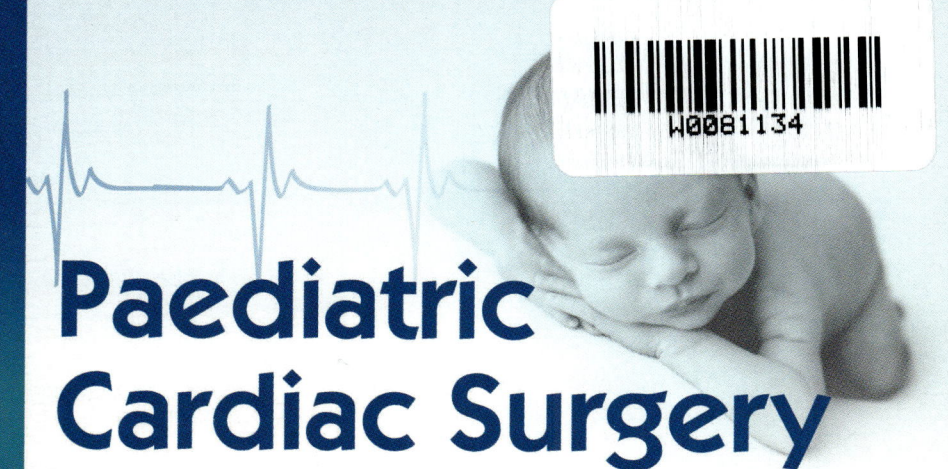

# Paediatric Cardiac Surgery

## Manual for Perioperative Nurses

*Contributors*

**Hani Najm** MD, MSc, FACC
Chairman, Paediatric and Congenital
Heart Surgery at Cleveland Clinic,
King Saud University,
Riyadh, Saudi Arabia

**Munir Ahmad** MD, BSc, FRCS
Cardiac Surgeon at National Guard Health Affairs
Royal College of Surgeons in Ireland,
Riyadh, Saudi Arabia

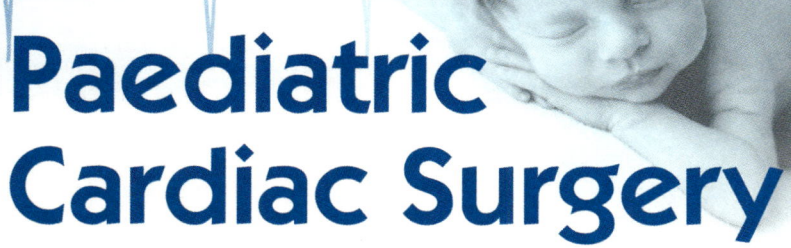

# Paediatric Cardiac Surgery

# Manual for Perioperative Nurses

**Edith D Jonkman** BSc, RN

Assistant Nurse Manager
Heart Vascular Institute
Perioperative Services
Cleveland Clinic
Abu Dhabi, UAE

**CBS**

## CBS Publishers & Distributors Pvt Ltd

New Delhi • Bengaluru • Chennai • Kochi • Kolkata • Mumbai
Bhubaneswar • Hyderabad • Jharkhand • Nagpur • Patna • Pune • Uttarakhand

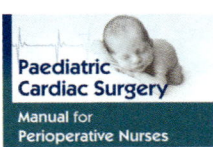

**ISBN:** 978-93-86827-93-7

Copyright © Author and Publisher

## First Edition: 2019

Published by Satish Kumar Jain and produced by Varun Jain for

**CBS Publishers & Distributors** Pvt Ltd

4819/XI Prahlad Street, 24 Ansari Road, Daryaganj, New Delhi 110 002, India.
Ph: 23289259, 23266861, 23266867          Website: www.cbspd.com
Fax: 011-23243014          e-mail: delhi@cbspd.com; cbspubs@airtelmail.in.
**Corporate Office:** 204 FIE, Industrial Area, Patparganj, Delhi 110 092
Ph: 4934 4934          Fax: 4934 4935          e-mail: publishing@cbspd.com;
publicity@cbspd.com

### Branches

- **Bengaluru:** Seema House 2975, 17th Cross, K.R. Road,
  Banasankari 2nd Stage, Bengaluru 560 070, Karnataka
  Ph: +91-80-26771678/79          Fax: +91-80-26771680          e-mail: bangalore@cbspd.com
- **Chennai:** 7, Subbaraya Street, Shenoy Nagar, Chennai 600 030, Tamil Nadu
  Ph: +91-44-26680620/26681266          Fax: +91-44-42032115          e-mail: chennai@cbspd.com
- **Kochi:** 42/1325, 1326, Power House Road, Opp KSEB, Power House,
  Ernakulam 682 018, Kochi, Kerala
  Ph: +91-484-4059061-65          Fax: +91-484-4059065          e-mail: kochi@cbspd.com
- **Kolkata:** 6/B, Ground Floor, Rameswar Shaw Road, Kolkata-700 014, West Bengal
  Ph: +91-33-22891126, 22891127, 22891128          e-mail: kolkata@cbspd.com
- **Mumbai:** 83-C, Dr E Moses Road, Worli, Mumbai-400018, Maharashtra
  Ph: +91-22-24902340/41          Fax: +91-22-24902342          e-mail: mumbai@cbspd.com

### Representatives

| | | | | | |
|---|---|---|---|---|---|
| • **Bhubaneswar** | 0-9911037372 | • **Hyderabad** | 0-9885175004 | • **Jharkhand** | 0-9811541605 |
| • **Nagpur** | 0-9021734563 | • **Patna** | 0-9334159340 | • **Pune** | 0-9623451994 |
| • **Uttarakhand** | 0-9716462459 | | | | |

*Printed at:* Nutech Print Services, Faridabad, India

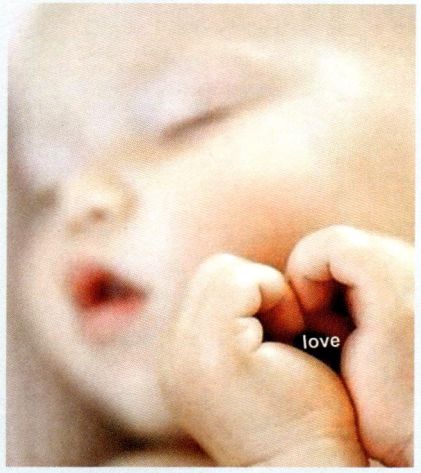

**Caring is the art of nursing**

# *Preface*

This book is a guide to the most common and some uncommon congenital heart disease and associated surgical interventions as practiced on newborns and children. It is the result of many years of clinical practice as a paediatric cardiac perioperative nurse and is designed to explain and reveal both the complex surgical procedures, the nature and variety of cardiac defects.

The text of this edition has been modified and refined through discussions with surgeons, consultant surgeons, anaesthesiologists, perfusionists, medical students, and nurses in the hospitals where I have worked.

The research and writing began at the King Faisal Hospital in Jeddah, Saudi Arabia, where I saw intense and complex surgical procedures being performed on infants with such skill and grace that I felt that new or re-skilling nurses in a paediatric context would benefit from seeing and reading about the deployment of such surgical ability.

I began taking notes, photographs and interviewing the surgeons, reading operative reports, and the information grew to an informal 'how-to-assist' manual; a way of being an expert paediatric cardiac nurse, able to anticipate the surgeon's needs through education and understanding.

I gradually added more procedures and illustrations and my Manual became in demand by not only nurses working in the cardiac operating theatres but also by medical students, perfusionists and anaesthesiologists.

This book, therefore, is the result of research and observation over many years of assisting in paediatric cardiac operations, and it aims to make complex surgical procedures more accessible to perioperative nurses. If it helps them be more responsive to surgeons and their tiny patients, where seconds saved are further chances of life, it will have succeeded.

The utmost care has been taken to confirm the accuracy of the information presented. However, in view of ongoing research in congenital heart disease and surgical treatment, approaches of individual cardiac surgeons may vary from the surgical procedures presented in the book.

This book is dedicated to the surgeons who carry out these complex and life-saving procedures, without whose expertise, many alive today would never have reached adolescence.

**Edith D Jonkman**

# *Acknowledgements*

First and foremost I would like to express my sincere gratitude to Robert Vance, academic editor, psycho-analyst and history writer, for editing the book and for his brilliant idea of adding 'Nursing Observations' throughout the book. I am deeply thankful for his encouragement, personal support and professional expertise.

A very special thank you to Dr. Hani Najm MD, Chairman, paediatric and adult cardiac surgeon at the National Guard Hospital, Riyadh, Kingdom of Saudi Arabia, whom I troubled on many occasions to let me take pictures while he was operating on complex cardiac procedures, and to whom I am forever grateful to let me take a rare picture of a native aortic valve during the 'Nikaidoh' operation, a procedure that was not previously performed in Saudi Arabia!

My deepest gratitude to Dr. Munir Ahmad MD, associate consultant paediatric and adult cardiac surgeon at the National Guard Hospital, Riyadh, Kingdom of Saudi Arabia, for reading the entire book and for writing the 'Surgeon's Comments', which in my opinion is the icing on the cake!

I would like to thank Dr. Ahmed Jamjoom MD, Chairman, paediatric and adult cardiac surgeon at the King Faisal Specialist Hospital and Research Centre—Gen. Org, Jeddah, Kingdom of Saudi Arabia, for always being demanding, which taught me that paying attention to detail with regards to surgeon's preferences, is fundamental to the best surgical outcomes of the patients. I can still hear him say: 'don't give me what I ask, give me what I need'.

I would also like to thank Dr. Ghassan Baslaim MD, paediatric and adult cardiac surgeon for teaching me the finer skills of assisting with complex paediatric cardiac surgery and forever emphasizing that keeping my eyes on the field, especially at crucial moments, was more important than being concerned with tidying surgical instruments, counts, and whatever else was going on in the operating theatre.

A very special thank to Dr. Mohamad Burhani MD, paediatric cardiac surgeon for believing in me and for his continuous support from wherever he worked around the globe!

Thank you Dr. Zohair Al-Halees MD, paediatric and adult cardiac surgeon at the King Faisal Specialist Hospital and Research Centre—Gen. Org, Riyadh, Kingdom of Saudi Arabia, for letting me take pictures of the 'Fontan' procedure, which displays this fascinating operation in colourful photos in the book.

A special thanks to Karen Clarke and her team from the SickKids Hospital, Toronto, Ontario, Canada, for inviting me and giving me an inside in the surgical care provided to paediatric cardiac patients in a North American health care setting as compared to an European and Middle Eastern health care setting.

Thank you Dr. Ahmad Omran MD, FACC, FESC, FASE. Consultant Cardiologist, Head of Non-Invasive Cardiology Laboratory. KAMC, National Guard Hospital, Riyadh, Kingdom of Saudi Arabia for reading Chapters 1 and 2 to confirm its accuracy, and for his encouragement.

A special thank you to Dr. Carlos Mestres, staff Physician, Consultant at the Department of Cardiac Thoracic and Vascular Surgery, Cleveland Clinic, Abu Dhabi, UAE.

My special thanks are due to Mr YN Arjuna (Senior Vice President Publishing, Editorial and Publicity); Mrs Ritu Chawla (AGM Production); Mr Neeraj Prasad, Mr Kshirod Kumar, Mr Parmod Kumar and Mrs Jyoti, for their skillful service and immense help in editing and figure work of the manuscript.

**Edith D Jonkman**

# Contents

*Preface*                                                                     *vii*

*Introduction*                                                                 *xv*

## 1. Congenital Heart Disease and its Risk Factors                             1

Introduction                                                                    1
Incidence and Causes                                                            3
Adverse Genetic Risk Factors                                                    3
Adverse Environmental Risk Factors                                             4
Congenital Heart Disease in More Detail                                         6
Foetal and Newborn Circulation and its Implications for
    Infants Born with Congenital Heart Disease            10
Diagnostic Tests                                                              15
Non-Genetic Risk Factors                                                      19
Summary of Treatment for Paediatric Congenital
    Heart Disease—Non Surgical Treatment                  24
Surgical Treatment                                                            26
Prognosis                                                                     27

## 2. Understanding Congenital Heart Disease Diagnosis and Classification       29

Diagnosis                                                                     29
Sequential Segmental Classification                                           30
Determining the Situs                                                         31
Identifying the Cardiac Position                                              32
Key Points of the Sequential Segmental Classification                        38

## 3. Nursing the Young Patient in Paediatric Cardiac Surgery                   47

Introduction                                                                  47
Preoperative Nursing Care                                                     47
Newborns and Infants                                                          48
Toddlers                                                                      49
Preschool Age                                                                 50
School Age                                                                    50
Adolescent                                                                    51
Nursing and Premedication                                                     52

## 4. Perioperative Nursing in the Cardiac Operating Room   54

| | |
|---|---|
| Introduction | 54 |
| Assisting the Surgeon | 54 |
| Positioning the Patient | 56 |
| Cardiopulmonary Bypass Preparation | 65 |
| Incision | 68 |
| Cannulation and Cardiopulmonary Bypass | 73 |
| Going on Bypass | 85 |
| Coming off the Bypass Machine | 87 |
| Sequence for Assisting the Surgeon with Placing a Child on Cardiopulmonary Bypass | 91 |
| Sequence for Assisting the Surgeon with Discontinuation of Cardiopulmonary Bypass | 95 |
| Effects of Cardiopulmonary Bypass on Neonates and Infants | 97 |
| Peritoneal Dialysis Catheter | 104 |
| Ultrafiltration and Modified Ultrafiltration | 104 |
| Cardioplegia and Hypothermia | 105 |
| Circulatory Arrest | 105 |
| Defibrillation Paddles | 106 |
| Pacing the Heart | 108 |
| Delayed Chest Closure | 112 |
| Extracorporeal Membrane Oxygenation (ECMO) | 112 |
| Emergency Chest Reopening in the Neonatal Intensive Care Unit | 115 |

## 5. Nurses' Overview of Paediatric Cardiac Anomalies, Surgical Procedures and Techniques for Congenital Heart Defects   117

| | |
|---|---|
| Introduction | 117 |

**Section 1: When Chambers and Valves are in Normal Sequence and Normal Position and Shunting is Predominant**   118

| | |
|---|---|
| Patent Ductus Arteriosus (PDA) | 121 |
| Patent Ductus Arteriosus Repair—Technique | 127 |
| Patent Foramen Ovale (PFO) | 132 |
| Atrial Septal Defect (ASD) | 135 |
| Atrial Septal Defect Repair—Technique | 144 |
| Ventricular Septal Defect (VSD) | 149 |
| Ventricular Septal Defect Repair—Technique | 157 |
| Atrioventricular Septal Defects (AVSDs) | 161 |

Common Types of Atrioventricular Septal Defects 164
Atrioventricular Septal Defect Repair—Technique 166

**Section 2: When Chambers and Valves are in Normal
Sequence and Normal Position and Stenosis or
Obstruction is Predominant** 169

Univentricular Heart 169
Blalock-Taussig Shunt, Glenn and Fontan Procedure 171
Blalock-Taussig Shunt Procedure—Technique 174
Glenn Shunt Procedure—Technique 178
Extracardiac Fontan Procedure—Technique 185
Tricuspid Valve Stenosis or Atresia (Obstructed or
    Absent Atrioventricular Connection) 193
Ebstein Anomaly 195
Pulmonary Valve Stenosis or Atresia (Obstructed or
    Absent Ventriculoarterial Connection) 198
Pulmonary Stenosis/Atresia with a Ventricular
    Septal Defect 203
Pulmonary Stenosis /Atresia with Intact Ventricular
    Septal Defect 209
Mitral Valve Stenosis or Atresia (Obstructed or Absent
    Atrioventricular Connection) 210
Aortic Valve Stenosis or Atresia and Subaortic Membrane
    (Obstructed or Absent Ventriculoarterial Connection) 210
Subaortic Membrane (SAM) 215
Ross Procedure—Technique 220
Bentall Procedure—Technique 234
David Procedure—Technique 236

**Section 3: When Chambers and Valves are not in Normal
Sequence and Normal Position—Atrioventricular
Discordance and Ventriculoarterial Discordance** 240

Double Inlet Left ventricle and Double Inlet Right Ventricle
    (Atrioventricular Discordance) 240
Congenitally Corrected Transposition of the Great Arteries
    (Atrioventricular and Ventriculoarterial Discordance) 244
Tetralogy of Fallot (Ventriculoarterial Discordance) 251
Tetralogy of Fallot Repair—Technique 256
Double Outlet Right Ventricle (Ventriculoarterial
    Discordance) 260
Double Outlet Left Ventricle (Ventriculoarterial
    Discordance) 265

Truncus Arteriosus (Ventriculoarterial Discordance) 266
Truncus Arteriosus Repair—Technique 271
Transposition of the Great Arteries (Ventriculoarterial
 Discordance) 277
Transposition of the Great Arteries Repair—Technique 283
Rastelli Procedure—Overview 290
Nikaidoh Operation—Technique 294
DKS Procedure—Technique 301

**Section 4: Anomalies of the Great Arteries (Anomalies
of the Pulmonary Artery and Aorta)** 302

Anomalous Origin of the Left Coronary Artery from the
 Pulmonary Artery 302
ALCAPA Repair—Technique 305

*Section 4.1: Anomalies of the Aorta* 311

Coarctation of the Aorta (CoA) 312
Coarctation of Aorta Repair—Technique 315
Interrupted Aortic Arch (IAA) 323
Aortopulmonary Window (APW) 329
Aortopulmonary Window Repair—Technique 331
Hypoplastic Left Heart Syndrome 332
Norwood Procedure—Technique 337

*Section 4.2: Anomalies of the Venous Connections
  Anomalies of Pulmonary Veins* 355

Partial and Total Anomalous Pulmonary Venous Return
 or Drainage (PAPVD, TAPVD) 355
PAPVD Repair—Technique 361
TAPVD (Supracardiac and Infracardiac) Repair—
 Technique 362
TAPVD (cardiac) Repair—Technique 363
Scimitar Syndrome 364
Repair of Scimitar Anomaly—Technique 365

**Section 5: Other Cardiac Anomalies** 367

Cor Triatriatum 367
Vascular Rings/Slings 368
Ectopia Cordis 372

*References* 373
*Index* 382

# *Introduction*

It has been said that nursing is both the art of caring and the application of science. In nursing, knowledge is the key to success and involves the mutual application of compassion and technology in the process of healing. In this book, I hope to show how both can assist in paediatric cardiac surgery, where focussed care and acute attention by both surgeon and nurse can mean the difference between life and death.

In the operating theatre where the patient is either newborn or in infancy, the caring attention of the nurse must shift from a therapeutic overall understanding of the patient's needs, to a focus on the needs of the surgeon and surgery, thereby saving precious minutes through anticipation and understanding of the surgical procedures involved. By understanding paediatric cardiac surgical needs, we, the nurses, can assist the surgeon more competently, more quickly and more efficiently.

Nursing is the first and foremost intimate physical contact with the patient and this is accentuated when the patient is in many cases, fragile and newborn. The infant patient however, cannot interact with the nurse and in paediatric cardiac surgery, it is usually the surgeon who has the closest contact. But through understanding the procedures, the nurse may become reconnected to the patient, resulting in a sense of relationship and empathic caring, creating a more alert attention to the tiny patient's needs. If the nurse cannot meet the emotional needs of the paediatric patient, she can certainly provide the technical resources that give the level of care that is needed. The procedures illustrated and explained in this book will help in that vital work.

The nurse in many ways is a physical resource for the surgeon and her job is to ensure that the equipment, from scalpels to cannulae, pieces of ready, appropriate and to hand. If caring is the hallmark of good nursing, understanding the technical demands of the procedures and sequence of the surgery, will give the nurse confidence and a feeling of active participation. Nurse/physician relationships can be challenging at times, especially during complicated heart surgery, where it sometimes

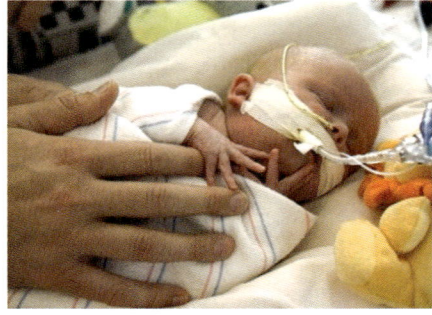

may seem that the surgeon's stress levels are so high that he/she takes it out on the surgical team, including the nurses, to relief some of his/her stress and displays inappropriate behaviour, which may result in fear of ever wanting to assist during surgery with this particular surgeon again!

Nurses can work towards improving working relationships with surgeons by staying up-to-date with advances in their specialty; nurses can take pride in their expertise. Continuing education, specialty certification, clinical research, and conferences are good ways to stay in touch with development in their field; 'knowledge is power'.

Improving communication with surgeons can be accomplished when nurses feel empowered to approach surgeons as equal professional colleagues. This means that nurses must assume responsibility for the quality of their relationships with surgeons. As perioperative nurses we cannot let negative behaviour by surgeons push us into angry communication, or discourage us, in the worst scenario, from assisting with surgery.

Through this book, I bring my twenty years of cardiac nursing experience to print for the benefit of all, so that through photographs, explanations and case samples, nurses can become familiar with the many presenting problems their careers may involve. It is a paradox that the tiniest patients can teach us all so much. Their intimate caring needs for surgical skill forces us to be compassionate, their minute suffering makes us aware how fragile and universal is humanity.

# Congenital Heart Disease and its Risk Factors

## INTRODUCTION

To begin with, **congenital** means *inborn* or *existing* at birth. Congenital heart disease (CHD) is more accurately a type of birth defect, where the heart and/or blood vessels near the heart, develop abnormally during the foetal stage. It is responsible for more deaths in the first year of life than any other birth defect.[1] In addition, many of these defects need to be carefully monitored and most require treatment. Not all of these days children reach adulthood, despite the improved treatment available today. Even those with successful operative repair may have late complications. Children born with congenital heart disease often require lifelong medical attention.

The term 'congenital heart disease' refers to a fundamental problem with the heart's structure and function due to abnormal heart development before birth. Many types of heart defects exist, and most either obstruct blood flow in the heart or vessels near it, or cause blood to flow through the heart in an abnormal pattern. More rarely, only one ventricle may be present, or the right or left side of the heart may fail to form properly. A baby's heart begins to develop early and begins beating just 22 days after conception. Between days 22 and 24, the heart begins to bend to the right and fold itself into a loop. By day 28, the tube has a general heart shaped form with structures of the chambers and blood vessels in place (Fig. 1.1). Medical science believes that it is during this time of development these structural defects can occur. These defects can affect different parts of the heart as well as how it functions.[2] It is worth remembering that the heart of a newborn with congenital heart disease is tiny, around the size of a walnut. To repair such a vital, yet delicate organ requires surgical and nursing skills of the highest order.

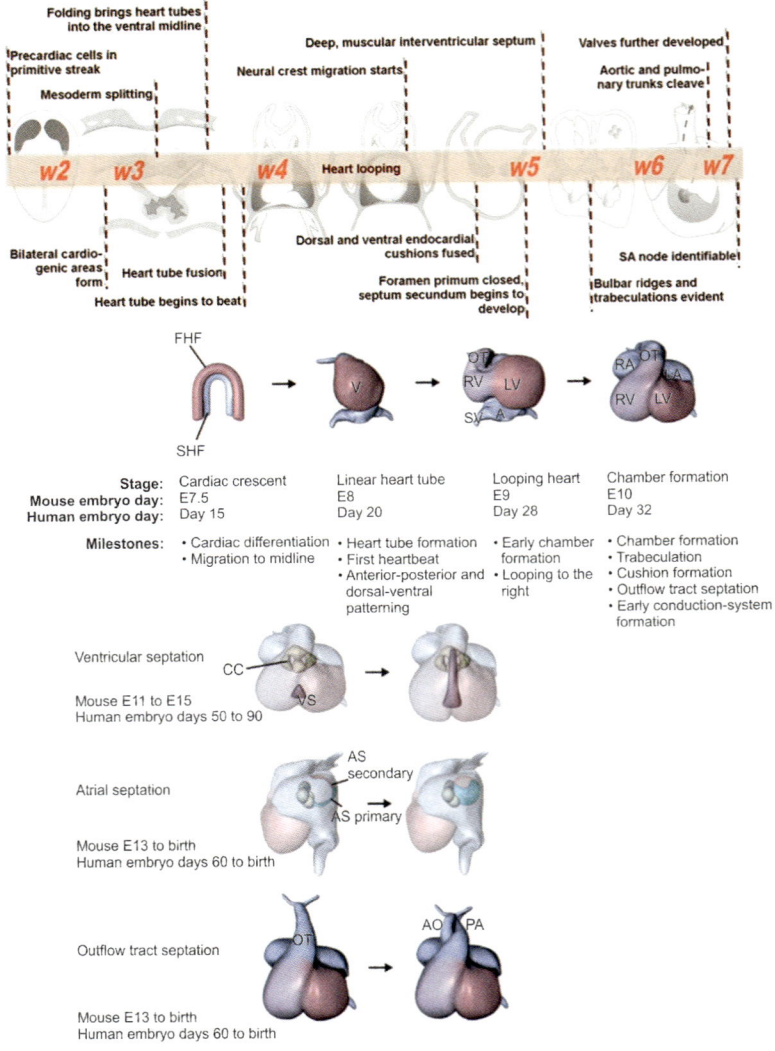

**Fig. 1.1:** Heart development-timeline—during week 4 and week 5 (between days 28 and 32 of pregnancy) the heart begins to loop and fold in on itself, creating the chambers. Medical science believes that most cases of congenital heart disease occur when something disrupts, in particular, this crucial third stage of the heart's development

## INCIDENCE AND CAUSES

Approximately 8 per 1,000 live birth babies are born with a congenital heart defect. Each year, there are about 1.5 million new cases worldwide (Table 1.1).[3] In general, heredity is recognised as playing a part in the various forms of congenital heart disease, although in many cases, the cause is unknown. The cause of congenital heart disease may be genetic, viral or environmental.

No single cause can be identified for most congenital heart defects. These defects are thought to be caused by a combination of genetic inheritance and adverse response to environmental factors or simply by chance. On the other hand, if there is a strong genetic predisposition present, even a mild environmental factor can contribute to its development. However, if there is no genetic predisposition, a few factors can produce congenital heart disease.

## ADVERSE GENETIC RISK FACTORS

There are a number of chromosome abnormalities that are associated with congenital heart defects. The most common are Down's syndrome[5] and Marfan syndrome[6].

| **Table 1.1:** Incidence of some congenital heart disease | |
|---|---|
| *Lesion* | *Frequency* |
| Ventricular septal defect | 1:280 |
| Atrial septal defect | 1:1062 |
| Atrioventricular canal | 1:1372 |
| Tetralogy of Fallot | 1:2375 |
| Transposition of the great arteries | 1:3175 |
| Tricuspid atresia | 1:12,658 |
| Ebstein's anomaly | 1:8772 |
| Pulmonary atresia | 1:7576 |
| Hypoplastic left heart syndrome | 1:3759 |
| Truncus arteriosus | 1:9346 |
| Double-outlet right ventricle | 1:6369 |
| Total anomalous pulmonary venous connection | 1:10,638 |

**Source:** *Adapted from Hoffman and Kaplan, 2002[4]*

## ADVERSE ENVIRONMENTAL RISK FACTORS

Several environmental factors can have a detrimental effect on the development of congenital heart disease. The most common factors are:

### Direct Inheritance

The incidence of mothers with congenital heart disease having affected children is between 2.5 and 18%, and the incidence of fathers with congenital heart disease having affected children is between 1.5 and 3.0%. Both figures are significantly higher than for the general population.[7] It is unusual for more than one child in the same family to have congenital heart disease.

### Consanguinity

In Saudi Arabia and surrounding Middle Eastern countries, first-cousin marriage may be a significant risk factor for specific types of congenital heart disease in a consanguineous[i] population. Inbreeding studies suggest an autosomal recessive[ii] component is

---

[i]Relationship by blood or by a common ancestor, e.g. brother, sister, first-cousin.

[ii]Autosomal recessive is one of several ways that a trait, disorder, or disease can be passed down through families. An autosomal recessive disorder means two copies of an abnormal gene must be present in order for the disease or trait to develop. Genes come in pairs. Recessive inheritance means both genes in a pair must be defective to cause disease. People with only one defective gene in the pair are considered carriers. However, they can pass the abnormal gene to their children. If you are born to parents who both carry an autosomal recessive change (mutation), you have a 1 in 4 chance of getting the malfunctioning genes from both parents and developing the disease. You have 50% (1 in 2) chance of inheriting one abnormal gene.

This would make you a carrier. In other words, if four children are born to a couple who both carry the gene (but do not have signs of disease), the statistical expectation is as follows:

- One child is born with two normal genes (normal),
- Two children are born with one normal and one abnormal gene (carriers, without disease);
- One child is born with two abnormal genes (at risk for the disease).

In a consanguineous population, the risks of inheriting abnormal genes are much higher.

the cause of some congenital heart defects. Research in Saudi Arabia suggests first-cousin consanguinity is significantly associated with ventricular septal defect, atrial septal defect, atrioventricular septal defect, pulmonary stenosis, and pulmonary atresia. However, the study showed there is no relationship between consanguinity and tetralogy of Fallot, tricuspid atresia, aortic stenosis, coarctation of the aorta, and patent ductus arteriosus.[8]

## Diabetes Type I and Type II

Women with diabetes are five times more likely to give birth to a baby with congenital heart disease than women who do not have diabetes. It is estimated that 3 to 6% of pregnant women with diabetes will give birth to a baby with a heart defect, most commonly ventricular septal defect and transposition of the great arteries.[9, 10]

## Rubella

Rubella during pregnancy is the most well-known infectious disease causing congenital heart disease in the foetus.[11] Rubella is not usually a serious infection for adults or children. However, it can have a devastating effect on an unborn baby if a mother develops the infection during the first 8 to 10 weeks of pregnancy. The foetus contracting rubella has a high risk of being born with a patent ductus arteriosus, pulmonary valve stenosis, aortic valve stenosis or a ventricular septal defect.[12]

## Alcohol Use

Alcohol can have a poisonous effect on the tissue of the foetus. Foetal alcohol syndrome refers to a range of birth defects caused by the pregnant woman drinking too much alcohol before coming to term. It is estimated that as many as half of all children with foetal alcohol syndrome will have congenital heart disease, most commonly an atrial septal defect.[13]

## Drug Use

Some prescription and over-the-counter medications and street drugs used during pregnancy increase the risk of heart defects. Medications such as lithium (used to manage bipolar disorder) may cause Ebstein anomaly[14] and accutane (used for acne treatment) may also increase the risk of some congenital heart disease.[15]

## Smoking

Although the mechanism for how smoking might be associated with heart defects is unknown, research suggests a strong link between maternal smoking and the development of congenital heart disease.[16, 17]

## CONGENITAL HEART DISEASE IN MORE DETAIL

### Symptoms

As in most diseases, symptoms depend on the specific condition. Even when the disease is present at birth, the symptoms may not be immediately obvious. The severity of symptoms often depend on whether the defect causes cyanotic or acyanotic heart disease. Cyanosis is a bluish discolouration of the skin due to less than normal amounts of oxygen in the blood. With these defects, cyanosis is the major symptom because the blood that is circulated is not oxygenated adequately. Many of these babies at birth will appear healthy because the circulation is still following the foetal circulation path. This circulation path provides adequate communication of oxygenated blood with unoxygenated blood to perfuse the body. Once these foetal structures begin to close, the infant becomes seriously ill and requires immediate interventions to keep oxygen saturation levels adequate to supply the body. Defects such as coarctation of the aorta, which is classified as an acyanotic heart disease since it does not cause cyanosis, may remain asymptomatic and not be diagnosed for many years. Other acyanotic heart disease, such as a small ventricular septal defect, may never cause any problems, and some children with a ventricular septal defect enjoy normal physical activity and a normal lifespan. However, pulmonary atresia, which causes cyanosis, can lead to severe symptoms and even death, if not treated immediately after birth.

The most common symptoms in newborns include: heart murmer, cyanosis, rapid breathing/shortness of breath, poor feeding and poor weight gain (Table 1.2).

**Table 1.2:** Most common symptoms of congenital heart disease

1. Heart murmur
2. Cyanosis
3. Rapid breathing/shortness of breath
4. Poor feeding
5. Poor weight gain/failure to thrive

## Heart Murmur

Normal heartbeats make a characteristic sound as the heart valves open and close as blood moves through the heart. A heart murmur is an extra or unusual heartbeat sound, detected by a stethoscope. This extra or unusual sound is created by an abnormal blood flow in the heart, and may indicate heart disease. Heart murmurs are very common in neonates and small children and are usually benign. A heart murmur is a common finding in the newborn period, particularly in the first 24 hours following delivery. In asymptomatic infants, turbulent blood flow resulting from the closure of foetal shunts results in a functional or innocent murmur. Any murmur accompanied by cyanosis, respiratory distress, or signs of congestive heart failure warrants urgent investigation. The presence or absence of a heart murmur does not imply either the presence or absence of congenital heart disease. However, if a heart murmur is detected in newborns, further investigation should be initiated to rule out congenital heart disease.

## Cyanosis

Oxygen is carried in the blood by haemoglobin. While oxygenated haemoglobin is bright red, reduced haemoglobin and thus reduced oxygen levels, is dark blue or purple in colour, and is what produces the dusky or blue colour of the skin and mucous membranes. Cyanosis can either be peripheral or central. Peripheral cyanosis is common in newborns, and is a bluish discolouration of hands and feet due to lack of oxygen, caused by peripheral vasoconstriction, as a result of transient hypothermia (Fig. 1.2).

Central cyanosis is present throughout the body and is evident as a bluish discolouration of mucous membranes such as lips, tongue, skin, and nail beds (Fig. 1.3). It may be a symptom of congenital heart disease, which should always be considered if such a child is presented to the emergency department. Central cyanosis indicates the presence of potentially serious and life-threatening disease and needs immediate medical attention.

Congenital heart disease, which causes cyanosis is related to heart lesions that allow blood to flow or shunt from the pulmonary circulation to the systemic circulation. In other words, desaturated blood from the right side of the heart, is not flowing to the lungs to become saturated but instead, is flowing or shunted to the systemic circulation, bypassing the lungs.

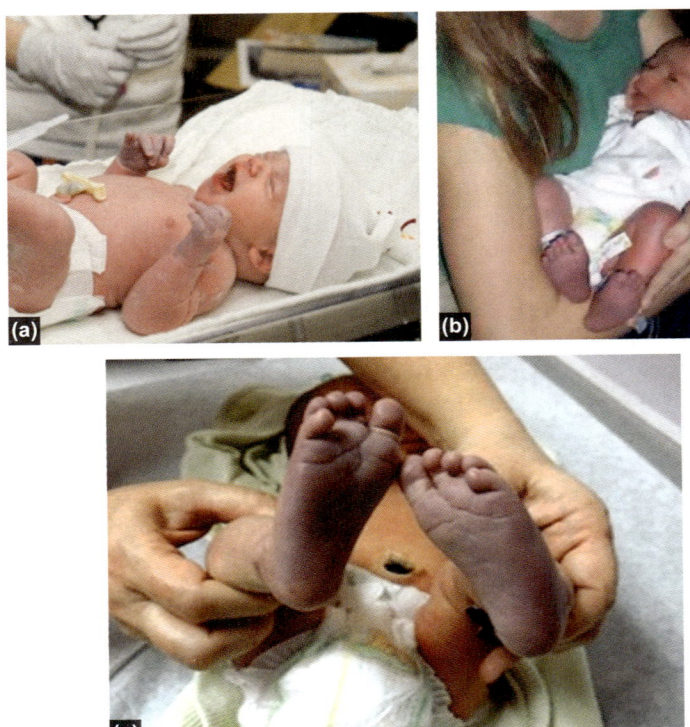

**Fig. 1.2:** (a–c) A newborn often has blue hands and feet, known as peripheral cyanosis. This is normal and should clear within minutes after birth

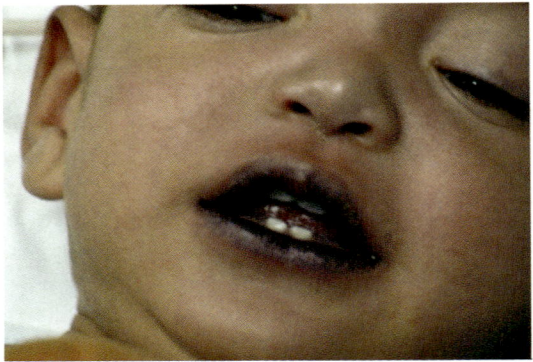

**Fig. 1.3:** A blue baby with central cyanosis just before heart surgery

Infants are naturally pink. Abnormal colouring is easily detected. If a baby is suffering from a weakened heart, especially when too little blood is pumped through to the lungs, the baby will have a bluish tint (cyanosis). Both an excessively pale or blue tint of a newborn's skin is an indicator that a newborn may be suffering from a congenital heart condition.

The most common cyanotic lesions are shown in Table 1.3.

**Table 1.3:** Most common cyanotic congenital heart disease

1. Tetralogy of Fallot
2. Total anomalous pulmonary venous return
3. Transposition of the great arteries
4. Tricuspid stenosis/atresia
5. Pulmonary stenosis/atresia
6. Ebstein anomaly
7. Truncus arteriosus

## Rapid Breathing or Shortness of Breath

In cyanotic heart lesions or lesions with low cardiac output, (e.g. obstructive lesions), the neonate or infant may at first compensate with rapid breathing (tachypnoea), particularly, on exertion, (e.g. when feeding or crying). They then become tired quickly and shortness of breath follows. A newborn's heart rate is normally between 120 and 150 beats a minute with a breathing rate of between 35 and 60 breaths per minute. If a newborn appears to be struggling to breathe, panting or gasping, coupled with a rapid or slowed heartbeat, this may indicate congenital heart disease.

## Poor Feeding

As a result of rapid breathing, the neonate or infant will tire easily, become short of breath and may not be able to take a full feeding. Difficulty feeding is a symptom that is easy for most parents to recognize in their newborn. A newborn should be hungry about every hour and a half during the first six weeks of life, moving to every two to three hours in the first year. A baby who is struggling to feed, or showing a lack of interest in feeding, may have underlying congenital heart disease.

### Poor Weight Gain/ Failure to Thrive

In addition, rapid breathing will reduce the time to swallow-resulting in failure to gain weight. An infant naturally loses 5 to 10% of his or her birth weight during the first week and this is regained within the first three weeks of life. But if a newborn continues to lose, or not gain weight, this indicates that something is amiss and it can be a symptom of heart disease (Fig. 1.4).

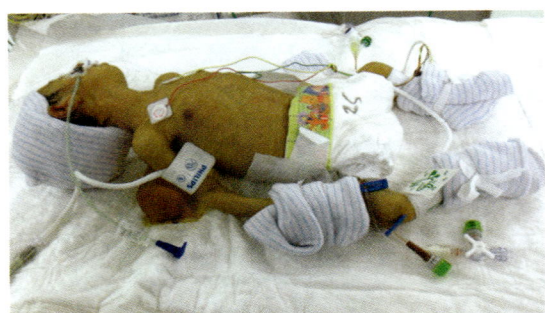

**Fig. 1.4:** Poor weight gain in a baby (3-month-old) with pulmonary atresia. *(Photo by EDJ, courtesy of KAMC, National Guard Hospital, Riyadh, Saudi Arabia)*

## FOETAL AND NEWBORN CIRCULATION AND ITS IMPLICATIONS FOR INFANTS BORN WITH CONGENITAL HEART DISEASE

It is important to have some knowledge of the transition from foetal to newborn circulation and its implications for infants born with congenital heart disease. Understanding the foetal and newborn circulation and their different functions explain, why many infants with significant congenital heart disease are asymptomatic in the immediate newborn period, but may quickly deteriorate within a few hours or days depending on the type and severity of the underlying heart condition.

The normal circulation of a foetus follows a slightly different path than after a baby is born (Fig. 1.5). The placenta acts as the lung, therefore, less blood passes through the foetal lungs. There are two structures within a foetal heart that allow this bypass. One is the patent ductus arteriosus or PDA. The PDA allows mixing between the pulmonary artery and the aorta, as it is a passageway between these two major vessels. The other is the patent foramen ovale (PFO). The PFO is an opening between the

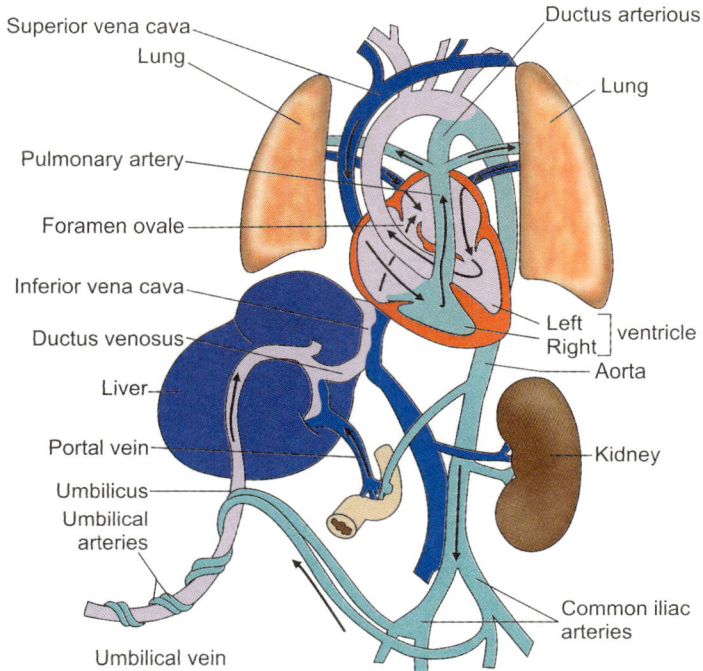

**Fig. 1.5:** Foetal circulation—the normal circulation of a foetus follows a slightly different path than after a baby is born

right and left atrium. It allows mixing of blood between the two atria.

In more detail, the unborn baby receives oxygenated blood and nutrients from the placenta through the umbilical vein. Most of this blood bypasses the liver through the ductus venosus and enters the inferior vena cava (the amount of blood directed towards the liver increases with increasing gestational age). Again, most of this blood returning to the heart bypasses the right ventricle and the lung circulation and flows through the patent foramen ovale (PFO) into the left atrium, left ventricle, and into the aorta. This blood, high in oxygen and nutrients, supplies the brain and upper body of the unborn child. Some of the blood that enters the right atrium via the inferior vena cava mixes with the blood returning to the right atrium via the superior vena cava, then enters the right ventricle and pulmonary artery. Most of this blood (about

90%) bypasses the lungs and instead is pumped through the patent ductus arteriosus (PDA) into the descending aorta. This happens because of increased resistance in the pulmonary arteries (pulmonary vascular resistance or PVR[iii] in the unborn child is high). This blood supplies the lower body and returns to the placenta via the umbilical arteries. Some blood from the right ventricle (about 10%) reaches the lungs, to meet metabolic needs. With increasing gestational age, this amount of blood flowing to the lungs increases in preparation for birth.

Thus, the foetal circulation is characterized by the presence of three shunts; the ductus venosus, the patent foramen ovale, and the patent ductus arteriosus. In the foetus, the gas exchange takes place in the placenta. In order to supply deoxygenated blood to the placenta and return oxygenated blood to the systemic organs, these shunts (ductus venosus, foramen ovale, and ductus arteriosus) are necessary. When a baby is born, and the umbilical cord is clamped, blood flow through the umbilical vein to the ductus venosus ceases. The ductus venosus constricts, with functional closure occurring immediately. When the baby takes his or her first breath, the lungs will expand, causing the pulmonary venous return to the left atrium to increase causing elevated left atrial pressure. The left atrial pressure, eventually, exceeds the right atrial pressure. This results in the functional closure of the patent foramen ovale. After closure of the patent foramen ovale, blood from the right atrium is pumped through the right ventricle and into the lungs, rather than through the patent foramen ovale (Fig. 1.6).

During foetal life, blood pumped through the pulmonary artery is shunted through the patent ductus arteriosus and into the descending aorta as the result of high pulmonary vascular resistance (PVR). In the newborn circulation, a reversal of blood flow occurs as the PVR drops and blood is shunted from the aorta, through the patent ductus arteriosus into the pulmonary arteries and into the lungs (Fig. 1.7a, b). Thus, if the ductus arteriosus

---

[iii]Pulmonary vascular resistance is the resistance in the pulmonary vascular bed against which the right ventricle must eject blood. The cause effect relationship of the onset of breathing and pulmonary vascular resistance is not completely understood. However, increased $PaO_2$ in the breathing neonate compared to the foetus lowers pulmonary vascular resistance and allows more blood to flow to the pulmonary circulation.

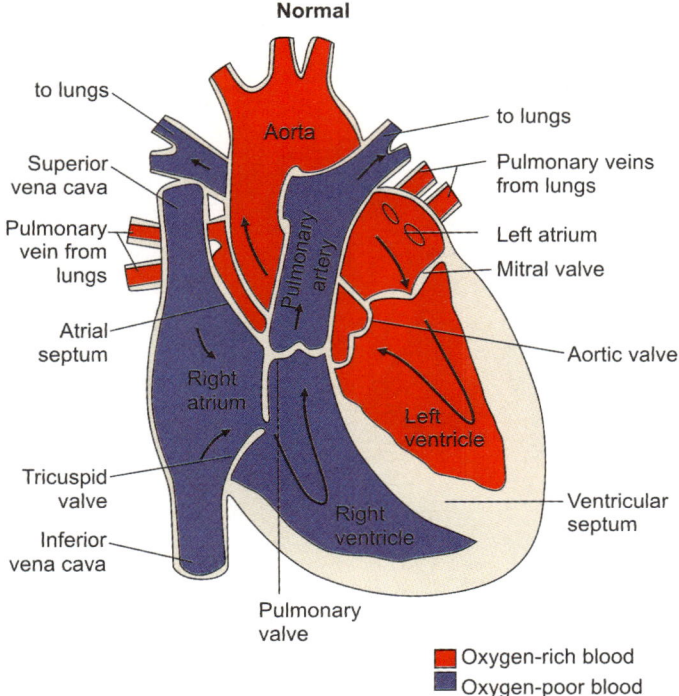

**Fig. 1.6:** After closure of the patent foramen ovale, blood from the right atrium is pumped through the right ventricle and into the lungs, rather than through the patent foramen ovale

remains patent after birth, some oxygenated blood (depending on the size of the ductus arteriosus) is pumped through the ductus back into the lungs instead of being pumped to the aorta and rest of the body and the baby, especially, premature infants struggle to maintain adequate oxygen levels.

*In utero*, the patency of the ductus is maintained by high levels of prostaglandin and a low foetal $PO_2$. Prostaglandin is secreted by the placenta. When the placenta is clamped, prostaglandin levels decrease and the ductus arteriosus closes. Another major contributing factor to the closure of the ductus is a rise in oxygen levels in the blood, which occurs after the baby is born. When a baby is born with congenital heart disease, which is 'shunt dependant' as is the case in transposition of the great arteries, tricuspid and pulmonary stenosis, prevention of closure of the

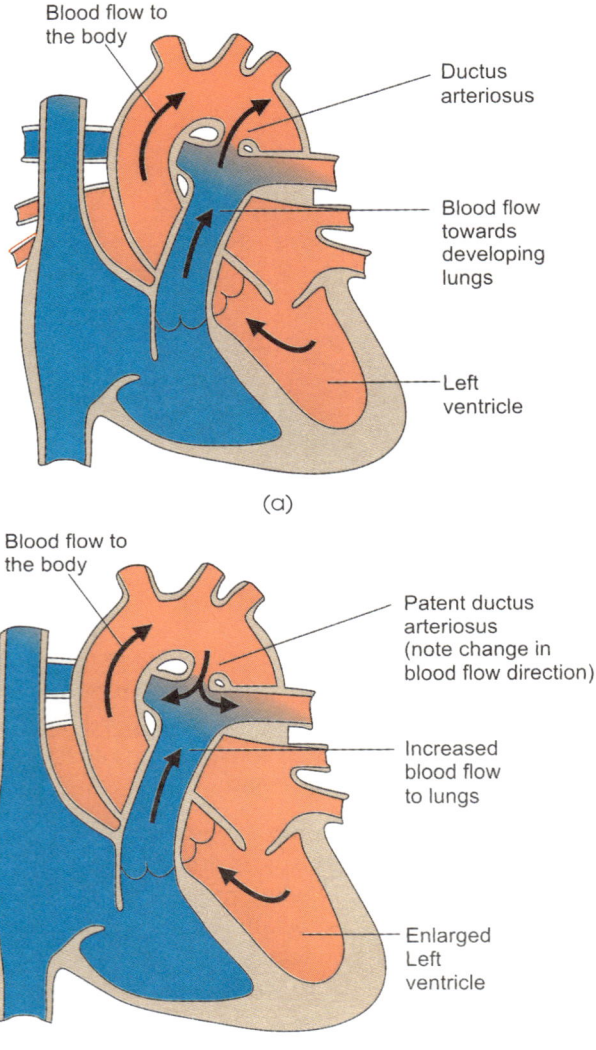

(a)

(b)

**Fig. 1.7:** (a) During foetal life, blood pumped through the pulmonary artery is shunted through the patent ductus arteriosus and into the descending aorta as the result of high pulmonary vascular resistance. (b) In the newborn circulation, a reversal of blood flow occurs as the PVR drops and blood is shunted from the aorta, through the patent ductus arteriosus into the pulmonary arteries and into the lungs

ductus by means of administrating prostaglandin is of paramount importance for the survival of the infant.

In summary, the transition from the foetal to the neonatal circulation includes elimination of the placental circulation, lung expansion, and increase in lung blood flow and closure of the foramen ovale, ductus arteriosus, and ductus venosus. With birth, the function of gas exchange is transferred from the placenta to the lungs, and therefore from the systemic circulation to the pulmonary circulation. The venous and arterial circulations are separated, and not only are the foetal shunts unnecessary but their persistence may lead to circulatory compromise. However, in certain congenital heart disease, a foetal shunt (ductus arteriosus and/or foramen ovale) is necessary for the survival of the child. For most congenital structural heart disease, the foetal shunt pathways allow redistribution or mixing of desaturated venous and saturated arterial blood so that systemic blood flow is adequate. For example, in a foetus with severe left heart obstruction, the systemic blood flow is transferred to the right ventricle, through the foramen ovale, and almost entirely transmitted via the ductus arteriosus. This 'ductal-dependent' systemic circulation is tolerated in the foetus, but poorly tolerated in the newborn because normal closure of the ductus arteriosus progressively decreases systemic blood flow and progresses to circulatory failure and shock. Severe right heart obstruction is also well-tolerated in the foetus, because the combined foetal cardiac output can be transferred to the aorta, with the ductus arteriosus supplying predominantly lung blood flow. After birth, such 'ductal-dependent' pulmonary blood flow can lead to critically low levels of pulmonary blood flow and severe cyanosis when the ductus arteriosus closes.

An understanding of foetal haemodynamics and the acute and chronic changes that occur with transition to the newborn circulation are important for the care of normal newborns and are crucial to the recognition, diagnosis, and management of the newborn with significant congenital heart disease.

## DIAGNOSTIC TESTS

Diagnostic tests, like symptoms, depend on the specific condition. Some parents know that their unborn child has a heart condition. In other cases, the diagnosis is made at birth. It can also occur that the presence of congenital heart disease is discovered some time later. One of the most common signs of congenital heart disease is the detection of a heart murmur during routine physical examination of an infant with a stethoscope (Fig. 1.8). This 'murmur' or low noise from abnormal blood flow may lead the physician to seek further tests. Further evaluation for heart disease includes a chest X-ray, and electrocardiogram (ECG).

In developed countries, many congenital heart anomalies are now diagnosed by detailed antenatal scans before delivery. Several diagnostic tests are used to confirm the presence of a defect after

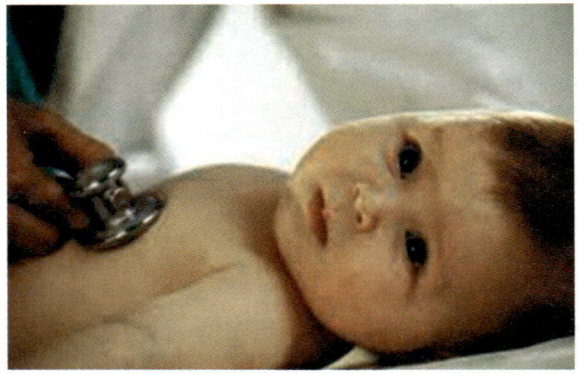

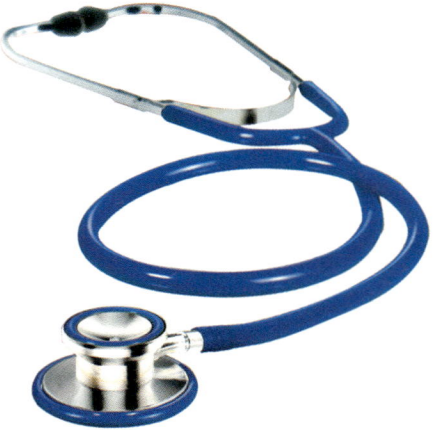

**Fig. 1.8:** Routine physical examination of an infant with a stethoscope

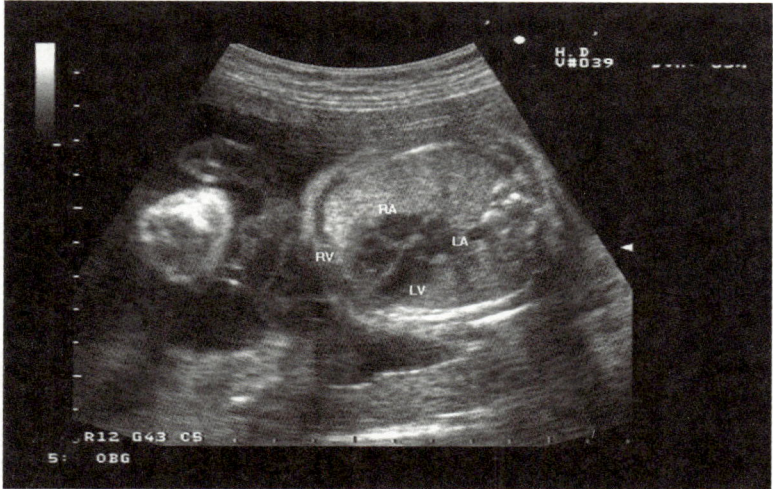

**Fig. 1.9:** Echocardiography showing normal 4-chamber view of the foetal heart

birth, including cardiac catheterization, echocardiogram (heart ultrasound), (Fig. 1.9), electrocardiogram, magnetic resonance imaging (MRI), computed tomography (CT) and chest X-ray. Investigations in general include a thorough health and development history of the infant or child as well as a history of the pregnancy, in addition to the mother's health and drug use during the pregnancy, and a family history of cardiac abnormalities.

## Cardiac Catheterization and Assessment

Cardiac catheterization has long served as the 'gold standard' for the anatomic and physiological assessment of patients with congenital heart disease. Although it still serves as an invaluable diagnostic tool, it is an invasive procedure, requiring anaesthesia and other associated risks of inserting a catheter into the femoral artery of an infant. Advancing it into the heart, especially in the newborn, can cause vascular injury, perforations or tears, cardiac perforation, cardiac valve injury, or blood loss that requires transfusion. Arrhythmias are also risks. Many surgeons now prefer non-invasive alternatives for data collection.

Fortunately, advances in non-invasive imaging have allowed cardiac catheterization to become increasingly a catheter-based therapeutic option rather than a diagnostic tool. Echocardiography, magnetic resonance imaging (MRI), and computed tomography (CT) scan, in many cases replace the need for cardiac catheterization.

## Echocardiography

Nowadays, the initial investigation of choice, in most centres, is echocardiography, which has gained particular importance in paediatric cardiac disease because of the excellent descriptions of intracardiac structures that can be obtained with high-resolution transducers. Transthoracic echocardiography is the most widely used echocardiogram in small infants.

Transoesophageal echocardiography (TEE) is done through the oesophagus with the ultrasound transducer positioned behind the heart. Transoesophageal probes are available for children as small as 3 kilograms. This technique is routinely used in the operating room to evaluate and plan procedures (Fig. 1.10).

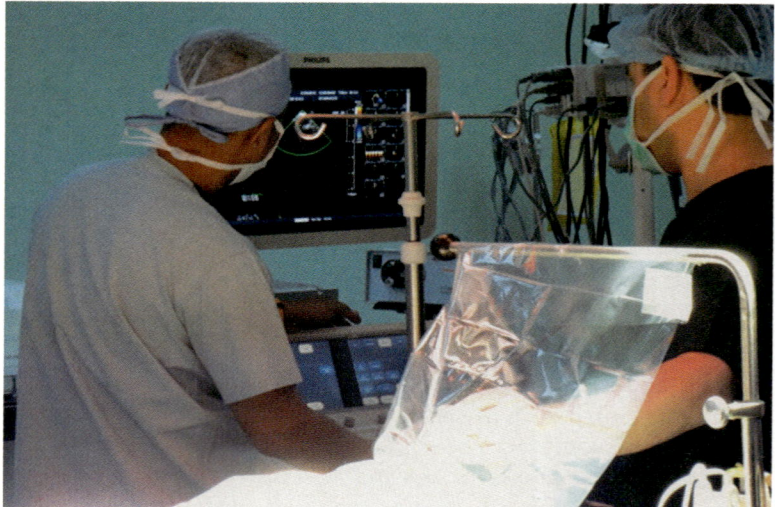

**Fig. 1.10:** Transesophageal echocardiography (TEE) performed in the operating room. (Photo by EDJ, courtesy of KAMC, National Guard Hospital, Riyadh, Saudi Arabia)

## DIAGNOSTIC TESTS IN SUMMARY

**Chest X-ray:** *A diagnostic test, which uses invisible electromagnetic energy beams to produce images of internal tissues, bones, and organs onto film.*

**Electrocardiogram (ECG or EKG):** *A test that records the electrical activity of the heart, shows abnormal rhythms (arrhythmias or dysrhythmias), and detects heart muscle stress.*

**Echocardiogram (echo):** *A procedure that evaluates the structure and function of the heart by using sound waves recorded on an electronic sensor that produces a moving picture of the heart and heart valves.*

**Cardiac catheterization (cath):** *A cardiac catheterization is an invasive procedure that gives very detailed information about the structures inside the heart. Under sedation, a small, thin, flexible tube (catheter) is inserted into a blood vessel in the groin, and guided to the inside of the heart. Blood pressure and oxygen measurements are taken in the four chambers of the heart, as well as the pulmonary artery and aorta. Contrast dye is also injected to more clearly visualize the structures inside the heart.*

**Computed tomography (CT) scan:** *A computed tomography, more commonly known as a CT or CAT scan, is a non-invasive diagnostic medical test that, like X-rays, produces multiple images of the inside of the body. The cross-sectional images generated during a CT scan can be reformatted in multiple planes, and can even generate three-dimensional images. These images can be viewed on a computer monitor, printed on film or transferred to a CD or DVD. CT images of the heart provide greater detail than X-ray, particularly of soft tissue and blood vessels.*

**Magnetic resonance imaging (MRI):** *Magnetic resonance imaging is a test that uses strong magnetic fields and radio waves to form high quality cross-sectional images of organs and body structures without the use of X-ray radiation. Cardiac MRI is often complementary to other imaging techniques, such as echocardiography and cardiac CT as it provides an even clearer picture of the heart and vessels than a CT scan.*

## NON-GENETIC RISK FACTORS

The following known risk factors may occur in infants born with congenital heart disease, who receive delayed medical or surgical treatment:

### Endocarditis

Bacterial endocarditis (BE, also called infective endocarditis) is an infection of the heart valves or the heart's inner lining (endocardium). Bacterial endocarditis occurs when germs (especially bacteria but occasionally fungi and other microbes) enter the bloodstream and attack the lining of the heart or the heart valves. Bacterial endocarditis causes growths (vegetation) or holes on the valves or scarring of the valve tissue, most often resulting in a leaky heart valve. Without treatment, bacterial endocarditis can be a fatal disease. Endocarditis is a major concern in almost all unrepaired congenital heart defects as well as in most repaired defects with a few exceptions. It is rare in complete repaired ventricular septal defect and patent ductus arteriosus repair.

Normally, bacteria can be found in the mouth, on the skin, in the intestines, respiratory system, and the urinary tract and cause no harm. The most common procedures causing endocarditis are dental procedures where bacteria in the gums are released into the bloodstream. Tonsillectomy and adenoidectomy, common procedures performed in small children, may also be a source of bacteria that produce endocarditis, whereas, ear tube insertion, a common procedure performed in children, presents less risk of infection.

While all forms of congenital heart disease carry a risk of infective endocarditis, related to abnormal blood flow or abnormal valves, it is most common in tetralogy of Fallot, transposition of the great arteries, ventricular septal defects, patent ductus arteriosus, coarctation of the aorta, bicuspid aortic valves, and mitral valve prolapse with mitral valve regurgitation. It is not common in isolated secundum atrial septal defect and pulmonary stenosis.

Bacterial endocarditis safety guidelines from the American Heart Association (2014) state[18]: The highest risk group for bacterial endocarditis includes those with:

1. An artificial (prosthetic) heart valve, including bioprosthetic and homograft valves
2. Previous bacterial endocarditis
3. Certain congenital heart diseases, including:
   - Complex cyanotic congenital heart disease such as single ventricle, transposition of the great arteries, tetralogy of Fallot.
   - Unrepaired cyanotic congenital heart disease, including patients with palliative shunts and conduits.

- Congenital heart disease that is completely repaired by surgery or with a transcatheter device. Endocarditis prevention is reasonable for at least 6 months following the device implant. According to the American Heart Association, after 6 months, there is insufficient data to make recommendations for preventive antibiotic therapy.
- Repaired congenital heart disease with defects still remaining at the site or next to the site of a prosthetic patch or prosthetic device.

---

**NURSING OBSERVATION**

*The perioperative nurse receiving the child in the holding bay, must ensure, that prophylactic antibiotics for all children undergoing cardiac surgery are prescribed according to current hospital policies.*

## Embolism

Under normal circumstances, a small blood clot dislodged from the venous circulation would be trapped in the lungs and dissolve. However, a right-to-left shunt can permit paradoxical embolism (the clot material paradoxially enters the arterial circulation instead of going to the lungs) and ultimately may cause a stroke, or necrosis of a distal extremity, i.e. finger or toe (Fig. 1.11).

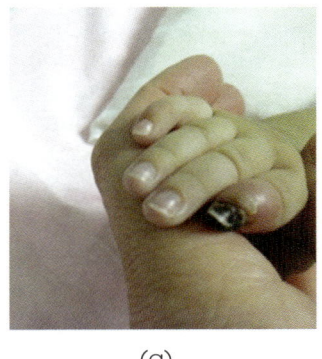 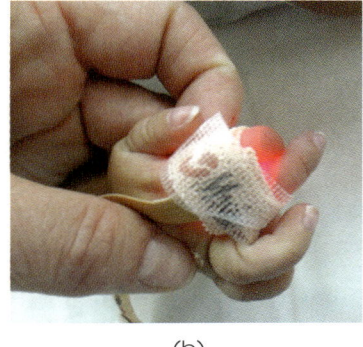

(a)                                        (b)

**Fig. 1.11:** A right-to-left shunt can permit paradoxical embolism and ultimately may cause a stroke or necrosis (a) and subsequently loss (b) of a distal extremity, i.e. finger or toe. *(Photo by EDJ, courtesy of KAMC, National Guard Hospital, Riyadh, Saudi Arabia)*

## Pulmonary Hypertension

Elevated pulmonary artery pressure, in congenital heart disease is caused by pulmonary overcirculation, pulmonary vasoconstriction, and pulmonary vascular disease, either alone or in combination. One of the most common defects associated with elevated pulmonary pressure is a large ventricular septal defect. Pulmonary vascular disease with morphologic alterations of the pulmonary vasculature is one of the most serious complications of congenital heart disease. Once established, it is progressive and leads to premature death. Pulmonary vascular disease can occur in children with unrepaired or partially repaired congenital heart disease, as well as in children with appropriately corrected heart malfunctions. Late secondary pulmonary hypertension has been reported in adults who have had appropriately repaired congenital heart surgery, such as adults with transposition of the great vessels who underwent an arterial switch procedure as newborns. Why these children or adults develop this condition is unclear. The risk of developing irreversible pulmonary vascular disease (referred to as Eisenmenger syndrome[iv])[19] depends on the specific physiology of each lesion, including the degree of pulmonary overcirculation, the pressure on the pulmonary arteries, and the degree of hypoxia. One important factor is the degree of pulmonary overcirculation. The age at which specific lesions cause irreversible pulmonary vascular disease varies. For example, children with large ventricular septal defects who have increased pulmonary blood flow and elevated pressures generally do not develop irreversible pulmonary vascular changes before one or two years of age, while children with truncus arteriosus can develop pulmonary vascular disease in infancy. Other defects, such as an atrial septal defect, do not produce irreversible pulmonary vascular disease until adulthood.

## Congestive Heart Failure (CHF)

Congestive heart failure (CHF) is a condition in which the heart cannot effectively meet the oxygen needs of the body's other organs.

---

[iv]Eisenmenger syndrome refers to any untreated congenital cardiac defect with intracardiac communication that leads to pulmonary hypertension, reversal of flow, and cyanosis. The previous left-to-right shunt is converted into a right-to-left shunt secondary to elevated pulmonary artery pressures and associated pulmonary vascular disease.

It actually is not as much a specific diagnosis but rather a collection of symptoms that can be the result of a variety of different heart problems. The most common type of CHF in children is caused by a structural abnormality in the heart and may not affect the pumping action. Heart defects that allow too much blood to flow to the lungs as with a child with a ventricular septal defect can cause CHF. These are called **left-to-right shunt** problems because blood from the left side of the heart is allowed to pass back to the right side of the heart and go through the lungs again instead of going out to the body. Children (like adults) can also have CHF due to weakness or abnormality of the heart muscle. Many factors can cause CHF and treatment depends on the specific problem.

Symptoms of CHF are different for children at different ages. In neonates, significant CHF results in poor growth due to the fact that a significant amount of energy is used by the heart as it has to work harder to do its job, since in left-to-right shunting, blood from the left ventricle is flowing back through the shunt into the pulmonary circulation instead of flowing through the body. Because the pulmonary circulation is *flooded* as a result, the neonate is also having breathing difficulties. They breathe faster than normal and often have an increased heart rate. The breathing difficulties can be observed by the perioperative nurse as the neonate will use more of their chest muscles and belly to compensate. Sometimes, the heart is pumping so hard the perioperative nurse can feel or even see the pumping heart through the chest. There may be puffiness of the eyes or feet due to CHF.

On the other hand, these symptoms may not occur as soon as the baby is born, because the pressure in the lungs (pulmonary vascular resistance or PVR) of all babies is higher than the pressure in the heart, thus, preventing excessive blood flow to the lungs. It can take from two days to eight weeks before the pressure in the lungs falls to normal levels. When this happens, the lungs will become flooded in heart defects with left-to-right shunting and CHF will gradually develop. Cardiac anomalies that present with severe CHF and cyanosis in the neonatal period include hypoplastic left heart syndrome, severe aortic stenosis, interrupted aortic arch, and transposition of the great arteries. This is because these lesions are ductal dependent. As soon as the patent ductus arteriosus closes, these newborns will present with cyanosis and shock and need immediate medical attention.

Older children with congestive heart failure are beyond the time of rapid growth, and therefore, do not have major growth problems like infants. Their symptoms are usually related to their inability to tolerate exercise. They become short of breath more quickly compared to their peers and need to rest more often.

## SUMMARY OF TREATMENT FOR PAEDIATRIC CONGENITAL HEART DISEASE—NON SURGICAL TREATMENT

Treatment of congenital heart disease depends on the specific condition. Some congenital heart diseases can be treated with medication alone, while others require one or more surgeries. Medications include diuretics, which aid the baby in eliminating water and salts, and digoxin for strengthening heart contraction, by slowing the heartbeat and removing fluid from tissues. Interventional cardiology now offers neonates and infants minimally invasive alternatives to surgery. Device closures for patent ductus arteriosus, patent foramen ovale, and atrial septal defects can now be performed with a standard transcatheter procedure using a closure device mounted on a balloon catheter.

The survival of neonates or infants with certain forms of CHD (e.g., tricuspid valve atresia, transposition of the great arteries, hypoplastic left heart) depends on unrestricted communication between the left and right atria. The presence of an interatrial shunt may be important to increase cardiac output in obstructive lesions of the right side of the heart (e.g., tricuspid atresia, severe pulmonary valve stenosis or atresia). It may be needed to enhance mixing of blood, especially in infants with transposition of the great vessels and with the absence of a patent ductus arteriosus. Furthermore, the interatrial shunt may increase cardiac output to 'off-load' the right side of the heart in pulmonary vascular obstructive lesions, or relieve left atrial hypertension in left-sided obstructive lesions (e.g., hypoplastic left heart); and to decompress the right atrium in postoperative right ventricular failure. Balloon atrial septostomy is probably the oldest interventional cardiac procedure, first performed by Rashkind and Miller in 1966 on a neonate with transposition of the great vessels and severe desaturation (Fig. 1.12).[20]

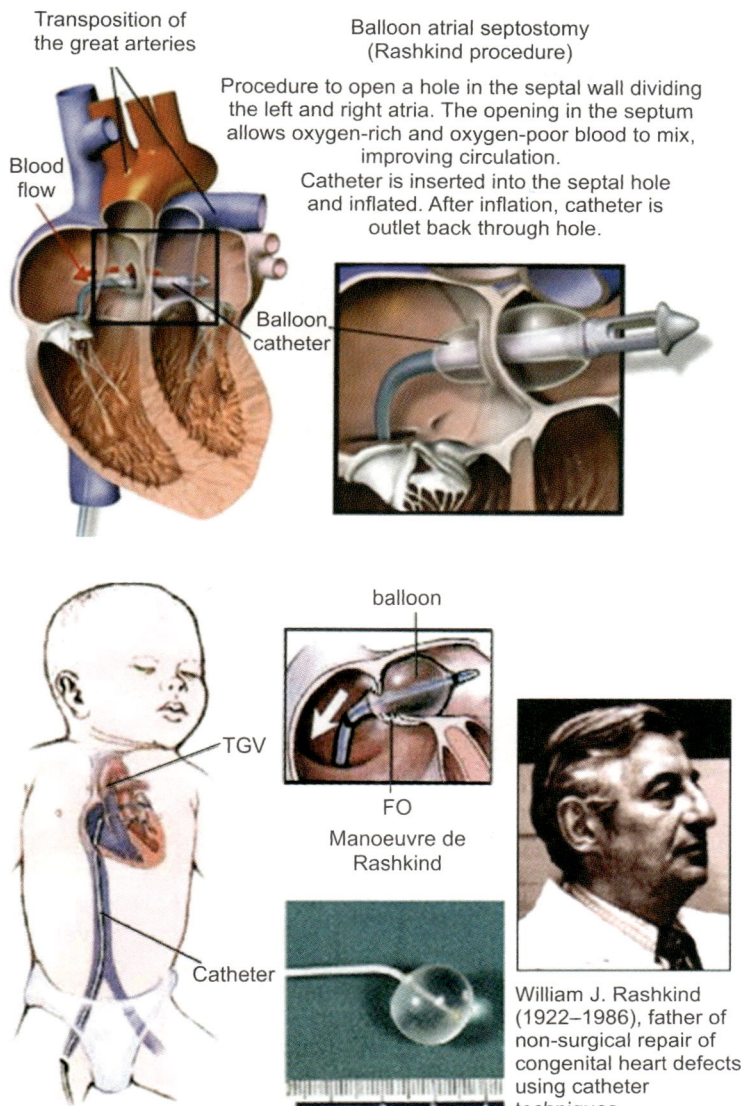

Transposition of the great arteries

Balloon atrial septostomy (Rashkind procedure)

Procedure to open a hole in the septal wall dividing the left and right atria. The opening in the septum allows oxygen-rich and oxygen-poor blood to mix, improving circulation.
Catheter is inserted into the septal hole and inflated. After inflation, catheter is outlet back through hole.

Blood flow

Balloon catheter

balloon

TGV

FO

Manoeuvre de Rashkind

Catheter

William J. Rashkind (1922–1986), father of non-surgical repair of congenital heart defects using catheter techniques.

**Fig. 1.12:** Balloon atrial septostomy (Rashkind procedure)

**Table 1.4:** A summary of interventional cardiac catheterization

| Lesion | Procedure performed |
|---|---|
| Transposition of the great arteries, tricuspid atresia, and hypoplastic left heart | Atrial septostomy—for a septostomy, an opening is made either by a balloon or blade in the atrial septum to allow blood to mix between the left and right side of the heart. This procedure is generally used in transposition of the great arteries if the patent ductus arteriosus is very small and there is no other communication between the left and right side of the heart to allow mixing of blood. Septostomy may also be performed for tricuspid atresia and hypoplastic left heart |
| Patent ductus arteriosus, atrial and ventricular septal defect | Closing the defect with a device (coil, Amplatzer device) |
| Pulmonary valve and aortic valve stenosis | Balloon valvoluplasty—a small balloon is inflated in a heart valve, widening the valve |
| Coarctation of the aorta | Balloon angioplasty—a balloon is inflated in the aorta to widen it |
| Patent ductus arteriosus, pulmonary artery branch and aorta stenosis | Stent insertion—small wire mesh coils (stents) can be placed in arteries to keep them open. Stents for treatment of CHD are often placed in arteries outside the heart, e.g. pulmonary and aorta. They can also be used to keep a ductus arteriosus, or a Blalock–Taussig shunt patent. |

Types of interventional cardiac catheterization are varied and individualized to each child. Most commonly, interventions are used in certain lesions where the valves are narrowed (e.g., pulmonary or aortic valve stenosis) or arteries causing obstruction of blood flow (e.g., coarctation of the aorta) (Table 1.4.)

## SURGICAL TREATMENT

The goal of surgery is to repair the defect as much as possible, restore circulation to as close to normal as possible, reduce symptoms, improve survival and improve quality of life. Sometimes, multiple surgical procedures are necessary. Surgery for most congenital cardiovascular defects has low risk of death (less than 2%), compared to 80 to 100% in the 1940s. Most children with cardiac lesions require lifelong specialized cardiac care, first with a paediatric cardiologist and later with an adult congenital cardiologist. There are more than 1.8 million adults living with congenital heart defects worldwide.

## PROGNOSIS

How well a child does depends on the specific defect. Fifty years ago, the risk of death from congenital heart surgery was 30% compared to 5% today. In the 1980s, 60% of deaths from congenital heart disease occurred in the first year of life, whereas in the 1990s the majority of deaths occurred in adults over the age of twenty. It is predicted that 78% of children born with congenital heart disease will survive into adulthood. In the United Kingdom there are close to 1,50,000 adults living with congenital heart disease. Added to this number are an estimated 1,600 cases with complex or significant congenital heart lesions and many more with simple lesions entering the adult age group each year. These figures will continue to increase over time due to the ongoing development of techniques for the diagnosis and improved management of CHD. A number of large scale, long-term studies are available that predict the outcomes in some congenital heart lesions. Among the most important of these, is a report from the paediatric cardiac surgical database of 6461 children operated on, in Finland between the years 1953 and 1989 (Table 1.5).

**Table 1.5:** Prognosis for adults with congenital heart disease

| Good | Intermediate | Uncertain or poor |
|------|--------------|-------------------|
| Atrial septal defect | Aortic stenosis | Transposition of the great arteries |
| Patent ductus arteriosus | Tetralogy of Fallot | Post arterial switch procedure |
| Pulmonary stenosis | Transposition of the Great Arteries | Congenitally corrected transposition |
| Ventricular septal defect | Post-Senning/Mustard procedure | Ebstein's anomaly of tricuspid valve |
| Coarctation of aorta | | Single ventricle physiology |

**Source:** *Adapted from Nieminen, Jokinen, and Sairanen, 2001.*

Among the lesions with a good prognosis are atrial septal defect and patent ductus arteriosus, especially if repaired at a young age and before the development of pulmonary hypertension. Likewise, pulmonary stenosis has near normal mortality, with early age at operation predicting a better outcome. Children with ventricular septal defects also have a good prognosis when repaired early, especially in the absence of pulmonary hypertension or complete heart block. Coarctation of the aorta carries a known potential for increased late mortality, primarily due to coronary artery disease. However, when not associated with a ventricular septal defect and when operated early (age less than 9 years of age) and when postoperative hypertension is absent, long-term prognosis is not far from normal. Coarctation patients with residual stenosis, or additional lesions such as mitral valve abnormalities, ventricular septal defects, aortic valve disease, as well as those with risk factors for atherosclerosis may have a less favourable prognosis. Lack of published data of long-term follow-up for a number of congenital heart defects makes prognoses difficult. Since the introduction of the Jatene procedure in 1975, the arterial switch has replaced atrial redirection procedures for correction of transposition of the great arteries. Although it is hoped the child's outcome will be improved, insufficient numbers of children have entered the adult age group to make accurate prognoses. Similarly, accurate predictions of mortality are impaired in uncommon lesions such as congenitally corrected transposition, complex transpositions, Ebstein's anomaly of tricuspid valve and univentricular hearts where relatively small numbers of children have been studied for long-term outcomes. Unfortunately, published data as well as experience suggests that outcomes with these lesions will remain substantially poorer than in the general population.

# Understanding Congenital Heart Disease Diagnosis and Classification

## DIAGNOSIS

Before operating on congenital heart defects cardiac surgeons need the most precise diagnosis possible. Since 1960, the Cardiac Registry at Children's Hospital, Boston, (USA) has been where pathologists, cardiologists and cardiac surgeons have gained specialized knowledge of the anatomy of heart defects. Its collection of over 3,600 specimens, some dating back to 1944, is irreplaceable, since large, intact examples of heart defects are no longer seen at autopsy in the United States.

The cardiac registry was founded in 1965 by Richard Van Praagh MD, with his wife Stella Van Praagh MD, who served as its directors until 2002 (Fig. 2.1). The registry became an invaluable research and teaching facility. Richard Van Praagh is still a professor of pathology and his wife Stella Van Praagh (1927–2006) was a world-renowned paediatric cardiologist and pathologist. They and their colleagues generated more than 280 publications detailing the anatomy of heart defects. In 1972, Richard Van Praagh published perhaps his most important paper, 'The Segmental Approach to Diagnosis in Congenital Heart Disease'.[23] This approach to heart disease allows cardiologists and cardiac surgeons all over the world to communicate in a common language. Over the years, Dr. Van Praagh and his wife discovered 13 new types of congenital heart disease—including a new type of tetralogy of Fallot—and developed five new surgical operations. In 2000, The International Nomenclature Committee for Paediatric and Congenital Heart Disease was established, based on both the Van Praagh approach to the diagnosis and classification of complex cardiac anomalies and the European school of sequential segmental

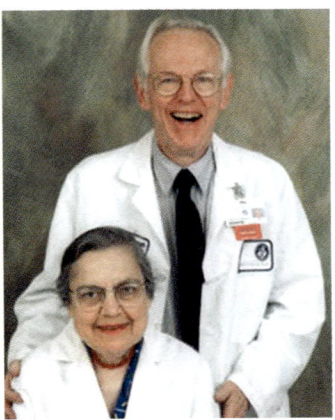

**Fig. 2.1:** Richard Van Praagh with his wife Stella Van Praagh, the founders of the Cardiac Registry

analysis. This committee eventually evolved into the International Society for Nomenclature of Paediatric and Congenital Heart Disease.

## SEQUENTIAL SEGMENTAL CLASSIFICATION

The sequential segmental approach is used to describe the anatomic structures of congenital heart disease. It is a systematic verification guide so that all the interconnected chambers and valves and their relationships will be documented. The system is based on following the blood flow into the heart (systemic and pulmonary venous), through the heart (the atrioventricular valves and ventricles) and then out the great vessels (semilunar valves and great vessels). It can be applied to patients of all ages using diagnostic procedures such as echocardiography, computed tomography (CT) scan and magnetic resonance imaging (MRI) scan.[24]

Although the sequential segmental approach is employed worldwide for the evaluation of congenital heart disease, not all aspects may be formally documented and the way they are documented may vary at individual health care institutions.

## DETERMINING THE SITUS

Before analyzing the intracardiac anatomy, the situs of the thoracic and abdominal organs are determined (referred to as the thoraco-abdominal situs) to provide an 'anatomic framework' for further analysis. The term **'situs'** means *'position, site,* or *location'* and, in the context of congenital heart disease, refers to the position of the atria (upper chambers of the heart) and viscera relative to the midline. **Viscera** refers to the *soft internal organs* of the body, especially those contained within the abdominal and thoracic cavities (stomach, liver, spleen, bronchi and lungs). Accurate determination of situs is essential because anomalies of situs are associated with an increased incidence of complex congenital heart disease.

## The Viscero-atrial Situs

Viscero-atrial situs refers to the position of the atria in relation to the thoracic and abdominal organs. The first step is to locate and identify the right and left atria. Typically, the right atrial appendage is broad and blunt; triangular (Fig. 2.2), whereas the left atrial

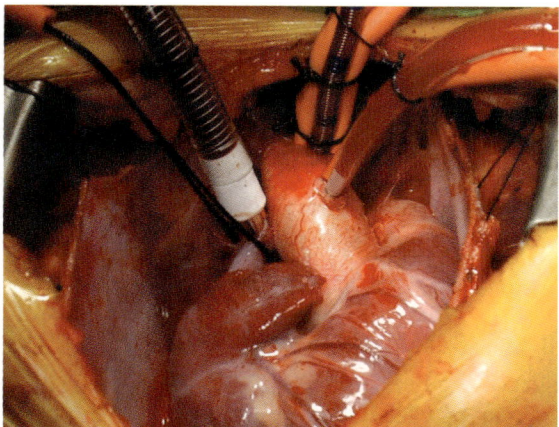

**Fig. 2.2:** Typically, the right atrial appendage is broad and blunt; triangular. *(Source: Photo by EDJ, courtesy of King Faisal Specialist Hospital, Jeddah, Saudi Arabia)*

appendage is narrow, pointed, and tubular (finger like). However, most of the time, radiological imaging is not reliable in identifying the anatomic differentiation of the right and left atria, and the localization of non-cardiac organs is more helpful for determining the situs. That is the supradiaphragmatic portion of the inferior vena cava (IVC) often provides a more reliable landmark for locating the anatomic right atrium (because of the rule of veno-atrial concordance; IVC always drains into the right atrium).

### Three Types of Situs

Thus, the cardiac situs describes the position or location of the cardiac atria in relation to the viscera. The cardiac situs is determined by the atrial location.[25]

1. **Situs solitus:** Situs solitus refers to the normal position, when the right atrium, the liver, the gallbladder, and the right lung, are situated on the right, whereas the stomach, spleen, the left lung and the aorta are situated on the left.

2. **Situs inversus:** In situs inversus, the anatomic configuration is an exact inversion of that of situs solitus (mirror image, Figs 2.3 and 2.4). Situs inversus is present in 0.01% of the general population. In situs inversus, the morphologic right atrium is on the left, and the morphologic left atrium is on the right. The normal pulmonary anatomy is also reversed so that the left lung has three lobes and the right lung has two lobes. In addition, the liver and gallbladder are located on the left, whereas the spleen and stomach are located on the right. The remaining internal structures are also a mirror image of the normal.

3. **Situs ambiguous:** When the situs is neither solitus nor inversus, it is referred to as situs ambiguous or heterotaxy; the heart is situated in the middle of the thorax. In these patients, the liver may be midline, the spleen absent or multiple, the atrial morphology unclear, and the bowel malrotated.

### IDENTIFYING THE CARDIAC POSITION

The position of the heart in the thorax and the orientation of the cardiac apex can be useful in determining the situs (atrial location) and are often described separately in echo reports. There are three types of cardiac positions within the thorax cavity and their positions are determined by the orientation of the base-apex axis of the heart and are independent of the cardiac situs. The direction in which the ventricles are aligned, defines the base-apex axis of the heart. The apex of the heart is the lowest superficial part of the heart. It is directed downward, forward, and to the left. The base is the opposite part of the apex (Fig. 2.5).

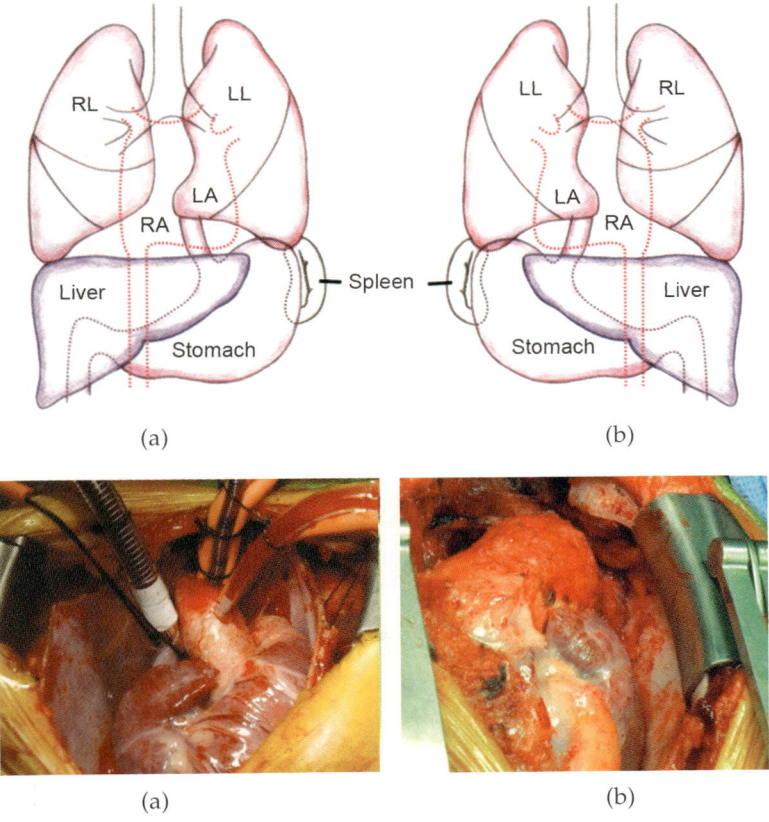

(a)                                    (b)

(a)                                    (b)

**Fig. 2.3:** Schematic drawings illustrate the standard anatomy of situs solitus (a) and the mirror image of situs inversus (b). The right lung (RL), left lung (LL), right atrium (RA), and left atrium (LA) are shown. Note the photo on the right (b) is of a 4-year-old child who had previous cardiac surgery, hence adhesions can be clearly seen as compared to photo (a), which is taken of the heart of a 3-year- old child who had first time surgery. *(Photos a, b by EDJ, courtesy of KAMC, National Guard Hospital, Riyadh, Saudi Arabia)*

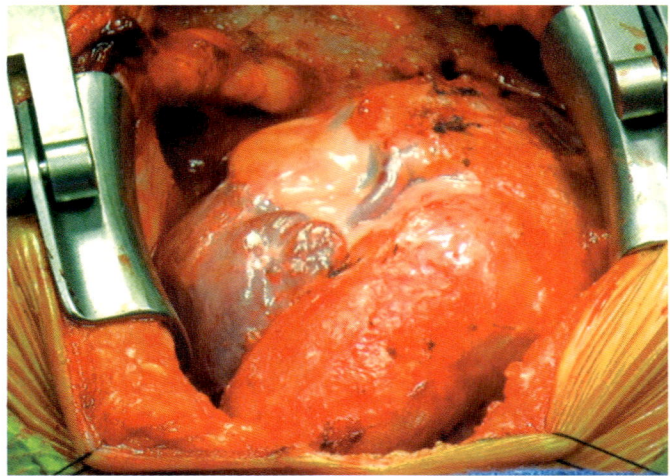

**Fig. 2.4:** In situs inversus, the morphologic right atrium is on the left (as seen in the picture), and the morphologic left atrium is on the right. Picture is taken standing at the head of the child. *(Photo by EDJ, courtesy of KAMC, National Guard Hospital, Riyadh, Saudi Arabia)*

## Three Types of Cardiac Position

The terms levocardia, dextrocardia and mesocardia indicate only the direction of the cardiac apex.

1. **Levocardia:** The heart is located mainly in the left chest, **levo** means *left* in Latin. This is the normal position of the heart (the direction of the cardiac apex is to the left) however, some or all of the thorax or abdomen viscera are transposed laterally (situs inversus). It is also known as situs inversus with levocardia (Fig. 2.6). This condition is often associated with severe heart defects and splenic abnormalities such as asplenia (absence of normal spleen function) or polysplenia (multiple small accessory spleens). Thus in levocardia, the position of the heart is normal but other viscera such as the lungs, liver, spleen, etc. are often transposed.

2. **Dextrocardia:** The heart is located predominantly in the right chest, **dextro** means *right* in Latin (Fig. 2.7). This is abnormal (the direction of the cardiac apex is to the right). It is commonly associated with defects of the heart. Dextrocardia is believed to occur in approximately 1 in 12,000 children. Dextrocardia situs

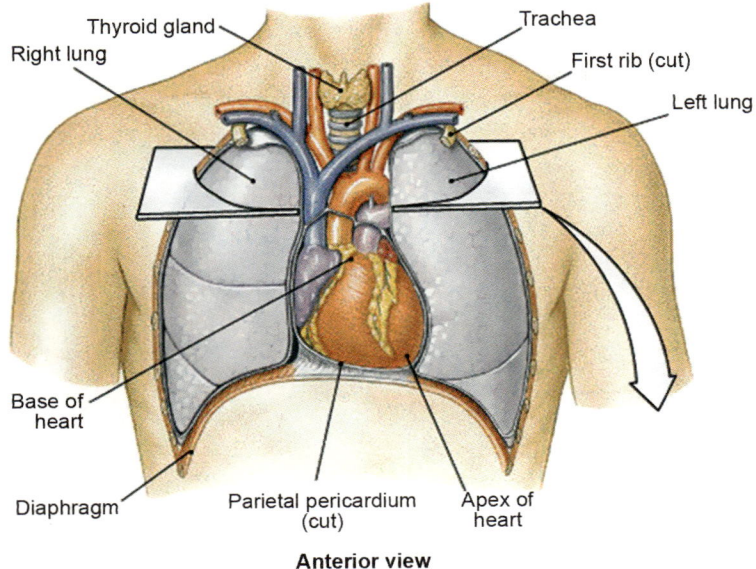

**Anterior view**

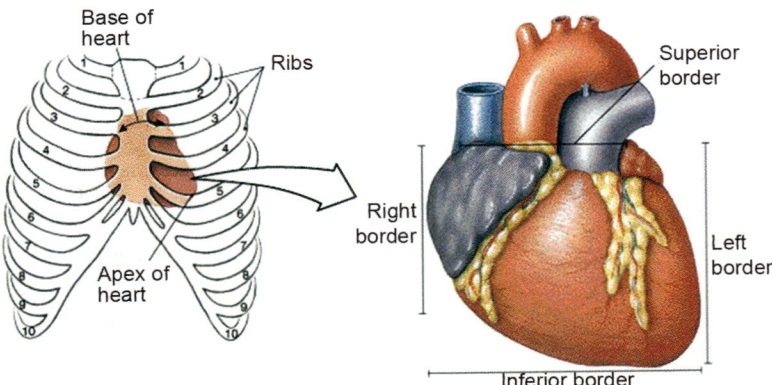

**Fig. 2.5:** The direction in which the ventricles are aligned defines the base-apex axis of the heart

inversus refers to the heart being a mirror image situated on the right side. For all visceral organs to be mirrored, the correct term is dextrocardia situs inversus totalis (Fig. 2.8). Situs inversus is more common with dextrocardia than with levocardia. A 3–5% incidence of congenital heart disease is common in situs inversus with dextrocardia, usually trans-position of the great arteries.[26] Situs inversus with levocardia is rare,[27] and is almost always associated with congenital heart disease.[28]

Normal organs                    Levocardia

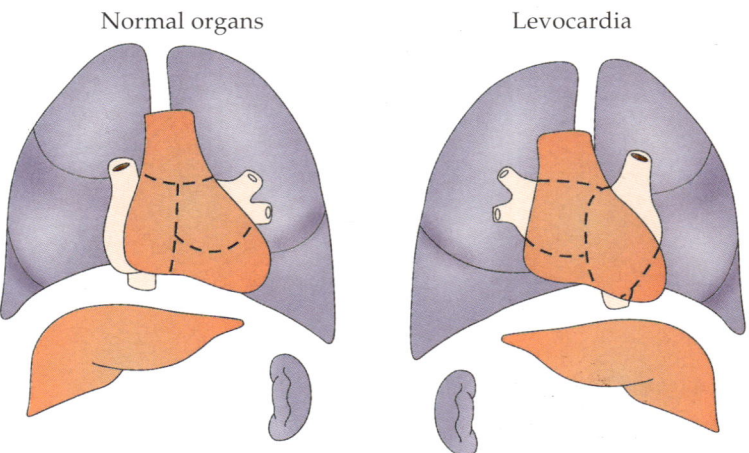

**Fig. 2.6:** Levocardia—normal position of the heart associated with transposition of other viscera (situs inversus)

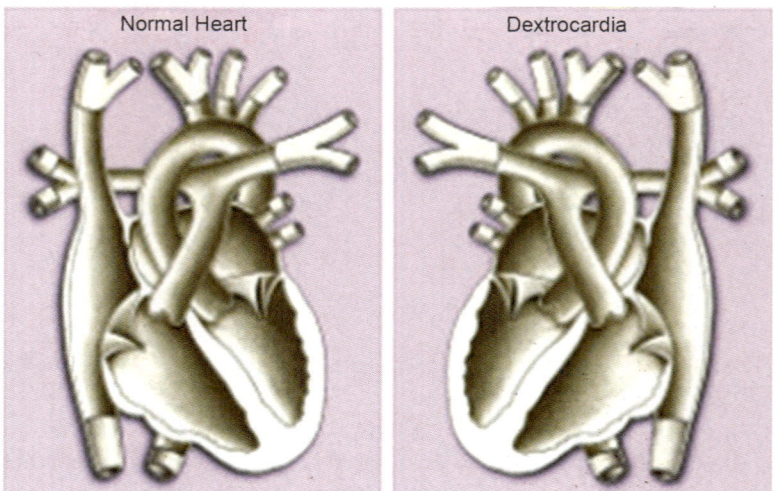

**Fig. 2.7:** Dextrocardia—the heart is located predominantly in the right chest. This is abnormal (the direction of the cardiac apex is to the right)

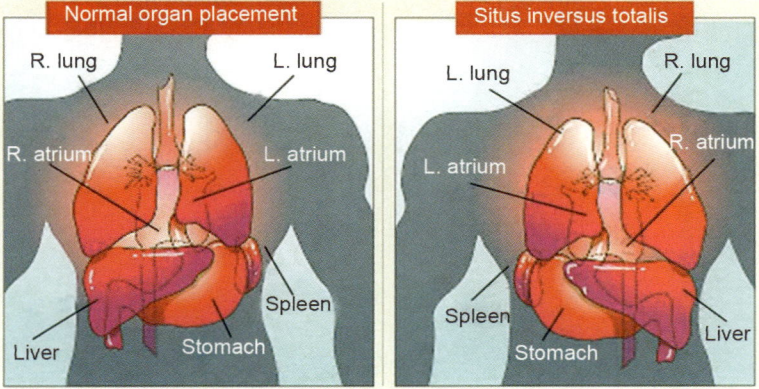

**Fig. 2.8:** Normal organ placement and situs inversus totalis.

Dextrocardia may be because a normally left-sided heart (levocardia) is displaced to the right side (either because of pressure from a mass in the left hemithorax, or collapse of the right lung drawing the heart to that side) or because the heart is *flipped* around and is anatomically inverted).

Dextrocardia with situs inversus (reversed abdominal contents) is essentially a mirror image of a heart, with a mirror image of the abdominal contents. In this situation, the cardiac anatomy and connections are usually (but not always) normal.

In dextrocardia with situs solitus (normally oriented abdominal contents), congenital cardiac disease is more likely. The lesions are frequently complex and often require surgical correction.

3. **Mesocardia:** The heart is located in the midline of the chest cavity, the apex of the heart is in the midline of the thorax. This is abnormal (Fig. 2.9).

---

**NURSING OBSERVATION**

*ECG leads may have to be placed in reversed positions on a child with dextrocardia situs inversus. In addition, when defibrillating a child with dextrocardia situs inversus, the pads may have to be placed in reverse positions. That is, instead of upper right and lower left, pads should be placed upper left and lower right.*

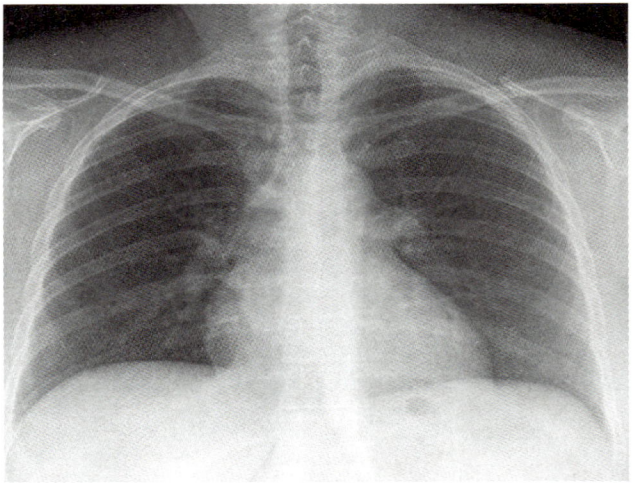

**Fig. 2.9:** The apex of the heart is in the midline of the thorax

## KEY POINTS OF THE SEQUENTIAL SEGMENTAL CLASSIFICATION
### Intracardiac Anatomy

In a normal heart, blood enters the heart via the right and left atria. The superior and inferior venae cavae carry blood from the upper and lower body into the right atrium. The pulmonary veins carry blood from the lungs back to the left atrium. In echo reports, the right and left atria are identified, with regards to the superior and inferior vena cava entering the right atrium and four pulmonary veins entering the left atrium. Following the normal sequence of flow, the atrioventricular valves and ventricles are identified. Normally there are two atrioventricular valves, tricuspid and mitral. The tricuspid valve is committed to the right ventricle and the mitral valve is committed to the left ventricle. Normally, both the atrial and ventricular septa are intact. Again following the normal sequence of flow, blood should emerge out of the ventricles into the great vessels. The pulmonary artery, taking blood to the lungs, is normally committed to the right ventricle while the aorta, taking blood to the systemic circuit, is normally committed to the left ventricle. The pulmonary artery emerges from the right ventricle and passes anterior to the aorta. The pulmonary artery then bifurcates and is differentiated from the aorta that forms an arch, giving off vessels to the head and neck. The pulmonary artery and aorta crisscross as they arise from their respective ventricles (Fig. 2.10).

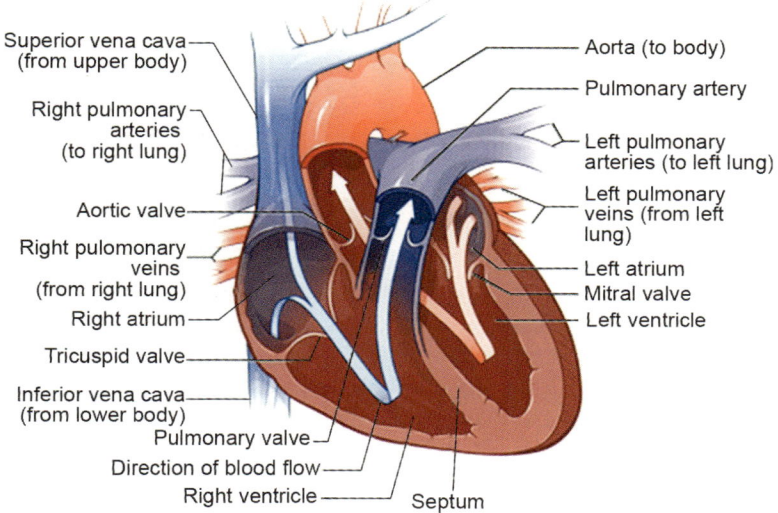

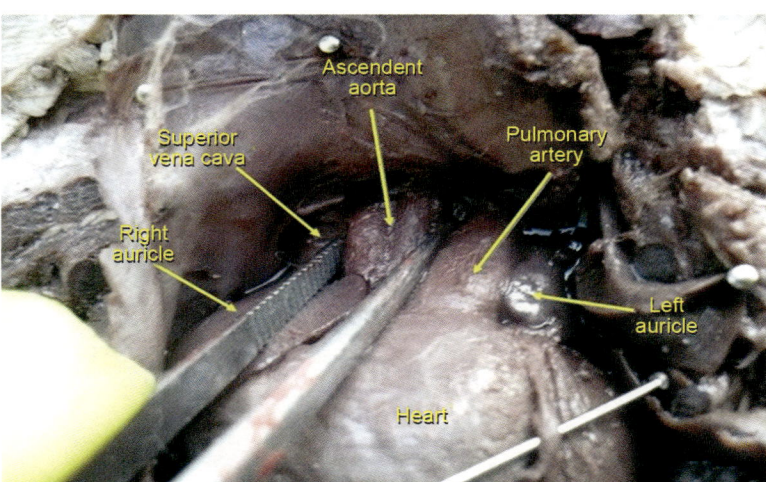

**Fig. 2.10:** Normal heart and normal blood flow through the heart. *Note:* The pulmonary artery and aorta crisscross as they arise from their respective ventricles and the normal position of the pulmonary artery is anterior (in front) of the aorta

Given these normal sequences and relationships the terms previously mentioned are then used to describe abnormal hearts. The following descriptions can be further interpreted in echo reports:

## Atresia and Hypoplastic

Chambers, valves, and vessels are described as absent (atretic) or small (hypoplastic) (Fig. 2.11).

## Concordant and Discordant

Relationships between chambers, valves and vessels are described as concordant (normal) or discordant. Concordant describes the relationship between the various chambers, valves, and great vessels. In the normal heart all the connections and relationships in the anatomic sequence are concordant. Discordant on the other hand, describes abnormal relationships between the various chambers and great vessels. For example, when the right atrium leads into the morphologic left ventricle and the left atrium into the morphologic right ventricle, the atrioventricular relationships are discordant

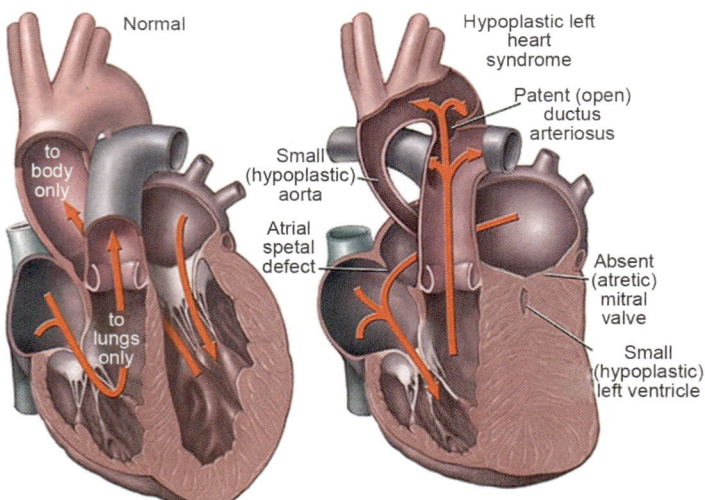

**Fig. 2.11:** Hypoplastic left heart syndrome is a good example to show what they mean by absent, or atretic (mitral valve), small or hypoplastic (aorta and left ventricle) and it also shows septal defects (atrial septal defect)

(Fig. 2.12). Likewise, the atrioventricular relationships may be concordant but the ventriculo-arterial relationships may be discordant where the aorta rises from the right ventricle and the pulmonary artery rises from the left ventricle (Fig. 2.13).

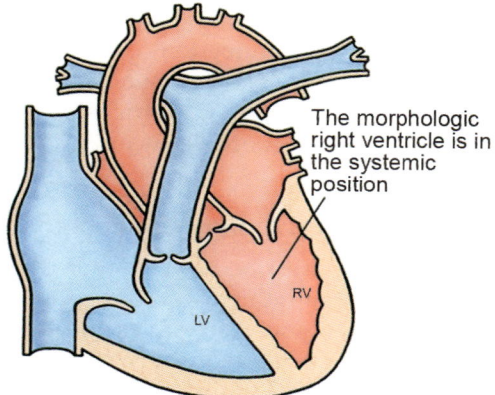

**Fig. 2.12:** The right atrium leads into the morphologic left ventricle and the left atrium into the morphologic right ventricle, the atrioventricular relationships are discordant (congenitally corrected transposition of the great arteries)

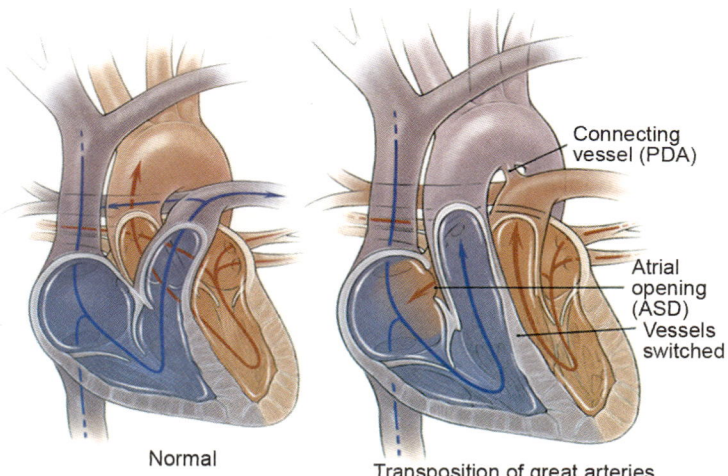

**Fig. 2.13:** The atrioventricular relationships are concordant but the ventriculo-arterial relationships are discordant where the aorta rises from the right ventricle and the pulmonary artery from the left ventricle (Transposition of the great arteries)

## Atrioventricular and Ventriculo-arterial Connections

Connection refers to the sequence of anatomic structures. Normally, the right atrium is connected to the right ventricle through the tricuspid valve. The right ventricle is then connected to the pulmonary artery through the pulmonary valve. Therefore, there are atrioventricular connections and ventriculo-arterial connections. Absence of right or left connection refers to both atrioventricular connection (absence of tricuspid or mitral valve) and ventriculo-arterial connection (absence of pulmonary or aortic valve).

## Normally Committed and Doubly Committed

Chambers or valves are described as being normally committed or doubly committed. Commitment describes possible abnormalities of flow through valves into ventricles and the great vessels. For example, in a child with tetralogy of Fallot, the atria, atrioventricular valves, and ventricles are positioned normally, and are concordant. Since the aorta overrides a ventricular septal defect, the aorta is doubly committed to both ventricles (Fig. 2.14). Likewise, in cases where there is only one ventricle (univentricular heart), both atrioventricular valves are usually doubly committed to the single ventricle.

## Inlet and Outlet

Inlet refers to anomalies of the structures and flow into the ventricle. Outlet, on the other hand, refers to anomalies of the structures and flow out of the ventricles into the great vessels.

## Septa

In the structurally normal heart, right and left sides are divided and are without communication. Shunting refers to those flow anomalies where there is an abnormal communication, such as an atrial or ventricular septal defect, that allows abnormal flow between the right and left sides of the heart. Since right-sided pressures are normally lower than those on the left side, when such defects are encountered abnormal flow, is usually left-to-right and results in increased flow into the lungs. Normally, the lungs can accommodate the increased flow without significant symptoms if the degree of shunting is small or moderate. When significant shunting is present and exceeds the ability of the lungs

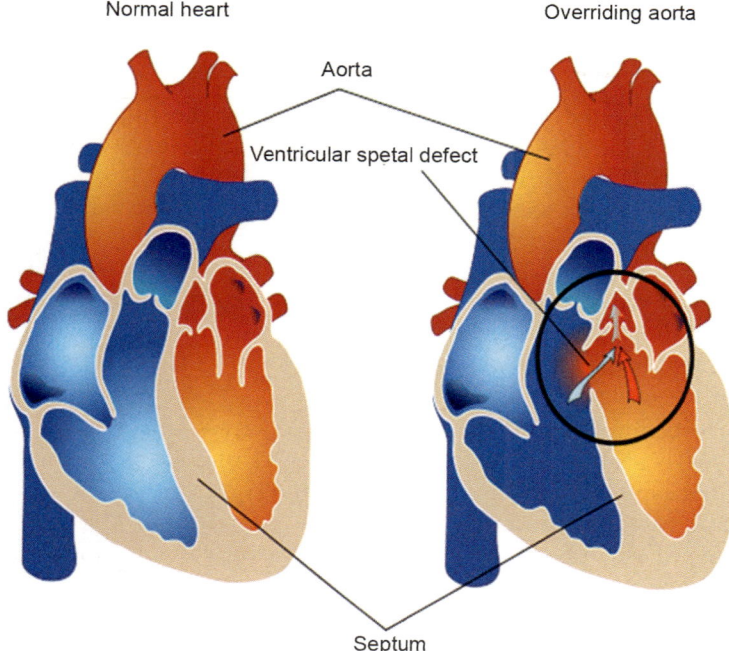

Normal heart          Overriding aorta

Aorta

Ventricular spetal defect

Septum

**Fig. 2.14:** Since the aorta overrides a ventricular septal defect, the aorta is doubly committed to both ventricles

to accept the increase, the lungs are literally flooded and symptoms of cardiac failure result.

## Cardiac Chambers and Ventricular Loop

Morphologic right and left ventricles refer to the anatomic characteristics of the chambers and not their positions, (e.g. the morphologic right ventricle is on the left in congenitally corrected transposition). The left or rightward orientation of the ventricular loop is evaluated by a cardiologist and the ventricles are identified on the basis of their internal morphologic features. D-loop refers to the rightward (dextro = D) loop or bend of the embryonic heart tube and indicates that the ventricles have looped normally during development. L-loop refers to a leftward (levo = L) loop or bend of the embryonic cardiac tube and indicates that the ventricles have looped abnormally, resulting in the right ventricle being located on the left and connected to the left atrium and the left ventricle being located on the right and connected to the right atrium. Sometimes, the term ventricular inversion is used (Fig. 2.15).

As mentioned before, the identification of the right and left ventricle is based on their specific morphologic features. In some cases, it may be difficult to determine which ventricle is which? Usually, in such cases, it is assumed that if the aortic valve is on the right side, the right ventricle is located to the right of the left ventricle, (D-loop). In a normal heart, the aortic valve is located posterior to (behind) and to the right of the pulmonary valve (Fig. 2.16). If the aortic valve is on the left side, the right ventricle is located to the left of the left ventricle (L-loop). This rule is referred to as the *loop* rule.

The position of the mitral and tricuspid valves (atrioventricular valves) is also in correlation with the ventricular loop. In general, the tricuspid valve is associated with the right ventricle and the mitral valve is associated with the left ventricle. In D-loop the tricuspid valve is on the right and the mitral valve is on the left (normal position), whereas in L-loop the tricuspid valve is on the left and the mitral valve is on the right, since the ventricles are reversed.

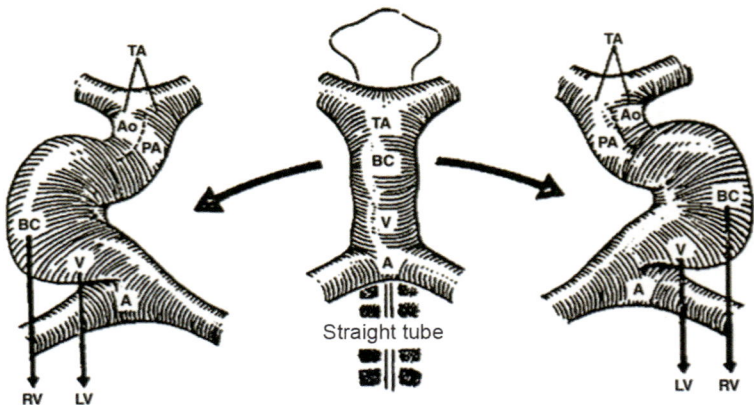

**Fig. 2.15:** Development of the heart. Diagram shows the formation of a D-loop (left) and an L-loop (right) from the embryonic cardiac tube (centre). A—atria, Ao—aorta, BC—bulbus cordis, LV—left ventricle, PA—pulmonary artery, RV—right ventricle, TA—truncus arteriosus, V—embryonic left ventricle

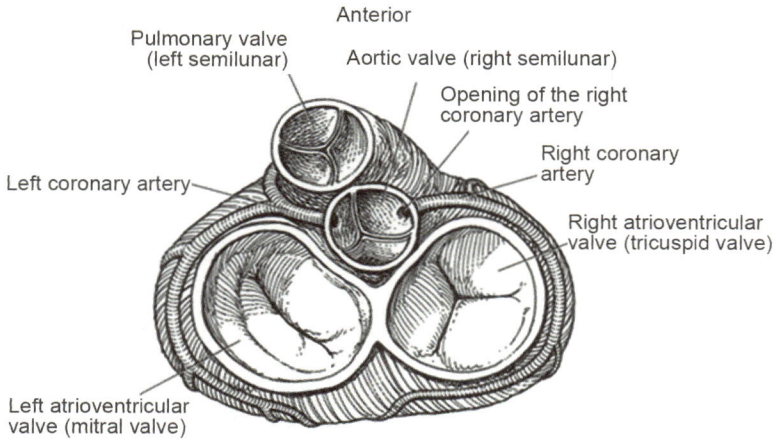

**Fig. 2.16:** Normal position of the aortic valve; located posterior and to the right of the pulmonary valve

## Position of the Aorta and the Pulmonary Artery

The position of the great vessels is determined by the cardiologist and described in the echo report (Fig. 2.17). Abnormalities in the origin of the great vessels, or conotruncal anomalies, are predo-minantly of three types: d-transposition (dextro-transposition), l-transposition (levo-transposition), and d-malposition with double outlet right ventricle. The pulmonary artery, taking flow to the lungs, is normally committed to the right ventricle while the aorta, taking blood to the systemic circuit, is normally com-mitted to the left ventricle.

## Crisscross Heart

A crisscross heart is a rare and complex congenital anomaly (8 in 1000,000 and less than 0.1% of all congenital heart defects). Many investigators have attempted to define the characteristics of this variance. A crisscross heart (CCH) almost never occurs as an isolated lesion, which makes it harder to define the nature of the defect. The term crisscross heart was introduced by Anderson et al (a British cardiac morphologist), in 1974, who described the anomaly in which the ventricular chambers are arranged in a superior-inferior fashion; the right ventricle is located superior or

**Cardiac Position**
Levocardia. Abdominal situs solitus. Atrial situs solitus.
D Ventricular Loop. S Normal position great vessels.

**Veins**
Normal systemic venous drainage. Normal pulmonary venous drainage.

**Atrium**
Normal left atrial size. Patent foramen ovale.

**Atrioventricular Valves**
Normal tricuspid valve. Normal mitral valve.

**Ventricles**
Intact ventricular septum.

**Semilunar Valves**
Normal pulmonic valve. Bicuspid aortic valve.

**Great Vessels**
Normal left aortic arch. Left pulmonary artery distal stenosis.

**Function**
Normal left ventricular systolic function.

**Outflow Haemodynamics**
Trivial aortic valve insufficiency.

**Fig. 2.17:** An example of an echo report

up and the left ventricle is located inferior or down. This is also referred to as an upstairs-downstairs heart. Most commonly, the ventriculoarterial connection is double outlet right ventricle (DORV) and less often discordant. Associated anomalies include right ventricular hypoplasia, overriding of the AV valves and subaortic or subpulmonary stenosis. A ventricular septal defect is almost always present.

In summary, a detailed study by means of echocardiography, executing a sequential approach during image review, the cardiologist can achieve a more accurate interpretation of congenital heart disease and ensures that no abnormalities are overlooked (Fig. 2.17). It is routinely executed by cardiologists and discussed with cardiac surgeons and decided which surgical procedure is in the best interest for the child. Also perioperative nurses have access to these reports and studying these reports is often extremely helpful to gain a better insight into the child's condition in order to give better nursing care.

# Nursing the Young Patient in Paediatric Cardiac Surgery

## INTRODUCTION

Unfortunately, but of preoperative necessity, children needing cardiac surgery undergo several invasive and painful procedures such as venous and arterial puncture to collect blood samples. By the time these children are ready for surgery, they may have gone through traumatic and stressful experiences and being exposed to many unfamiliar faces and several investigations, either invasive or non-invasive.

## PREOPERATIVE NURSING CARE

In most centres, the anaesthesia provider visits the child before the planned surgery to establish rapport and assess the child, preferably, with the parents present. Although encouraged in some centres, it is not common practice for perioperative nurses to visit children prior to their surgery. The preoperative assessment is established by ward nurses. Usually, the first interaction the perioperative nurse will have with the infant patient is when they are brought to the operating room and however short that interaction may be, it is nevertheless an important one as the perioperative nurse is often seen as taking the child from the parents. Therefore, the perioperative nurse should have an understanding of the individual physical and psychosocial needs

---

**NURSING OBSERVATION**

*Having knowledge of preoperative preparation of children will help the nurse in the cardiac operating theatre to better care for them, who may be visibly stressed and crying. Tender nursing care can alleviate some of their distress through being prepared technically and where possible, through soothing and emotionally caring attention.*

of infant patients regarding the natural stages of development. The plan of care should reflect considerations for age and the developmental stages of each child. Every child is a unique individual. Each child's age, past hospital experiences, temperament and coping techniques can affect how he or she deals with the upcoming procedure. It is difficult for young children to grasp the concept of surgery especially the words open-heart surgery.

---

**NURSING OBSERVATION**

The perioperative nurse should also be thoughtful of the accompanying parent(s), when their child is brought to the operating theatre. When parents plan a family they hope and expect to have normal healthy children. The birth of a child with congenital heart disease demands a major change in their daily life and their prospects for the future.

---

## NEWBORNS AND INFANTS

Newborns or neonates (birth to twenty-eight days) and infants (twenty-eight days to eighteen months) (Fig. 3.1), are too young to benefit from preoperative planning, education, and explanations. An infant younger than one year will not remember the experience of being brought to the operating room and undergoing cardiac surgery. Things that are stressful to older infants in the hospital may include separation from parents, having

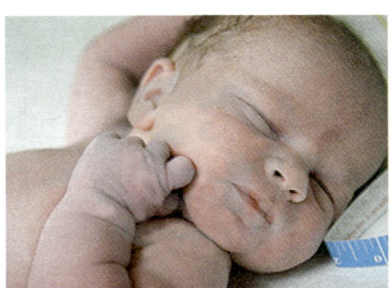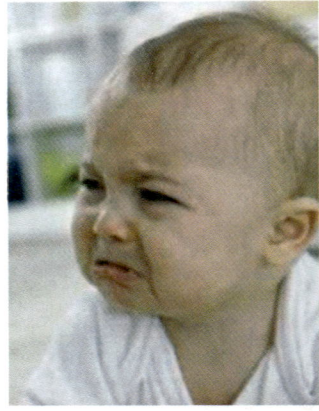

**Fig. 3.1:** Neonate and infant

many different caregivers, seeing strange sights, sounds and smells, new and different routines, and hunger due to fasting, to name but a few. Small infants learn to develop attachment to others; are dependent on others for warmth, nourishment, and stimulation and may view being taken from the security of the parents to the operating room as being abandoned by their parents. Recognizing what is stressful to newborns and infants can guide the perioperative nurse when receiving these children in the operating theatre in providing reassurance and emotional support to both parents and the child.

## TODDLERS

In general, separation from parents is traumatic for infants older than six months, and the parent's presence is necessary for the comfort of the toddler. A toddler (eighteen months to three years) is different from the neonate and infant since they are able to develop a two-way relationship with others, and may be able to communicate fears (Fig. 3.2). Yet while these young toddlers have a sense of self-will, they fear immediate threats and find it difficult to think beyond present situations. They may become aggressive through fear when taken to the operating room. A transitional object, such as a blanket or stuffed animal, can be very effective in soothing the infant during times of separation from parents. Parents should be encouraged to accompany an infant or child to the operating room and in many centres parents are allowed to stay with their child till induction of anaesthesia.

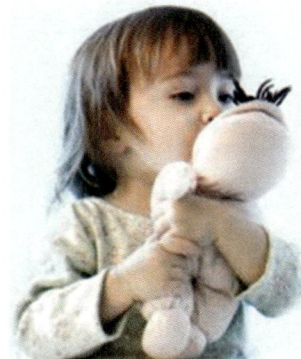
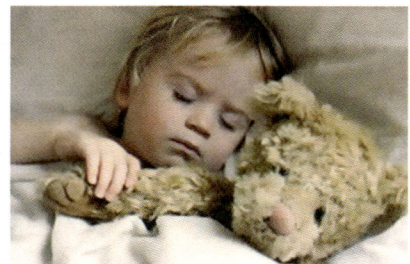

**Fig. 3.2:** Toddler

## PRESCHOOL AGE

Preschool age (three to five years) children begin to have fear of real or imagined situations and believe that every act has a purpose, often associating reward or punishment with their own and others actions. They may fear death, although may not always understand death as being permanent. Their imagination is developing (Fig. 3.3) and they may feel threatened by authoritative adults (doctors, nurses), they don't recognise. They may become aggressive through fear. Separation from parents at this age creates considerable anxiety.

## SCHOOL AGE

School age (six to twelve years) children prefer honest explanations (Fig. 3.4) and need reassurance. They do not want to be treated like babies. They may be able to distinguish between facts and in general, communicate well and want to be seen and treated as individuals. They also have a better understanding of death. The perioperative nurse should talk at the child's level about their fears and anxieties. They may have had previous cardiac surgery, and that experience will perhaps negatively influence subsequent surgery. Be careful with phrases like putting you to sleep when explaining general anaesthesia, as the child may associate this with a favourite pet they once had and was put to sleep. Separation from parents tends to be less of an issue in this age group.

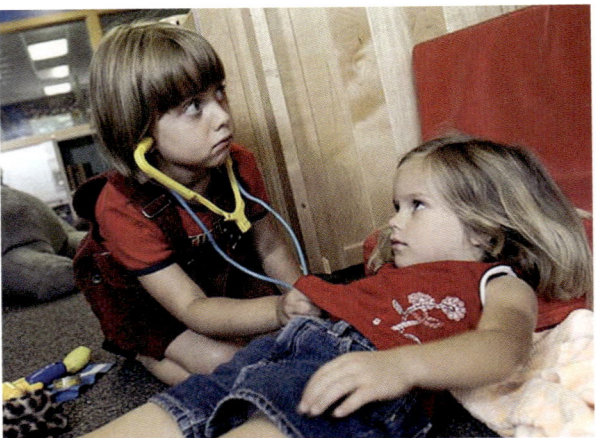

**Fig. 3.3:** Preschool age—their imagination is developing

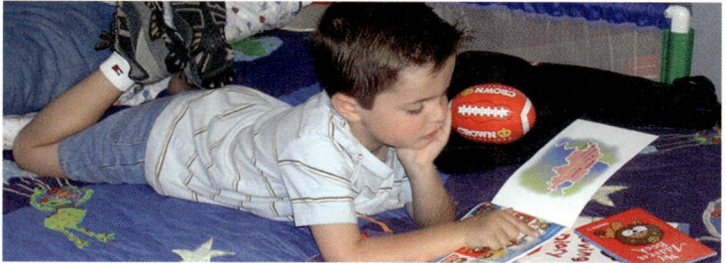

**Fig. 3.4:** School age children prefer honest explanations

## ADOLESCENT

The adolescent (twelve to sixteen years) is capable of reasoning and usually communicates well. These young adults prefer privacy and confidentiality, and are aware of opposite sex.

Not every patient of a particular age group will meet these broad psychological development criteria due to their illness. The attitude and adjustment of the parents towards children born with congenital anomalies will also greatly influence the child's mental state and acceptance of their illness. Remember, a significant proportion of survivors of open-heart surgery for congenital heart disease are at risk for psychological maladjustment and impaired quality of life. For some children, in particular for those with more severe congenital heart disease, research suggests psychological

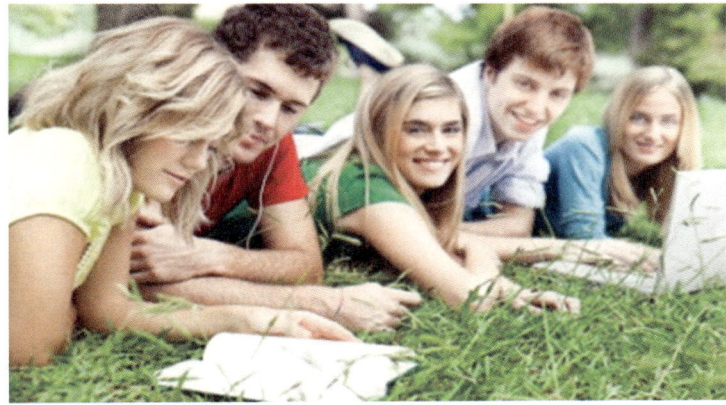

**Fig. 3.5:** A teenager, like one of these young people, is considered an adolescent

maladjustment is related to severity of the disease and develop-mental delay. Advanced diagnostic, medical and surgical manage-ment have extended and improved quality of life of many children born with congenital heart disease. Research into exploring subjective experiences and dilemmas of adolescents surviving into adulthood are small. Limited research on the subject identified dilemma of normality, dilemmas in disclosure, dilemmas in strategies for management of illness, the challenge of social integration versus social isolation, the challenge of dependence versus independence, the challenge of uncertainty, and strategies for coping. An understanding of these experiences by the perioperative nurse and other members of the healthcare team, can be beneficial in helping, in particular, the adolescent who has undergone multiple cardiac surgeries and help them to face the challenges of an uncertain, yet promising, future.

## NURSING AND PREMEDICATION

The perioperative nurse should have an understanding of premedication and its effects as most children having surgery, will have premedication prescribed. For infants younger than 1 year, however, it is usually not required. Premedication should be given at least 45 minutes to one hour before surgery, for it to be effective. It should make the child slightly sedated and calm and conse-quently facilitate smooth induction.

The perioperative nurse receiving the child in the holding bay of the operating room should stay with the child at all times, maintain a gentle touch, and be alert to the child's needs until the child is safely anaesthetized and intubated. Restraints, if necessary, should be loose. If the child is a newborn, infant or toddler, the perioperative nurse may hold the child in her arms during induction. Children may be induced by means of inhalation and today's facemasks for children are often scented with strawberry or banana to make them less gassy and traumatic for the child (Fig. 3.6). In most centres, however, intravenous induction is preferred and studies have shown this causes less psychological trauma then inhalation induction.

The optimal management of neonates, infants and small children undergoing repair of complex congenital cardiac lesions requires detailed knowledge by the anaesthesiologist of the anatomic and physiologic abnormalities and their consequences

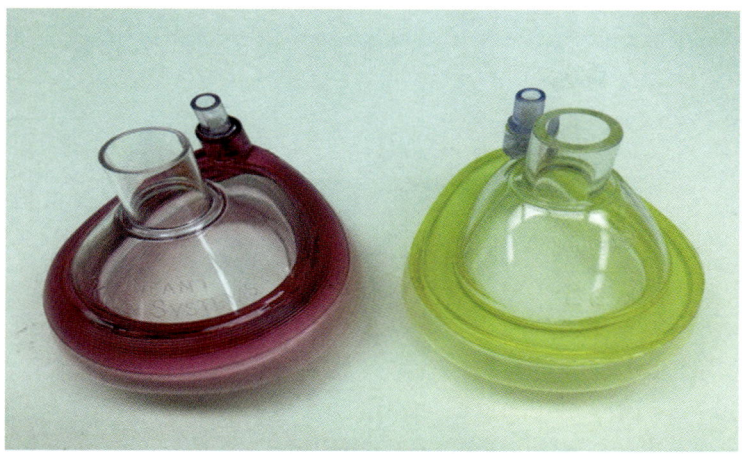

**Fig. 3.6:** Facemasks for children are often scented with strawberry or banana to make them less gassy and traumatic for the child. *(Photo by EDJ, courtesy of KAMC, National Guard Hospital, Riyadh, Saudi Arabia)*

on the perioperative course. Management of these children requires a team approach between the surgeon, anaesthesiologist, and the perfusionist. A perioperative nurse should have some knowledge and understanding of anaesthesia, and anaesthesia pharmacology to ensure the child safety outcomes.

# Perioperative Nursing in the Cardiac Operating Room

## INTRODUCTION

This chapter will promote the mastery of evidence-based perioperative nursing management of children born with complex heart disease. It aims to further develop knowledge, skills and understanding of the role of the surgical scrub nurses, so that they are equipped to work as a competent member of the multidisciplinary team. It aims to assist the perioperative nurse in utilising advanced knowledge and understanding of cardiac surgical procedures to ensure children safety outcomes.

Focused care and accurate attention by all members of the multidisciplinary team, including the scrub nurse, can mean a difference between life and death. It is worth bearing in mind that paediatric surgery is a specialty in itself and is not adult surgery scaled down to infant or child size. It is a specific skill, acquired over many years of observation, training and experience.

## ASSISTING THE SURGEON

In preparation for surgery, the perioperative scrub nurse prepares her instruments (Figs 4.1 and 4.2). This takes place usually from the time the child arrives in the operating room till the child is anaesthetized and all required monitoring devices are inserted by the anaesthetic team.

### NURSING OBSERVATION

*Many perioperative nurses, will, over time, move through one career specialism to the other. However, as cardiac centres are uncommon, few nurses will have the opportunity to work in a cardiac operating room during training. To nurse in paediatric cardiac surgery, it is essential to have two years minimum experience of general surgery scrub nursing before embanking on perioperative cardiac nursing training.*

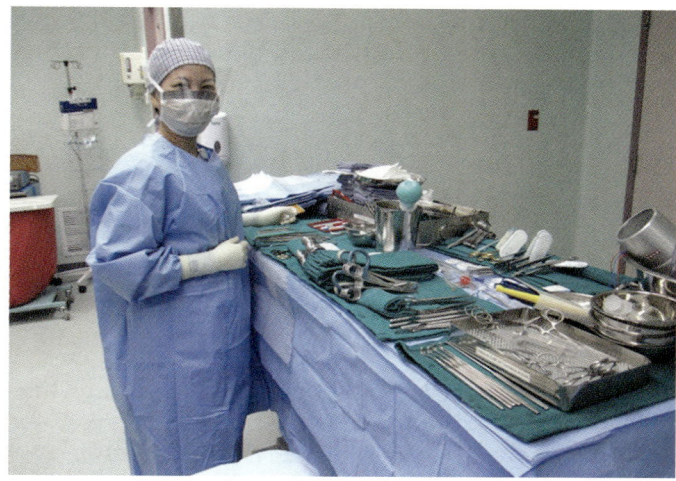

**Fig. 4.1:** A perioperative nurse preparing her instrument trolley. *(Photo by EDJ, courtesy of KAMC, National Guard Hospital, Riyadh, Saudi Arabia)*

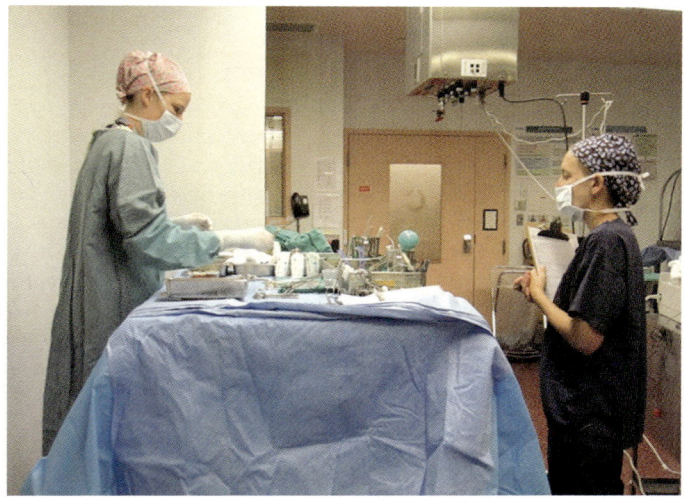

**Fig. 4.2:** A count of all instruments, sponges, needles and miscellaneous items is to be audibly and concurrently performed by the scrub nurse and circulating nurse before any cardiac procedure and be recorded on the count sheet labelled with the child's identification *(Photo by EDJ, courtesy of Sick Kids Hospital, Toronto, Canada)*

A count of all instruments, sponges, needles and supplementary items is performed and recorded for all surgical procedures to establish a baseline for subsequent counts (Fig. 4.2).[31]

**NURSING OBSERVATION**

*A count of all instruments, sponges, needles and miscellaneous items is to be audibly and concurrently performed by the scrub nurse and circulating nurse before any cardiac procedure and be recorded on the count sheet labelled with the child's identification and retained as part of the child's medical record. Perioperative nurses should be familiar with the departmental policies and procedures on the performance of surgical counts of the healthcare institution they work at.*

Assisting the cardiac surgeon is a highly skilled nursing task, and dealing with individual surgeons' stress levels as well as those of the supporting team can take its toll. Nurses on cardiac surgery duty should ensure adequate personal rest and be mentally prepared to commit to 100% effort, before taking on the responsibility of surgery support. There is probably no more demanding professional situation in the world, nor anywhere more crucial to life and death.

**SURGEON'S COMMENT**

*Paediatric cardiac surgery is a much more stressful task compared to adult surgery as the margin of error is very narrow and greater precision is required at many operative steps. Some of this stress is transmitted from the surgical team to the nursing team during the heat of the moment and is often spontaneous and abrupt. This may take the form of some harsh comments. As long as the limits of decency are not broken, these comments should never be taken as personal and should not affect one's performance during the surgical procedure. Often they are part of a high-risk game. Any excessive behaviour on the part of the surgeon, however, should be addressed through a dialogue after the end of the session.*

## POSITIONING THE PATIENT

Correct positioning of the child before surgery is the responsibility of all team members but is often the task of the perioperative nurse. The perioperative nurse must anticipate the equipment needed for the specific cardiac procedure. The child's position must provide optimum exposure for the procedure while providing access to intravenous lines and monitoring devices. The equipment

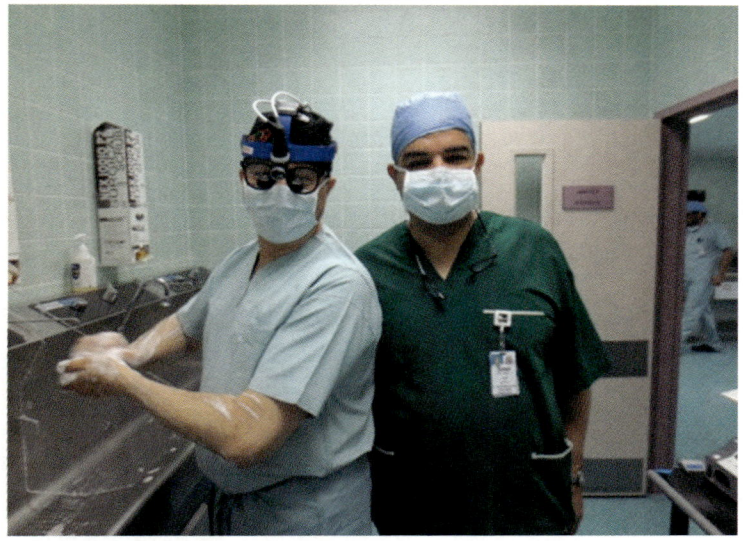

Dr. Hani Najm, Head of Cardiac Surgery and Dr. Mohamed Sallam, Consultant Cardiac Anaesthesiologist at the KAMC, National Guard Hospital, Riyadh, Saudi Arabia

to be used is based on the planned surgical procedure, surgeons' preference and the child's condition. The perioperative nurse must become aware of the procedure in advance of surgery. For cardiac surgery a full thoracotomy or a minithoracotomy, a median sternotomy or a ministernotomy incision may be necessary, depending on the type of the surgical intervention.

For the thoracotomy position, the child is either placed in a right lateral position for left thoracotomy (Fig. 4.3) and in a left lateral position for a right thoracotomy. Small towel rolls, pillows, and gel pads are used to protect pressure points and stabilize anaesthetized children (Fig. 4.4).

Complications of surgery associated with a thoracotomy incision include injury to the recurrent laryngeal nerve (Fig. 4.5), the phrenic nerve and the thoracic duct. Injury to the laryngeal nerve causes vocal cord paralysis and sometimes, is an important cause of acute or chronic respiratory distress in infants. Unilateral vocal cord paralysis normally causes more pronounced abnormalities of the infant's voice than bilateral vocal cord paralysis. Vocal cord dysfunction usually improves over time but

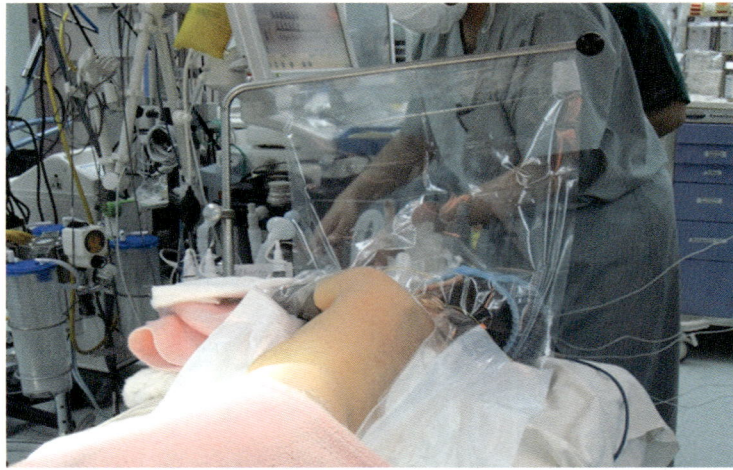

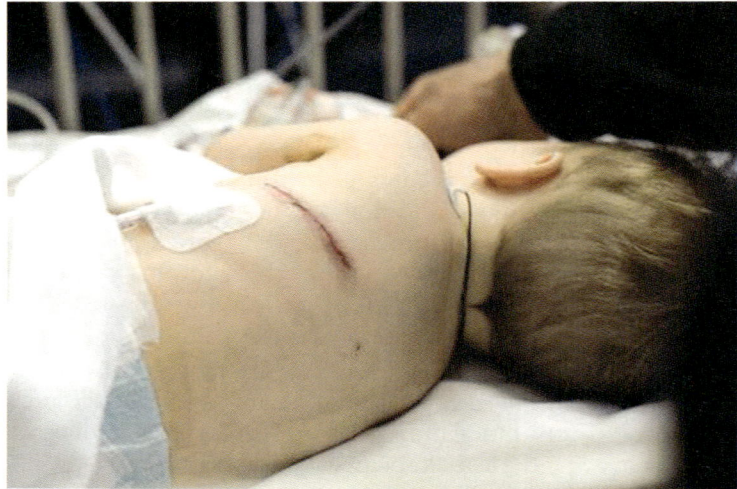

**Fig. 4.3:** A child in right lateral position for left thoracotomy incision. *(Photos by EDJ, courtesy of KAMC, National Guard Hospital, Riyadh, Saudi Arabia)*

may take years to resolve. Phrenic nerve damage is not uncommon and causes in most cases unilateral diaphragm paralysis, which may lead to respiratory distress, especially in neonates. The diaphragm is the main respiratory muscle in neonates and thus phrenic nerve injury can cause a delay in extubation and prolong

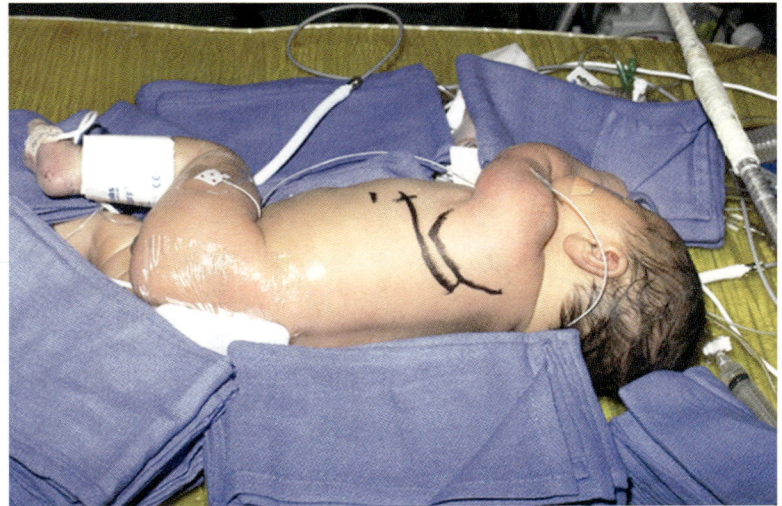

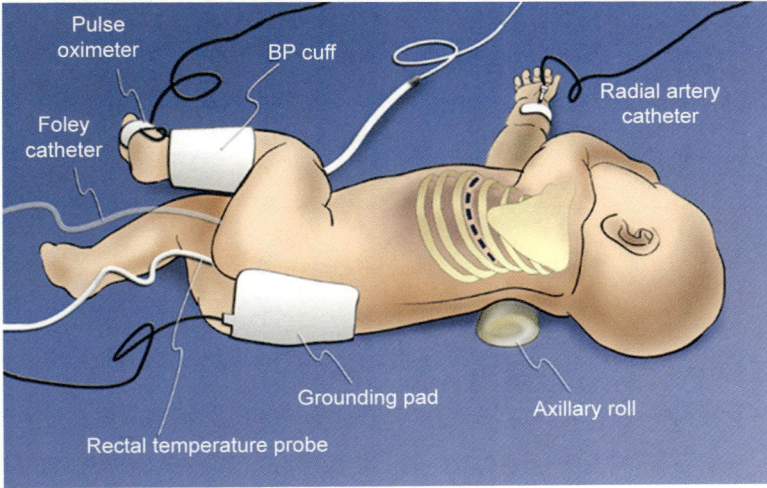

**Fig. 4.4:** Small towel rolls, pillows, and gel pads are used to protect pressure points and stabilize anaesthetized children

recovery of the child. The initial treatment is supportive, and spontaneous recovery occurs in most cases. If the neonate cannot be weaned off the ventilator, the infant is taken back to the operating theatre and surgical diaphragmatic plication is performed (Fig. 4.6).

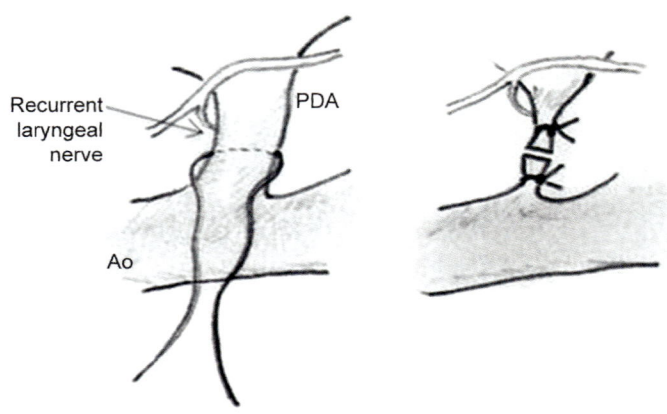

**Fig. 4.5:** Care should be taken by the surgeon to avoid injury to the recurrent laryngeal nerve

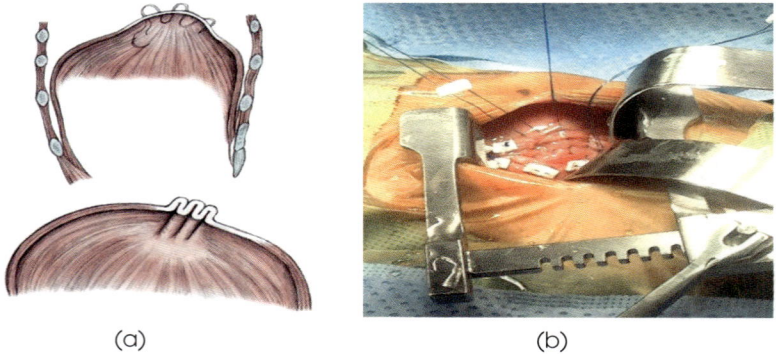

(a)                                              (b)

**Fig. 4.6:** Diaphragmatic paralysis (a) and diaphragmatic plication with a non-absorbable polypropylene suture  (b). *(Photo by EDJ, courtesy of KAMC, National Guard Hospital, Riyadh, Saudi Arabia)*

Chylothorax is a frequent and serious complication associated with thoracotomy. Chylothorax happens when chylus (lymph) leaks into the pleural cavity due to damage of the thoracic duct. This is referred to as pleural effusion. Chylothorax can also cause a delay in extubation and treatment is usually surgical ligation of the duct.

Most cardiac surgical procedures require cardiopulmonary bypass and the heart is accessed through a median sternotomy. The child is placed in a supine position. Some surgeons may prefer to mark the incision site (Fig. 4.7).

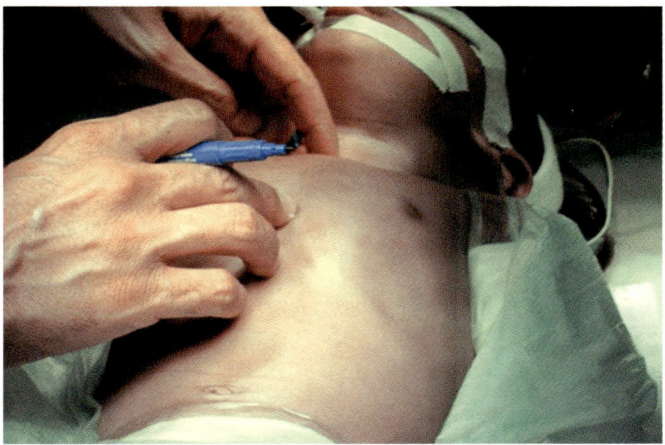

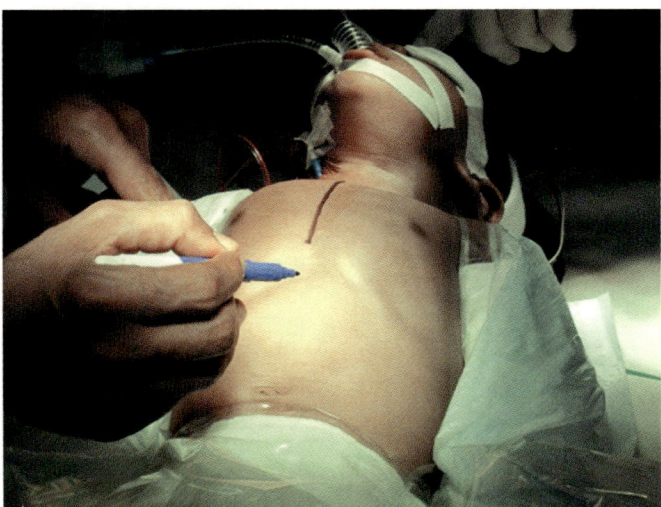

**Fig. 4.7:** A child in supine position and prepared for a median sternotomy. Some surgeons may prefer to mark the incision site. *(Photos by EDJ, courtesy of KAMC, National Guard Hospital, Riyadh, Saudi Arabia)*

After the child is placed on the operating table and all monitoring devices are secured, a protective screen is placed at the top of the table to protect the child from the weight of the drapes, allowing easy access to the child for both the surgeon and first assistant as well as for the anaesthesiologist (Figs 4.8 and 4.9).

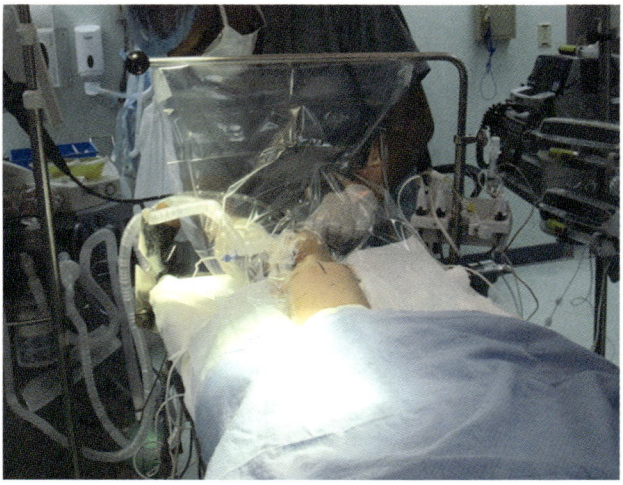

**Fig. 4.8:** A protective screen is placed at the top of the table to protect the child from the drapes and allow easy access for the anaesthesiologist. *(Photo by EDJ, courtesy of KAMC, National Guard Hospital, Riyadh, Saudi Arabia)*

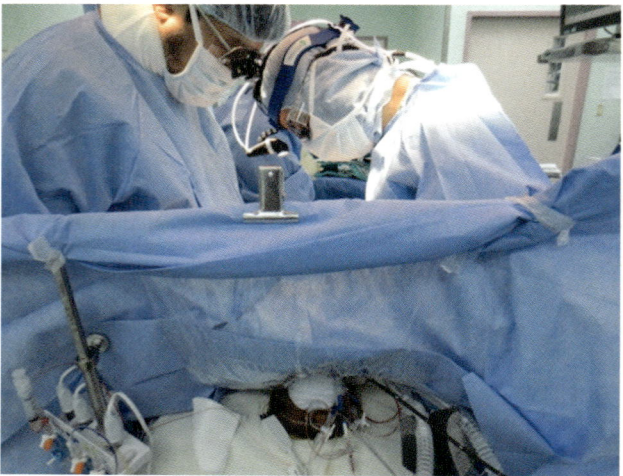

**Fig. 4.9:** A protective screen is placed at the top of the table to protect the child from the drapes and allow easy access to the child for both the surgeon and first assistant as well as for the anaesthesiologist. *(Photo by EDJ, courtesy of KAMC, National Guard Hospital, Riyadh, Saudi Arabia)*

*Neonates and infants are especially prone to becoming hypothermic on exposure to the operating room environment and hypothermia can lead to many complications including systemic acidosis, poor peripheral perfusion and depression of heart function. It is thus vital that infants should be covered with a heating lamp and older children with warm blankets throughout the time of positioning and anaesthetic preparation. It is also important to monitor the body temperature with a temperature probe to prevent hypothermia before the child is draped properly.*

The operating room lights should be positioned slightly above and to the left of the surgeon if he or she is right handed. The height of the operating table is adjusted so the surgeon's wrists are 1 to 3 cm below the elbows while operating. The first assistant and the assisting perioperative nurse adjust their positions to accommodate the surgeon. This sometimes means that nurses have to stand on a step during the procedure (Fig. 4.10).

Prior to surgery commencing, the neck, chest, and abdomen are prepped and sterile drapes placed around the operative field (Figs 4.11 and 4.12). In children the groins are not exposed, as is

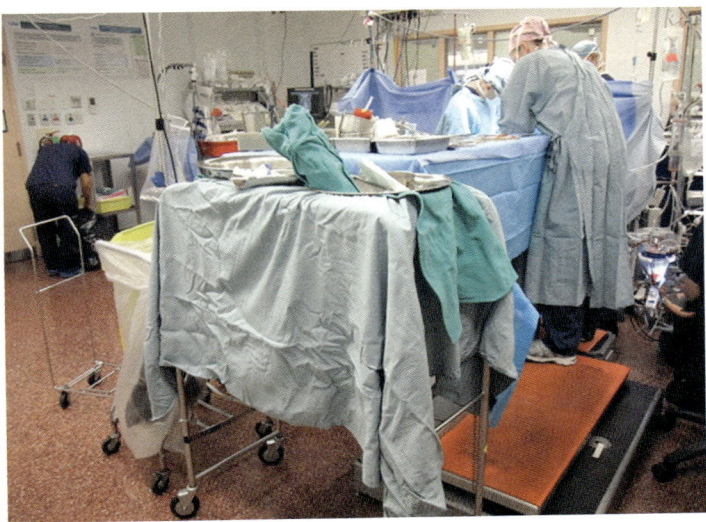

**Fig. 4.10:** A perioperative nurse standing on a step while assisting the surgeon. *(Photo by EDJ, courtesy of SickKids Hospital, Toronto, Canada)*

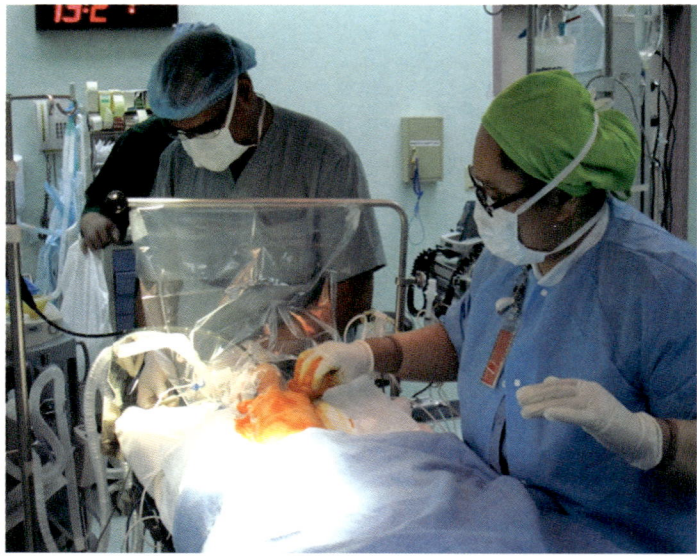

**Fig. 4.11:** Prior to surgery, the neck, chest and abdomen are prepped. *(Photo by EDJ, courtesy of KAMC, National Guard Hospital, Riyadh, Saudi Arabia)*

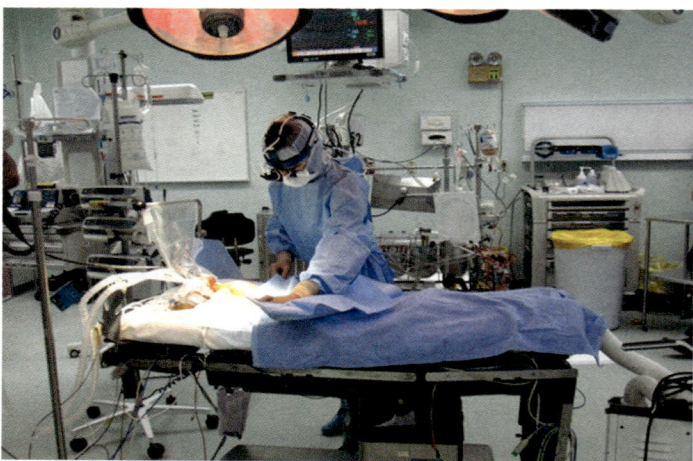

**Fig. 4.12:** Sterile drapes are placed around the operative field. *(Photo by EDJ, courtesy of KAMC, National Guard Hospital, Riyadh, Saudi Arabia)*

the case in adults for the purpose of femoral cannulation. In children and especially newborns, femoral cannulation is rarely done as this is technically not possible due to their tiny arteries and veins and no perfusion cannula would fit their femoral arteries and veins.

## CARDIOPULMONARY BYPASS PREPARATION

### History

The development of the heart-lung machine or cardiopulmonary bypass machine (CPB), made repair of intracardiac lesions possible. In 1953, John Gibbon (Fig. 4.13) performed the first successful open heart surgery using a heart-lung machine, which he had invented himself, while repairing an atrial septal defect on a young woman. Before that, surgeons had explored other roads like hypothermia, cooling the patient in a cold water tub and then rapidly performing the surgical correction of a heart lesion. After his first success, the following four patients of Gibbon died, which led him to abandon heart surgery and produced a generalized pessimism about extracorporeal circulation. However, a year later Walton Lillehei (Fig. 4.13) reverted this situation with the introduction of controlled cross-circulation in which a patient, usually, a child, was connected to a donor, usually the father or mother, whose heart and lung served as a pump and oxygenator, allowing the performance of open heart surgery. It was Lillehei again who, a year later introduced the bubble oxygenator, opening the doors to open heart surgery to all surgeons around the world. For this, and many other reasons, Walton Lillehei is considered by most surgeons as the 'Father of Open Heart Surgery'.[33]

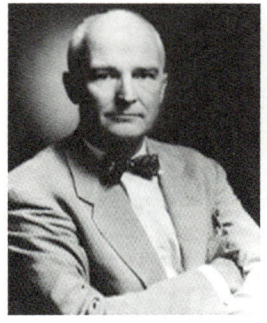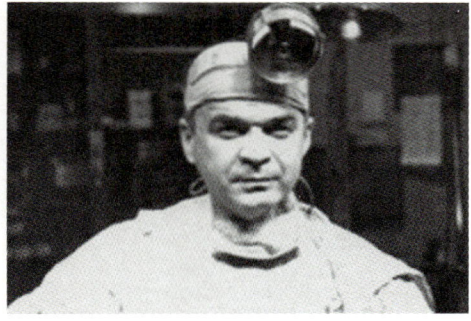

**Fig. 4.13:** John H. Gibbon (1903–1973) and C. Walton Lillehei (1918–1999)

Today, with the heart-lung machine, open heart surgery is routine. For most repairs of congenital cardiac lesions, the use of cardiopulmonary bypass (CPB) is necessary. CPB is a mechanical means of circulating and oxygenating the blood volume while diverting most of the circulation from the heart and lungs. It allows the surgeon to work on a blood free heart while preserving tissue perfusion and viability, particularly of the brain. CPB uses a pump, an oxygenator with reservoir function, a filter and plastic circuitry. Venous blood is drained into the oxygenator by one or two cannulae placed in the right atrium or vena cavae; arterial blood is returned to the patient via a single cannula normally placed in the ascending aorta. During CPB, the blood volume is circulated continuously between the patient and the CPB machine, where the blood is filtered, temperature regulated, and oxygenated.

It is the responsibility of a perfusionist to operate the heart-lung machine (Fig. 4.14). Ideally, the perfusionist should be opposite the surgeon to allow easy communication but in some centres the perfusionist and pump may be behind the surgeon, due to operating room design. Also, the assisting perioperative nurse may be standing next to or opposite the surgeon.

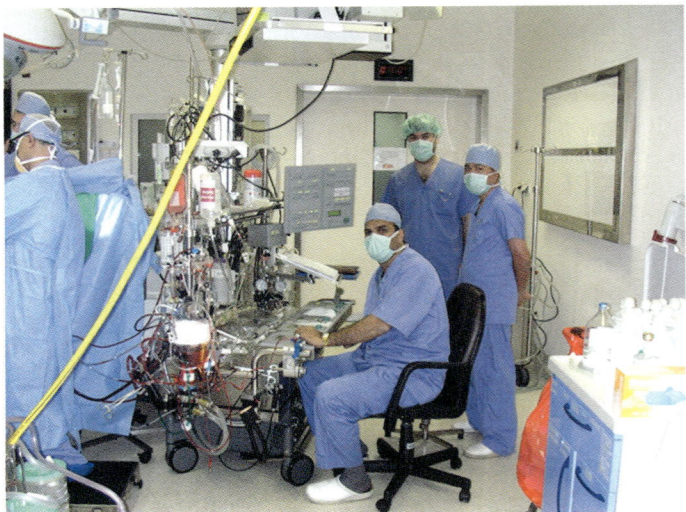

**Fig. 4.14:** Cardiopulmonary bypass (CPB) machine, or pump and perfusionists operating the CPB machine. *(Photo by EDJ, courtesy of King Faisal Specialist Hospital, Jeddah, Saudi Arabia)*

**PERFUSIONIST'S COMMENT**

*Perfusion as a field of study and practice by professionals has emerged during the history of cardiac surgery. In the 1950s and 1960s, physicians who had experienced and trained with the technology in the animal research laboratory often performed CPB. Much of the equipment used during that era was fabricated within the institution. Today, formal perfusion training programs teach clinical applications of extracorporeal technology for medical situations, where it is necessary to support or temporarily replace a patient's circulatory or respiratory function. The perfusionist is knowledgeable about applications of the technology and is educated to conduct CPB safely. There is a wide variety of cardiopulmonary equipments and supplies available, and there are many different ways in which these components can be assembled and used. Over the years, increased awareness of abnormal events (or the rare perfusion mishap) resulting in adverse clinical outcome has further helped define safe practices and codify institutional protocols and national practice guidelines.*

To commence the bypass, the lines of the cardiopulmonary bypass machine are passed to the operative field but must be secured in a way that does not interfere with the operative field, and located safely so they do not become dislodged (Fig. 4.15).

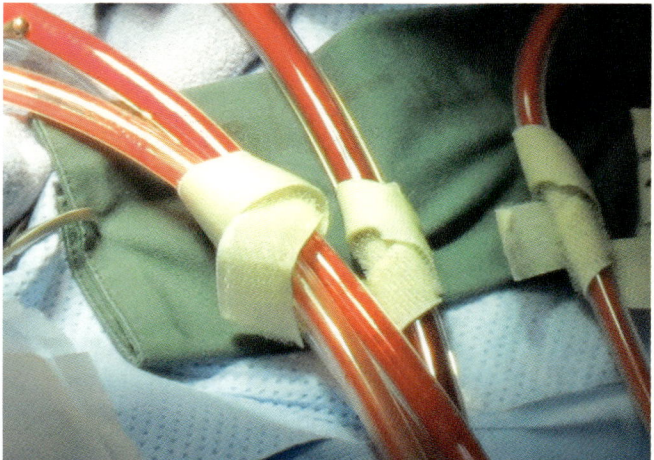

**Fig. 4.15:** The lines of the cardiopulmonary bypass machine are passed to the operative field but must be secured in a way that does not interfere with the operative field, and located safely so they do not become dislodged. *(Photo by EDJ, courtesy of KAMC, National Guard Hospital, Riyadh, Saudi Arabia)*

## INCISION

In first time median sternotomy, the sternum is divided with a reciprocating sternal saw (Figs 4.16 and 4.17a) and in neonates, some surgeons may use straight 'Mayo' scissors and cut the

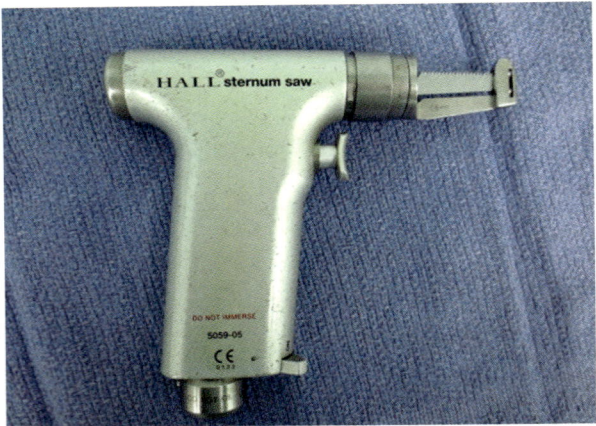

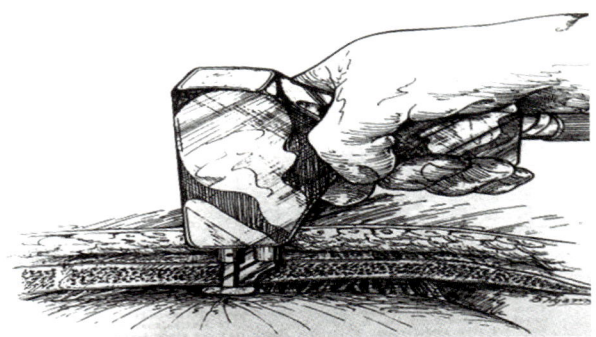

**Fig. 4.16:** In first time median sternotomy, the sternum is divided with a reciprocating sternal saw

sternum [Fig. 4.17b]. Any bleeding from the sternal edges is controlled with bone wax and/or cauterized. A sternal retractor is then inserted.

If there has been previous sternotomies, anterior and lateral chest X-rays are needed to determine the extent of adhesions and to count the number of chest wires that need to be removed (Fig. 4.18).

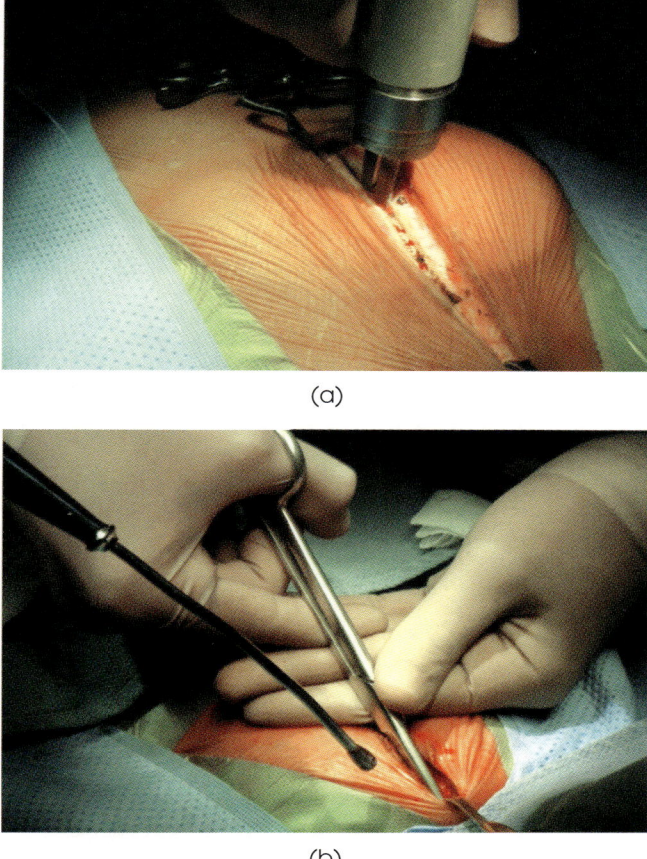

(a)

(b)

**Fig. 4.17:** The sternum is divided with a reciprocating sternal saw (a). In neonates, some surgeons may use straight Mayo scissors and cut the sternum (b). *(Photos a, b by EDJ, courtesy of KAMC, National Guard Hospital, Riyadh, Saudi Arabia)*

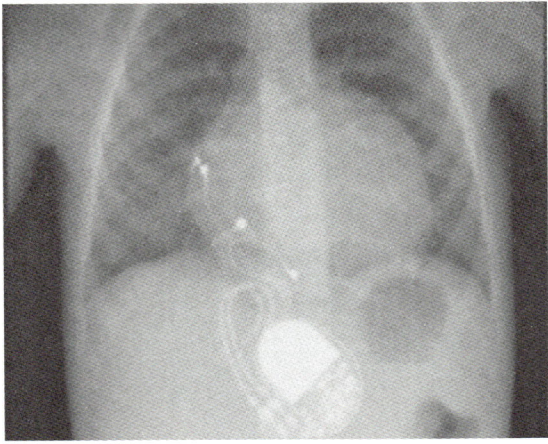

**Fig. 4.18:** Anterior and lateral chest X-rays are needed to determine the extent of adhesions and to count the number of chest wires that need to be removed. How many wires can be seen on this X-ray? On this X-ray a permanent pacemaker can also be noted

In redo or repeat sternotomy, the sternum is divided with an oscillating or vibrating sternal saw for safer access and adhesions from previous cardiac surgery must be dissected carefully (Fig. 4.19).

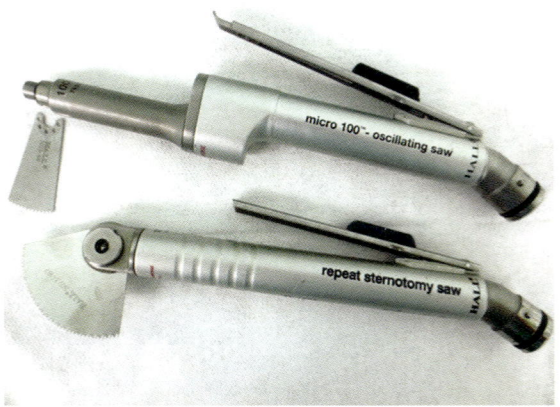

**Fig. 4.19:** In repeat sternotomy, the sternum is divided by an oscillating (vibrating) sternal saw. *(Photo by EDJ, courtesy of KAMC, National Guard Hospital, Riyadh, Saudi Arabia)*

### NURSING OBSERVATION

*In repeat sternotomies, external defibrillation pads should be placed on the child. The perioperative scrub nurse should be alert to increased risk of fibrillation from manipulation of the heart, bleeding and in some cases, laceration of the right ventricle. If the heart fibrillates during dissection, children can be defibrillated by means of the external defibrillating pads. NB: Division of the sternum is primarily a blind procedure and carries an increased risk of injury of major cardiac structures, such as the innominate vein, the right ventricle, and extracardiac conduits and grafts in the presence of adhesions, in particular, after first-time surgery.*

### SURGEON'S COMMENT

*Please always announce before you test the sternal saw for the information of the anaesthesiologist as they are normally supposed to stop patients' ventilation when the saw is being used.*

The thymus is a relatively large structure in young children and can present an obstacle to cannulation of the aorta. A portion or the entire thymus is almost routinely excised in children to improve exposure (Fig. 4.20). This procedure is not necessary in adults.

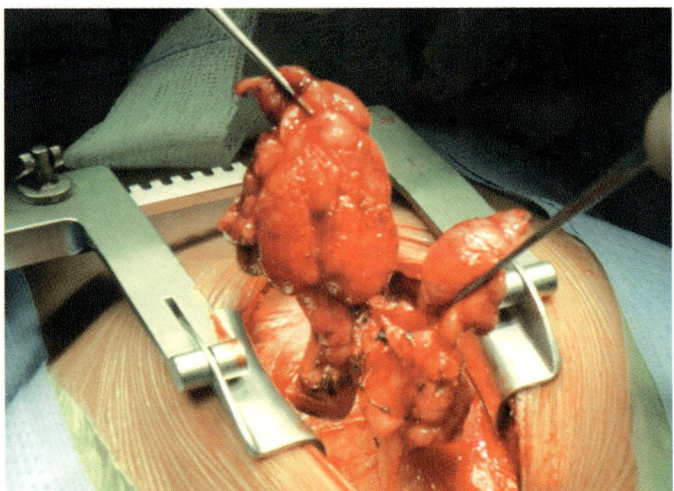

**Fig. 4.20:** A portion or the entire thymus is almost routinely excised in children to improve exposure. *(Photo by EDJ, courtesy of KAMC, National Guard Hospital, Riyadh, Saudi Arabia)*

**SURGEON'S COMMENT**

*There can be substantial blood loss when the sternum is split during sternotomy. A good supply of swabs, efficient suction and working diathermy should be ensured to expedite haemostasis and avoid unnecessary blood loss. In cases of re-sternotomy, the circulating nurse should also be fully attentive while the sternum is being opened so that extra help can be extended quickly and efficiently without wastage of time and efforts.*

Following the sternotomy, the pericardium is incised and retracted with silk sutures (Fig. 4.21).

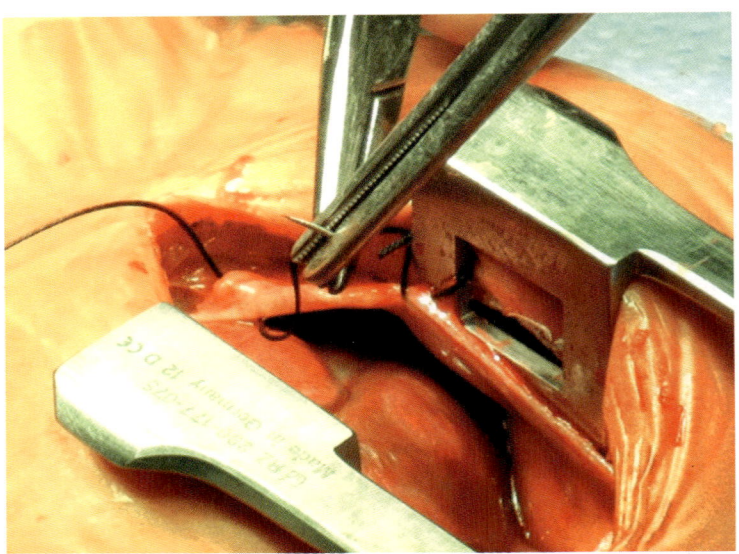

**Fig. 4.21:** Following the sternotomy, the pericardium is incised and retracted with silk sutures. *(Photo by EDJ, courtesy of KAMC, National Guard Hospital, Riyadh, Saudi Arabia)*

**SURGEON'S COMMENT**

*For some paediatric procedures, patients' own pericardium may be needed. Some surgeons prefer to harvest a piece of pericardium in the beginning of the operation, to be preserved in normal saline or be treated with glutaraldehyde as per individual preference.*

## CANNULATION AND CARDIOPULMONARY BYPASS

At the time of placing purse string sutures, the surgeon will ask the anaesthetist to administer heparin.[v] This is necessary to prevent clotting of blood in the heart-lung machine. When an adequate activated clotting time (ACT) is confirmed, the anaesthesiologist medically lowers the blood pressure to facilitate aortic cannulation.

The aortic cannula is always placed prior to the venous cannulae (and removed last), because in the event of an emergency, the perfusionist can temporarily initiate cardiopulmonary bypass via a single aortic cannula, (i.e. without venous cannulation). Crashing onto bypass is short-lived, however, as the CPB machine's reservoir is quickly depleted, thus the central veins need to be cannulated quickly and venous return to the pump established as soon as possible. Note that the aortic cannula does not have to enter directly via the aorta—an arterial cannula can be threaded into the aorta via the femoral artery (in adults) and in some instances, via the subclavian or innominate artery (in neonates, infants and children).

In newborns and infants one or two purse strings are placed on the aorta and the surgeon, using a scalpel with a No. 11 blade, makes an incision equal in length to the diameter of the cannula. The cannula is inserted and the purse strings are drawn tight with tourniquets and secured to the cannula with a silk tie (Fig. 4.22a, b].

After administration of systemic heparin and verification that the child is adequately anticoagulated, perfusate is recirculated through the CPB circuit one final time while the lines are tapped and inspected by the surgeon or an assistant to verify absence of any visible gas bubbles. Recirculation is stopped and the arterial

---

[v]An empirical loading dose of heparin at 300 to 400 U/kg is usually used, and maintaining the activated clotting time (ACT) greater than 480 seconds has been the gold standard for measuring adequate anticoagulation on bypass. The minimum safe ACT is in the region of 300 seconds based upon observations that above this level blood clots rarely occur in the extracorporeal circuit. The activated clotting time first came into clinical use in the mid-1970s to guide the administration and reversal of heparin during cardiopulmonary bypass procedures. Remember, neonates have a much greater variation of response to heparin administration and can show either a greater resistance or sensitivity to heparin than adults.

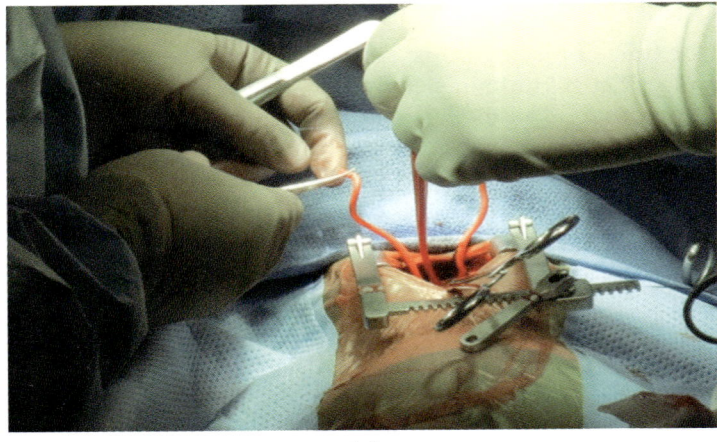

(a)

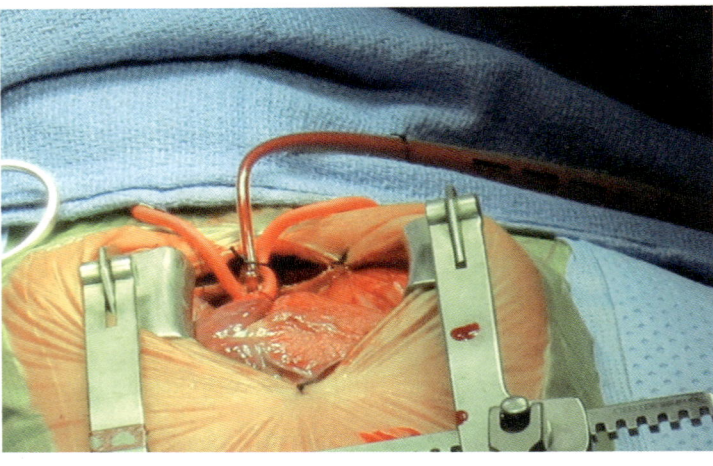

(b)

**Fig. 4.22:** The aortic cannula is inserted and the purse strings are drawn tight with tourniquets (a) and secured to the cannula with a silk tie (b). *(Photos a, b by EDJ, courtesy of KAMC, National Guard Hospital, Riyadh, Saudi Arabia)*

and venous lines are then clamped at the pump and table. The surgeon or assistant divides the arterial/venous recirculation loop. Most often, the surgeon connects the arterial cannula first after securing it in the ascending aorta with purse-string sutures. After the cannula is filled retrograde with the child's blood, an air-free connection is made between the CPB arterial flow line and the arterial cannula. Having the perfusionist slowly advance (come forward) the perfusate by activating the systemic flow pump will facilitate an air-free connection (Fig. 4.23); alternatively, an assistant

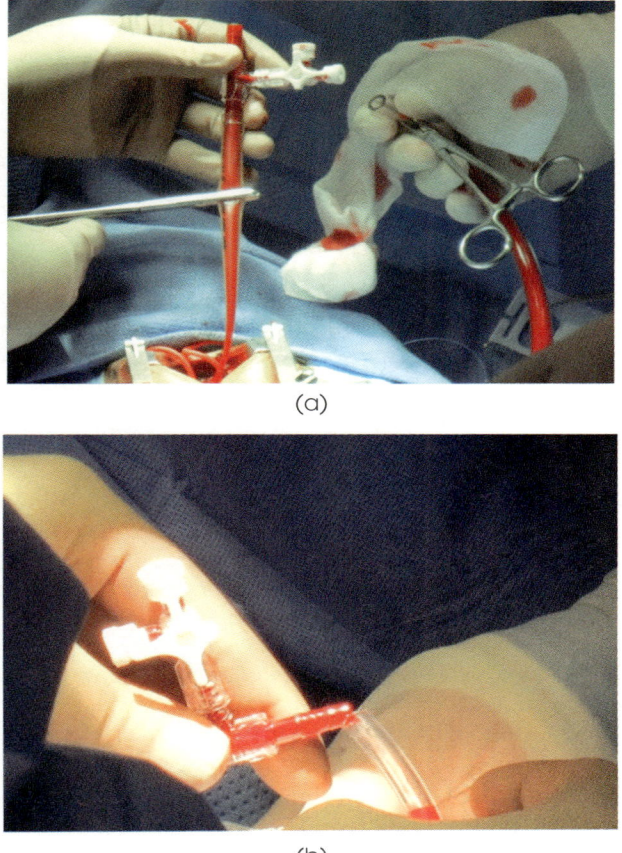

(a)

(b)

**Fig. 4.23:** After the cannula has been carefully de-aired by releasing the line clamp on the aortic cannula and the arterial pump line the perfusionist is asked to come forward, and the arterial cannula is then connected to the arterial pump line and secured to the drapes with a silk suture or towel clip to avoid unnecessary tension (Fig. 4.22b). *(Photos a, b by EDJ, courtesy of KAMC, National Guard Hospital, Riyadh, Saudi Arabia)*

can add sterile fluid from a syringe as the CPB line and cannula are joined. If the latter technique is used, the arterial flow line must be identified and distinguished from the venous drainage line to avoid the risk of reversed lines.

After the cannula has been carefully de-aired, it is connected to the arterial pump line (Fig. 4.23) and secured to the drapes with a silk suture or towel clip to avoid unnecessary tension (Fig. 4.22b).

---

**PERFUSIONIST'S COMMENT**

*The arterial cannula is generally placed into the ascending aorta; however, the great vessel anatomy of the child and the type of surgical procedure may influence arterial cannula placement. For example, in hypoplastic left heart syndrome, the ascending aorta is 1 to 5 mm in size, which is too small to accommodate a cannula capable of providing systemic perfusion. As an alternative, the arterial cannula is placed in the main pulmonary artery. Systemic perfusion is maintained from the pulmonary artery through the ductus arteriosus and down the descending aorta. Coronary perfusion is retrograde through the hypoplastic ascending aorta. The right and left pulmonary arteries are occluded with snares to prevent excessive perfusion of the pulmonary vascular bed. In newborns with transposition of the great arteries, the arterial cannula is placed in a more distal aspect of the ascending aorta because a large portion of the surgery is performed on the aortic root. Infants with interrupted aortic arch require two aortic cannulae, one in the ascending aorta to perfuse the head vessels and one in the descending aorta to perfuse the body. Cannulation of the femoral artery is not commonly used in neonatal or infant heart surgery because the femoral vessels are too small. In older children requiring reoperation, sternotomy is associated with a high-risk of inadvertently entering a conduit or a ventricular chamber. In these children, femoral or iliac arterial cannulation should be considered. The choice of cannula size depends not only on the lesion but also on the size of the child.*

---

After removal of the arterial line clamp at the field, the perfusionist should manually palpate or observe pulsation on an arterial flow line pressure monitor. The pressure transmitted from the aortic cannula through the arterial flow line will reasonably ensure that the cannula has been placed in the lumen of the aorta (or other arterial site). Absence of adequate pulsation may indicate malposition or insertion of the cannula into the vessel wall that could lead to arterial wall haematoma or dissection upon initiation of CPB (Fig. 4.24).

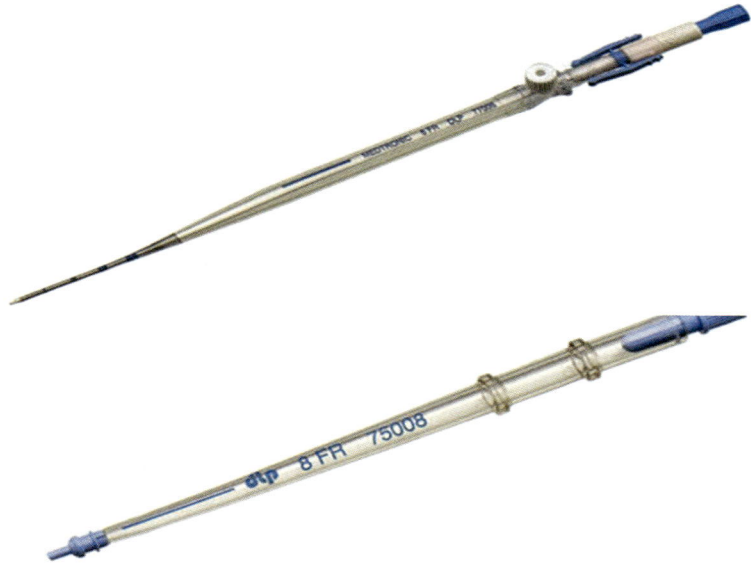

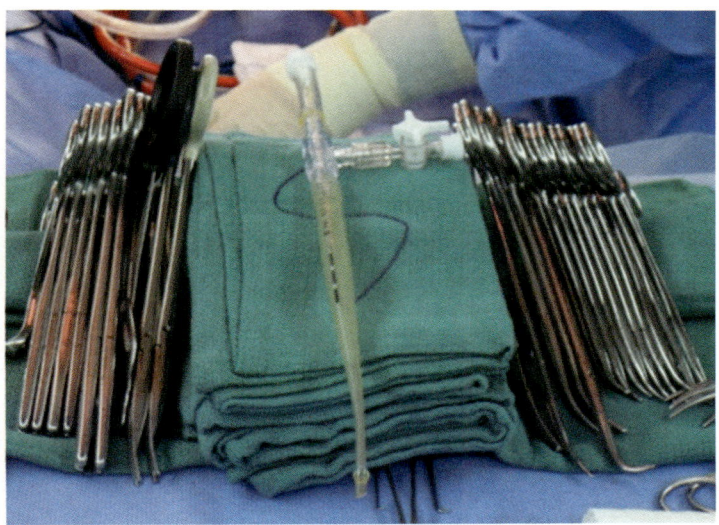

**Fig. 4.24:** Aortic cannulae used in paediatric cardiac surgery. *(Photo by EDJ, courtesy of KAMC, National Guard Hospital, Riyadh, Saudi Arabia)*

Depending on the needs of the surgeon and surgery, one or two venous cannulae may be placed. Most commonly two venous cannulae are placed into the right atrium and threaded into the inferior vena cava (IVC) and superior vena cava (SVC), or separate incisions are made into the SVC and IVC. The major advantages of a single cannula technique are speed and the use of fewer incisions. The major disadvantage of the single cannula is the inability to stop entire blood from passing through the heart and lungs, as well as physical interference with the right atrium. In instances entire in which a completely bloodless field is desired (e.g., valvular surgery), or in which access to the right atrium is necessary (e.g., atrial septal and ventricular septal defect repair), two cannulae are used.

When both venae cavae are to be cannulated, it depends on the surgeon's preference which vena cava is cannulated first. A purse string is placed in both the SVC and the IVC and subsequent cannulation is performed, again using a No. 11 scalpel for both. The cannulae are secured to their tourniquets in the same way as for the arterial cannula (Figs 4.25 and 4.26). Individual surgeons

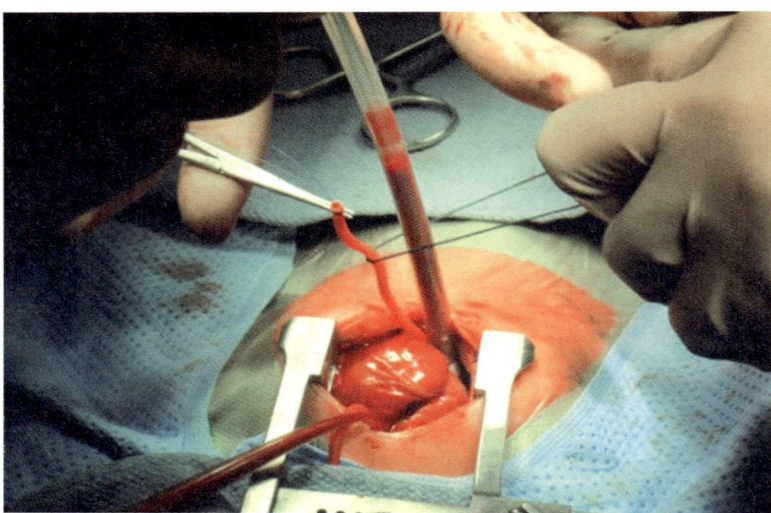

**Fig. 4.25:** The venous cannula (IVC) is secured to its tourniquet with a silk tie. *(Photo by EDJ, courtesy of KAMC, National Guard Hospital, Riyadh, Saudi Arabia)*

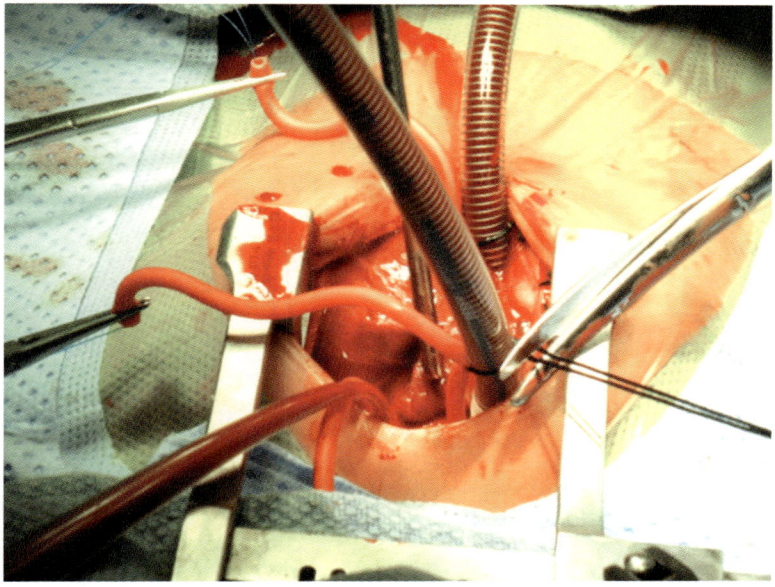

**Fig. 4.26:** The venous cannula (SVC) is secured to its tourniquet with a silk tie. *(Photo by EDJ, courtesy of KAMC, National Guard Hospital, Riyadh, Saudi Arabia)*

may place purse string sutures in the right atrium through which both the SVC and IVC are advanced.

If a single, two-stage venous cannula is used, it is inserted through a purse string suture in the right atrial appendage, the tip of which is incised with fine tipped scissors.

---

**SURGEON'S COMMENT**

*The optimal size and type of arterial and venous cannulae is declared by the perfusionist based on information from nomograms of patients' body weight/body surface area and also from consultant's preference card. Final selection of the cannulae should, however, be confirmed with the surgeon cannulating the patient before opening any cannula on the table. Selection may change due to variation in the anatomy and physiology of the underlying congenital anomaly.*

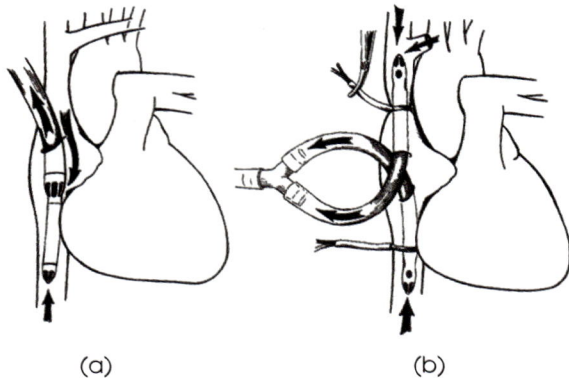

(a)           (b)

**Fig. 4.27:** Methods of venous cannulation. (a) Single cannulation of right atrium (RA) with a two-stage cavoatrial cannula. This is typically inserted through the right atrial appendage. Note that the narrower tip of the cannula is in the inferior vena cava (IVC), where it drains this vein. The wider portion, with additional drainage holes, resides in the RA, where blood is received from the coronary sinus and superior vena cava (SVC). The SVC must drain via the RA when a cavoatrial cannula is used. (b) Separate cannulation of the SVC and IVC. Note that there are loops placed around the cavae and venous cannulae and passed through tubing to act as tourniquets or snares. The tourniquet on the SVC has been tightened to divert all SVC flow into the SVC cannula and prevent communication with the RA

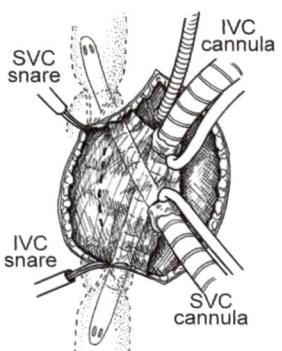

**Fig. 4.28:** Inferior vena caval (IVC) and superior vena caval (SVC) cannulae are advanced through pursestring sutures in the atrium. Both cavas are not yet snared. *Note:* The SVC cannula is placed through the lower pursestring and the IVC through the upper. The cannulae cross in the atrium. This is one method of venous cannulation

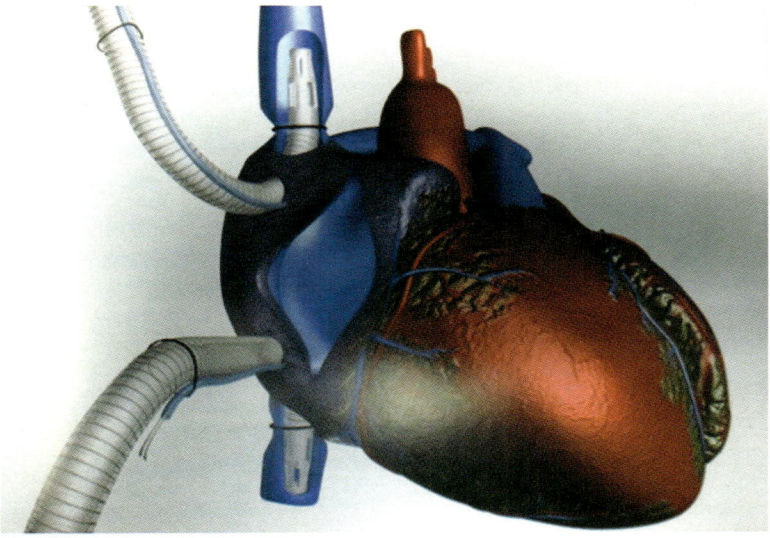

**Fig. 4.29:** In this picture, the SVC cannula is placed through the upper purse string and the IVC through the lower. The cannulae do not cross in the atrium. This is another method of venous cannulation

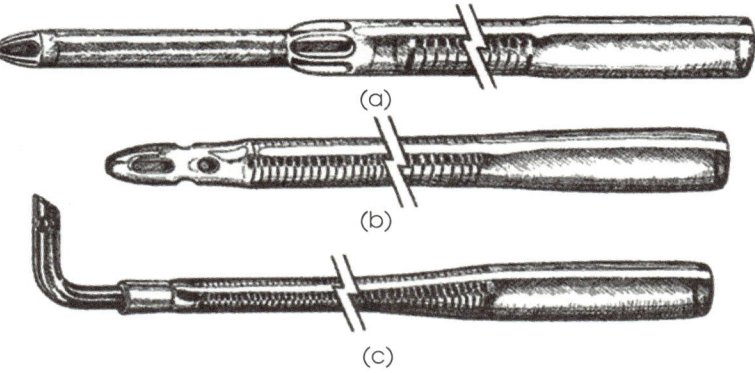

(a)

(b)

(c)

**Fig. 4.30:** Drawings of conventional venous cannulae. (a) Standard, tapered, two-stage cavoatrial cannula for insertion into the right atrium (RA) and inferior vena cava (IVC). (b) Wire-reinforced cannula for atrial or caval cannulation. (c) Cannula with right-angled tip (usually made of metal or hard plastic because the thin wall optimizes the ratio of internal to external diameters). This type of cannula is often used for congenital or pediatric cases and may be inserted directly into the vena cava near its junction with the RA

*Venous anatomy can be very complex. Bilateral superior venae cavae and inferior venae cavae that drain into an azygos vein or hemiazygous vein, or hepatic veins that drain directly into an atrial chamber, are common anatomic variations in the venous systems of patients with congenital cardiac defects. Venous cannulation must account for these variables if the repair is to take place during continuous-flow CPB.*

*If the repair is going to take place under deep hypothermic cardiac arrest (DHCA), CPB is used as a cooling modality. The repair occurs during the arrest period. Venous cannulation can, therefore, be simplified. A large single venous cannula is placed in the right atrium to achieve effective venous drainage. Once cooling has occurred, the cannulae are removed and surgery proceeds in a cannula-free field.*

*In the repair of defects associated with anomalies of systemic venous return, three venous cannulae may be required. Venous drainage is more effective and the cannulae are less obtrusive in the surgical field, if right-angle venous cannulae are used.*

*A third venous cannula may be required if a large left superior vena cava (SVC) with no bridging innominate vein is present. It is often easiest to place this cannula after the patient is on CPB. The venous tubing circuit can be constructed for these patients in a manner that will accommodate the addition of a third venous cannula.*

*To meet the surgical requirements, a large assortment of venous cannulae should be available. The type of venous cannula used and the amount of venous return it yields will vary depending on cannula size, child anatomy, site of insertion, and adequacy of cannula position.*

If a retrograde cardioplegia cannula is to be inserted, it is more easily inserted after placement of the venous cannulae but before cardiopulmonary bypass is instituted (Fig. 4.31). Retrograde cannulae are not used in infants and small children due to small size of coronary sinus[vi]. In young adults, a retrograde cannula can be inserted into the coronary sinus, usually, by means of a purse string suture and secured with a tourniquet. A pressure line is connected to the cannula and handed out to the anaesthesiologist to monitor the pressure at which cardioplegia is administered.

---

[vi] The coronary sinus drains most of the cardiac venous blood back to the right atrium. In cardiac surgery, this vein is used to give cardioplegia in a retrograde fashion.

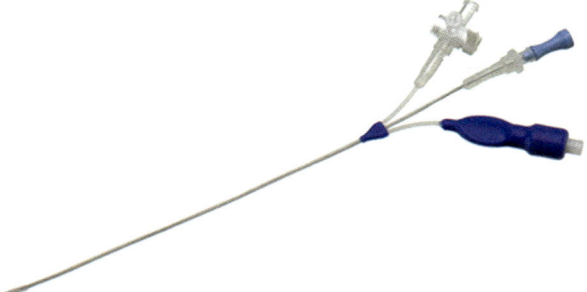

**Fig. 4.31:** Retrograde cannulae are designed to deliver cardioplegia solution to the heart through the coronary sinus in the reverse direction of normal blood flow (retrograde perfusion). These cannulae feature kink-resistant, wire-wound silicone bodies and smooth manual inflate cuffs with pressure monitoring lines. Cannulae come with either a guidewire stylet or without a stylet

Regardless of the cannulation technique selected, all cases of CPB will produce some blood flow return to the left ventricle (The right heart is normally drained or vented by the venous cannula(e). The normal sources of blood returning to the left ventricle during CPB include bronchial and Thebesian[vii] veins and blood returning to the right heart that gets by the CPB venous cannulae and passes through the pulmonary circuit. Abnormal sources include a left superior vena cava (LSVC), patent ductus arteriosus (PDA) or a systemic-to-pulmonary artery shunt (e.g., Blalock-Taussig shunt), major aortopulmonary collaterals, atrial or ventricular septal defects, anomalous systemic venous drainage into the left heart, and aortic regurgitation. Bronchial blood flow to the periphery of the lungs normally drains via the pulmonary veins and thus the left ventricle. On bypass the amount is influenced by the mean arterial pressure, which is one rationale

---

[vii]The smallest cardiac veins or Thebesian veins or veins of Thebesius are minute valveless veins in the walls of all four heart chambers. They are most abundant in the right atrium and least in the left ventricle. They drain the myocardium and pass through the endocardial layer to empty, mostly into the right atrium, but a few empty into the ventricles. The Thebesian venous network is considered an alternative (secondary) pathway of venous drainage of the myocardium. They are named after the German anatomist Adam Christian Thebesius, who described them in 1708.

for maintaining low perfusion pressure during CPB. Children with chronic lung infections and cyanotic congenital heart disease have exaggerated bronchial blood flow.

Coronary sinus flow into the right heart should greatly diminish with aortic crossclamping, except when cardioplegic solution is administered, and in the presence of an LSVC. Most coronary sinus blood should be removed if the venous cannulae are working properly, unless bicaval cannulae with caval tourniquets are used.

The purpose of left ventricular venting is to prevent distension of the ventricle, reduce myocardial rewarming, prevent cardiac ejection of air, and to facilitate surgical exposure. In order to minimize this, most paediatric CPB cases require a left ventricular (LV) vent (Fig. 4.32). Additionally, the bicaval cannulation

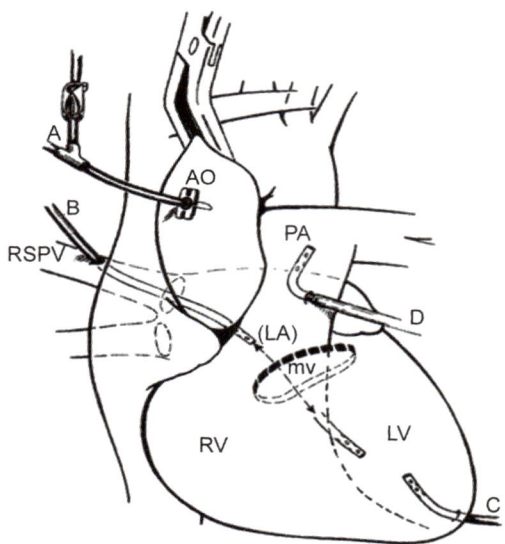

**Fig. 4.32:** Sites for venting the left ventricle. A: Aortic root cannula; one limb of the Y is connected to the cardioplegia administration system and the other limb to suction for venting left heart. B: Cannula inserted at the junction of the right superior pulmonary vein (RSPV) and left atrium and advanced through the left atrium and mitral valve (mv) into the left ventricle. C: Cannula is inserted directly into the apex of left ventricle. D: Cannula is inserted into the pulmonary artery. AO: Aorta; PA: Pulmonary artery; LA: Left atrium; RV: Right ventricle; LV: Left ventricle

technique may require the use of a second vent to capture coronary sinus blood that misses the IVC and SVC cannulae.

If an LV vent is needed, it is usually inserted before cardio-pulmonary bypass, although some surgeons may insert the LV vent after CPB. The surgeon makes an incision in the purse string suture at the junction of the right superior pulmonary vein and the left atrium and inserts the vent, which is then passed through the mitral valve and into the left ventricle. If the right atrium will be opened during the surgical procedure, an LV vent may also be inserted through the foramen ovale, through the left atrium, mitral valve and into the left ventricle.

## GOING ON BYPASS

Once all pump lines are inspected for security and correct placement, and upon instruction of the surgeon all line clamps are removed from the arterial and venous lines and cardiopulmonary bypass (CPB) commences. The perfusionist releases the arterial line clamp on the pump side first, and blood is transfused from the pump to the child. If this flow is unobstructed, the perfusionist releases the venous clamp, which ultimately diverts the child's venous blood into the cardio-pulmonary bypass circuit. This happens by gravity. The right heart should decompress (collapse).

The perfusionist then gradually increases the rate of arterial flow. This means that more and more blood will be transfused from the pump through the arterial cannula, to the child's body, and therefore, the ventricles will receive less and less blood. The arterial wave form on the child's monitor will become a flat line. The left heart (left ventricle) should collapse. To achieve a total decompressed left ventricle, tapes or silk ties are placed around both vena cava and tightened with tourniquets.

### NURSING OBSERVATION

*The scrub nurse must watch the CVP carefully, as a high CVP and poor venous drainage at the commencement of CPB, may indicate, a wrongly positioned venous cannula, perhaps a kinked venous line, or air in the venous line. The surgeon may need to re-adjust or re-insert the venous cannula to rectify the problem.*

Once total bypass (CPB) is achieved, an antegrade cardioplegia purse string is placed in the proximal ascending aorta, the cannula inserted and secured with a tourniquet (Fig. 4.33). This is commonly done after CPB. Cardioplegia is administered with re-dosing at 20 to 30 min intervals, and some surgeons may also use topical cold saline or *slush* on the heart to ensure proper cardiac arrest and preservation of the myocardium. The ECG waveform will become a *flat line*.

To reduce the metabolic and oxygen demands of the body, in particular the vital organs the moderate cooling of the child's body is commonly achieved with topical cold saline, although this is not uniform. All cardiopulmonary bypass machines have a heater/cooler device incorporated in the circuit, which allows for

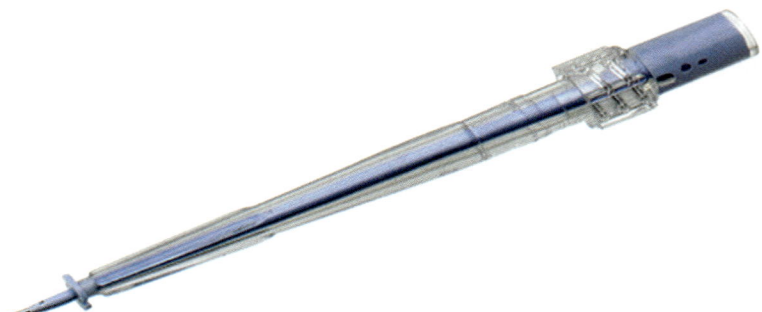

**Fig. 4.33:** Antegrade paediatric aortic root cannula (DLP)—antegrade cannulae are designed to deliver cardioplegia solution to the heart via the coronary ostia in the normal direction of blood flow (antegrade perfusion). Aortic root cannulae are intended to either aspirate air from the aorta or infuse cardioplegia directly into the aortic root near the aortic valve

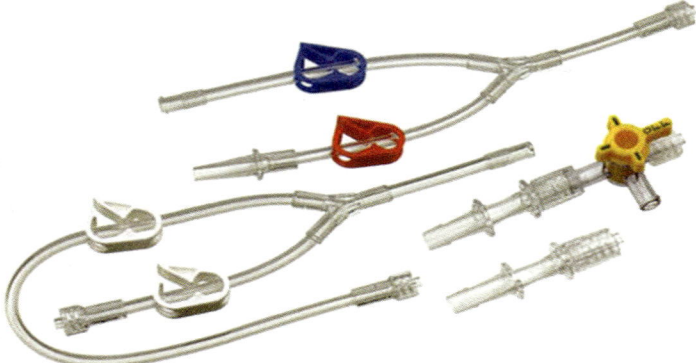

**Fig. 4.34:** Cardioplegia adapters are designed to permit customization of the cardioplegia circuit. Adapters can be used to switch between antegrade and retrograde delivery of cardioplegia. Additional adapters are available to extend the length of the cardioplegia circuit, recirculate the cardioplegia solution or provide an extension to the pressure monitoring line. All adapters are designed to be used in the perfusion circuit and are not patient size specific

cooling or warming the blood that is being transfused to the child. This will ultimately cool the child's core body temperature and reduce metabolic and oxygen demands. Other means of cooling a child is the use of cooling blankets, placed under the child or ice packs applied directly to the child (ice packs placed around the child's head is usually only needed when the procedure is performed with circulatory arrest and the child's core temperature is reduced to 18°C). Bladder and nasopharyngeal temperature probes must be present to continuously monitor the child's body temperature. Once the child's heart is on bypass, the heart stopped and cooled, surgery can begin.

## COMING OFF THE BYPASS MACHINE

Once the surgical repair has been carried out, and the aortic cross clamp removed, the body temperature of the neonate, infant or child is slowly increased. This is achieved by warming the blood from the heart-lung machine, by irrigating the heart topically with warm saline, and/or the use of heating blankets. These heating blankets are often placed underneath the child at the beginning of surgery, and can be heated as well as cooled.

### SURGEON'S COMMENT

*Surgeons vary in their routines to a greater or lesser extent but all cardiac surgeons tend to maintain a standard technique of sternotomy and cannulation in all their cases. This is meant to maintain a smooth flow of work, to reduce time required to go on cardiopulmonary bypass, especially, in emergency situations and to reduce the chances of complications during standard cannulation procedure. Each surgeon's techniques have in-built safety mechanisms to make cannulation and conduct of CP bypass safe for the patient. Nurses should endeavour to maintain this flow so that none of the standard steps are missed.*

*Sometimes, when there is no surgical assistant available, the surgeons cannulating the patient requests the help of the scrub nurse in the cannulation process. In this case, the priorities of the scrub nurse should change. It is preferable to make available all the requirements of cannulation including silk tie, scissors, dilator and clamps, etc. available within the reach of the surgeon. The scrub nurse should then completely concentrate on holding the cannula in position, till it is fully secured by the surgeon with the help of the tourniquets and silk tie. If the cannula comes out inadvertently before it is secured in place, re-insertion of the cannula becomes much more of a hazardous procedure.*

During all surgeries that require opening the heart, there is a chance that air may be *trapped* inside the heart. Once the child comes off bypass, this air may cause air emboli, especially, if present in the left side of the heart and once in the systemic circulation, may cause an infarct, either in the brain or other body organs. For this reason, air must be removed before coming off bypass and before the cross clamp on the aorta is released. With the aorta cross clamped, the child is placed in a 30° head-down position, the tourniquets on both vena cava are released and the perfusionist partly clamps the venous line, which restricts venous return to the pump and the right ventricle will fill with blood. The surgeon often says: 'fill up the heart'! To fill the left side of the heart with blood to remove air trapped in the left heart, the child is briefly ventilated, *'a few puffs to the lungs'*. This increases pulmonary venous return to the left heart and thereby removing any remaining air. This manoeuvre is referred to as Valsalva. At this point, the heart may be gently massaged to expel air (Fig. 4.35), with the vent in the left ventricle remaining in place and continuing to drain, removing potential air. The cardioplegia cannula may be left in place and placed on suction. There are

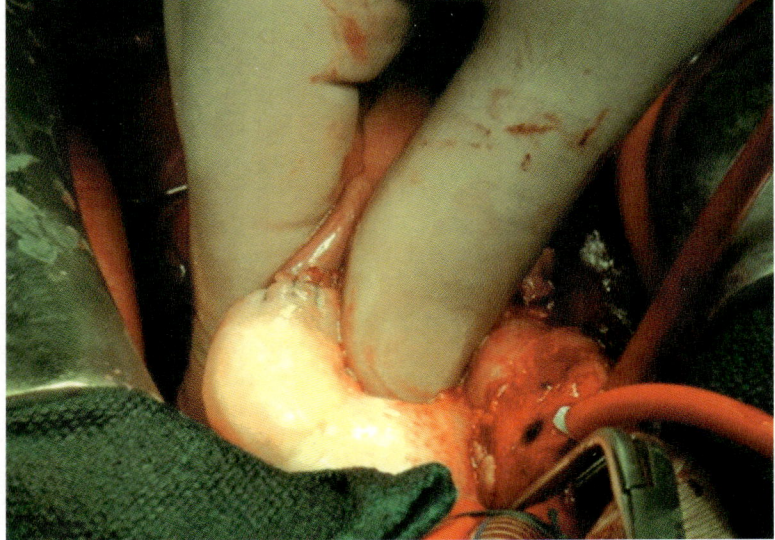

**Fig. 4.35:** The heart may be gently massaged to expel air. *(Photo by EDJ, courtesy of KAMC, National Guard Hospital, Riyadh, Saudi Arabia)*

several ways to remove air from the heart, but whichever method is used it is crucial to the outcome of surgery. Once all air appears to be removed, the aortic cross clamp is released, and the operating table is levelled to its normal position. The cardioplegia cannula, and/or retrograde cannula, and vent are removed. Transoesophageal echocardiography is used to assess the intracardiac repair and can also be used to determine whether there is residual air within the heart. When echocardiography confirms adequate repair, the surgeon is happy and the scrub nurse relaxes.

Postoperative monitoring lines, such as a left atrial line, are inserted, if necessary. Temporary pacing wires are almost always routinely inserted and are sutured to the right ventricle. Some surgeons may routinely attach pacing wires to the right atrium as well especially after complex cardiac repairs.

Discontinuation of CPB can be a crucial time and requires attention and alertness of all team members, including the scrub nurse. The perfusionist gradually occludes the venous line, which will restrict venous return to the pump and gradually fill up the heart with more and more blood. The perfusionist also gradually reduces the amount of blood being pumped into the aorta. This blood will flow through the right side of the heart and lungs. It will then return to the left side of the heart. When this blood volume is adequate, the aortic valve will open with each heartbeat, and a cardiac output will be observed. Gradually, the child's heart and lungs will take over the function of the heart-lung machine. If adequate arterial systolic pressure is achieved, cardiopulmonary bypass can be terminated. The venous cannula is removed, whereas, the arterial cannula remains in place, for the perfusionist to transfuse blood to the child to maintain an adequate systolic pressure. If the heart functions effectively and the child is stable and the echocardiogram shows satisfactory repair, protamine is given and the aortic cannula is also removed.

### NURSING OBSERVATION

*Once the child is stable, the venous and aortic cannulae are removed from the heart and the purse string sutures are tied. Usually, the venous cannulae are removed first. If there is still bleeding, the scrub nurse should be alert and be prepared with reinforcement sutures. If the child's heart does not pump effectively, the aortic and venous cannulae may have to be re-inserted and the child may have to go back on bypass. For the scrub nurse, it is essential to stay focussed at this time.*

If the child remains stable, chest tubes are inserted. At the same time, protamine is given by the anaesthetist to reverse the heparin action. The scrub nurse must ensure, that no blood be returned to the heart-lung machine, once half-dose of protamine has been administered. Final haemostasis and surgical closure of the sternal wound are performed according to surgeon's preference.

### NURSING OBSERVATION

*A surgical count of all instruments, sponges, needles, and miscellaneous items is to be audibly performed and recorded by the scrub nurse and circulating nurse, before closure of a cavity (heart) within a cavity (chest) and before wound closure (insertion of sternal wires) begins (second count). The third and final count is to be performed at skin closure. Perioperative nurses should be familiar with the departmental policies and procedures on surgical counts of the healthcare institution they work at.*

## SEQUENCE FOR ASSISTING THE SURGEON WITH PLACING A CHILD ON CARDIOPULMONARY BYPASS

### Aortic Cannulation

In newborns and infants, one or two purse strings are placed on the aorta. The surgeon and his assistant hold the two sides of the cannulation site with fine forceps and the surgeon, using a scalpel with a No. 11 blade, makes an incision equal in length to the diameter of the cannula. The aortic cannula is inserted and the purse strings are drawn tight with tourniquets and secured to the cannula with a silk tie.

### *Role of the Scrub Nurse*

1. Hand fine forceps to surgeon and a 5-0 polypropylene (prolene) suture, single mounted, for the first purse string. If a second purse string is required, this is usually handed to the surgeon double mounted, that is, both needles are mounted on two separate needle holders.
2. After handing the surgeon the purse string suture, have scissors, tourniquet with snugger and mosquito ready.
3. Hand tourniquet with snugger to assistant surgeon, suture is cut, purse strings are drawn tight with a tourniquet and held with a mosquito.
4. Then hand second purse string suture to surgeon if required.
5. Hand surgeon scalpel with a No.11 blade, followed by aortic cannula and silk tie to secure cannula to snugger.
6. Hand surgeon scissors for cutting silk tie, let him remove air from the cannula and connectors and then hand him the tubing clamp to clamp the aortic cannula. Cannula is connected to the arterial pump line.
7. Hand surgeon silk suture or blunt towel clip to secure the aortic cannula to the drapes.

### *Remarks*

1. Be familiar with the type of purse string suture; polypropylene or ticron, and the size of the needle; e.g. 5-0, 6-0. Also be familiar with the type of needle holder the surgeon uses; e.g. Castroviejo or Ryder needle holder.
2. Be familiar with the type and size of snuggers used; red rubber, size 8Fr or 12Fr.

Be familiar with type of mosquitos used; e.g. small, regular, curved, or straight mosquitos.

3. Be familiar with the routine of individual surgeons and their assistants; who cuts the suture, who places the tourniquet, etc. Often the surgeon will put the needle holder on both ends of the suture. So, when the needles are cut they are secure in the needle holder.

4. If a second purse string suture is required, this is usually double mounted.

5. Some surgeons may use a small artery forceps to hold the aorta before making the incision into the aortic root. Be familiar with the size of aortic cannula.

6. After the aortic cannula is filled retrograde with the child's blood, an air-free connection is made between the CPB arterial flow line and the arterial cannula. Having the perfusionist slowly advance (come forward) the perfusate by activating the systemic flow, pump will facilitate an air-free connection.

7. Be familiar with the connectors. Ensure the cannula fits the arterial pump line!

## Venous Cannulation

Depending on the needs of the surgeon and surgery, one or two venous cannulae may be placed. Most commonly two venous cannulae are placed into the right atrium and threaded into the superior vena cava (SVC) and inferior vena cava (IVC), or separate incisions are made into the SVC and IVC.

### Role of the Scrub Nurse

1. Hand fine forceps to surgeon and a 5-0 polypropylene suture. A purse string is placed in both the SVC and the IVC and subsequent cannulation is performed, again using a No. 11 scalpel for both. The cannulae are secured to their tourniquets in the same way as for the arterial cannula. Individual surgeons may place purse string sutures in the right atrium through which both the SVC and IVC are advanced. If a single, two-stage venous cannula is used, it is inserted through a purse string suture in the right atrial appendage, the tip of which is incised with fine tipped scissors.

2. Cannulae are connected to the venous pump line. Individual surgeons may ask the scrub nurse to fill-up the venous pump

line with saline. When handing the venous cannula to the surgeon, make sure to hold it up to prevent blood loss through the cannula. Individual surgeons may prefer to place a tubing clamp on the venous cannula prior to insertion.

## Remarks

1. Be familiar with the type of purse string suture; polypropylene or ticron, and the size of the needle. Usually, surgeons will use same type of suture, same needle size, and same needle holder for all purse strings. Be familiar with the way the surgeon likes the needle to be mounted; e.g. forehand, backhand, single mounted, double mounted, halfway, etc. For venous purse strings, usually, a single purse string suture is sufficient. When both venae cavae are to be cannulated, it depends on the surgeon's preference in which vena cava, a purse string suture is placed first; individual surgeons may place purse string sutures first in the SVC then IVC or vice versa.

2. Be familiar with the connectors. If two cannulae are used ensure to have a 3-way connector that fits both cannulae and fits the venous pump line!

   Often surgeons will use an extension (extra piece of tubing) for the SVC cannula.

NB: Individual surgeons may place aortic and venous purse string sutures first followed by cannulation. Other surgeons may place purse string suture in aorta followed by cannulation of the aorto, followed by placing a purse string suture in the SVC, followed by cannulation of the SVC, etc. Memorize individual surgeons preferences with regards to which sequence they use for placing an infant on the cardiopulmonary bypass machine.

## Cardioplegia

Once total cardiopulmonary bypass (CPB) is achieved, an antegrade cardioplegia purse string is placed in the proximal ascending aorta, the cannula (Fig. 4.33) is inserted and secured with a tourniquet. An appropriate size, aortic cross clamp is placed between the cardioplegia cannula and the aortic cannula.

Cardioplegia is administered with re-dosing at 20 to 30 min intervals and some surgeons may also use topical cold saline or cold slush on the heart to ensure proper cardiac arrest and preservation of the myocardium.

Before or after the cardioplegia cannula is connected, cardio-pulmonary bypass is commenced. Then an aortic cross clamp is placed and infusion of cardioplegia is commenced.

### Role of the Scrub Nurse

1. Hand fine forceps to surgeon and a 5-0 polypropylene suture for the purse string (single or double mounted).
2. After handing the surgeon the purse string suture, have scissors, tourniquet with snugger and mosquito ready.
3. Hand tourniquet with snugger to assistant surgeon. Suture is cut, purse strings are drawn tight with tourniquet and held with a mosquito.
4. Hand surgeon the cardioplegia cannula.
5. Hand surgeon mosquito to clamp cardioplegia needle prior to connecting.
6. Hand surgeon the aortic cross clamp. This is placed between the aorta cannula and the cardioplegia cannula.
7. The heart is arrested and cooled. Have cold saline ready.

### Remarks

1. Before or after the cardioplegia cannula is connected, cardiopulmonary bypass is commenced. Then an aortic cross clamp is placed and infusion of cardioplegia is commenced.
2. Cardioplegia is administered with re-dosing at 20 to 30 min intervals and some surgeons may also use topical cold saline or cold slush on the heart to ensure proper cardiac arrest and preservation of the myocardium.
3. Ensure the cardioplegia line is handed out to the perfusionist.
4. Cardioplegia solution is flushed into small kidney dish to prevent air entering the aorta when connecting to cardioplegia cannula.
5. Ensure to hand the surgeon an appropriate size cross clamp.
6. Be familiar with the technique individual surgeons use to cool the heart, e.g. further cooling of the heart with topical cold saline.

### Vent Insertion

A left ventricular vent (LV vent) is usually inserted before cardiopulmonary bypass (CPB), although some surgeons may insert the LV vent after CPB. The surgeon makes an incision in the purse string suture at the junction of the right superior pulmonary vein and the left atrium and inserts the vent, which is then passed through the mitral valve and into the left ventricle. If the right atrium will be opened during the surgical procedure, an LV vent may also be inserted through the foramen ovale, through the left atrium, mitral valve and into the left ventricle.

### Role of the Scrub Nurse

Hand fine forceps to surgeon and a 5-0 polypropylene suture. A purse string is placed in the RSPV and subsequent insertion of the vent is performed, using a No. 11 scalpel, followed by a dilator, which can be a mosquito, followed by the vent cannula. The vent is not secured to its tourniquet.

### Remarks

If the vent is placed through the foramen ovale, no purse string suture is required.

Be familiar to which pump line from perfusion the vent is connected—usually three lines which are colour coded, are part of a custom made pack which includes the aorta and venous pump lines and three additional pump lines, two for venting the heart and a third line for the cardiotomy sucker. Usually, the line with a yellow coding strip is for the cardiotomy sucker, and the red and blue lines are for the vents.

## SEQUENCE FOR ASSISTING THE SURGEON WITH DISCONTINUATION OF CARDIOPULMONARY BYPASS

### Discontinuation of CPB

Once the surgical repair has been carried out, the heart is de-aired.

Once all air appears to be removed, the aortic cross clamp is released and the operating table is levelled to its normal position. The cardioplegia cannula, and/or retrograde cannula, and vent(s) are removed. The body temperature of the neonate, infant or child is slowly increased. Postoperative monitoring lines, such as a left atrial line, are inserted, if necessary. Temporary pacing wires are almost always routinely inserted.

## Role of the Scrub Nurse

1. De-airing the right side of the heart and the Valsalva manoeuvre (de-airing the left side of the heart. Aortic cross clamp is removed and re-warming will begin. Have warm saline. The next step is removal of the venous cannula(e) and the aorta cannula.

2. Hand surgeon a tubing clamp to clamp the venous line, followed by a scalpel with a No. 11 or 15 blade to remove ties from tourniquet of venous cannula(e). Be ready to receive the venous cannula(e). Always have a jug full of warm saline ready on the table at this stage. The perfusionist may ask for the reservoir to be filled at this stage, which means the scrub nurse places the venous cannula into a jug with warm saline, removes the tubing clamp, the perfusionist releases the clamp on the venous pump line and the venous reservoir will fill up. Ensure to replace the tubing clamp on the venous cannula. The aortic cannula is removed in a similar fashion.

3. A surgical count of all instruments, sponges, needles and miscellaneous items is to be audibly performed and recorded by the scrub nurse and circulating nurse before closure of a cavity (heart) within a cavity (chest) and before wound closure (insertion of sternal wires) begins (second count).

4. Hand surgeon the pacing wires—be familiar whether the surgeon uses monopolar or bipolar pacing wires and if he/she prefers the needle to be removed from pacing wire prior to insertion. Have 6-0 polypropylene for attaching suture to right ventricle and silk suture for skin, if required.

5. If the child remains stable, chest tubes are inserted. At the same time, protamine is given by the anaesthesiologist to reverse the heparin action. Remove the cardiotomy sucker once half-dose protamine is announced by the anaesthesiologist.

6. Final haemostasis and surgical closure of the sternal wound are performed according to surgeon's preference.

## Remarks

1. During all surgeries that require opening the heart, there is a chance that air may be trapped inside the heart. Once the child comes off bypass, this air may cause air emboli and once in the systemic circulation, may cause an infarct, either in the

lungs or brain. With the aorta cross clamped, the child is placed in a 30° head-down position, the tourniquets on both vena cava are released and the perfusionist partly clamps the venous line, which restricts venous return to the pump and the right ventricle will fill with blood. The surgeon often says: fill up the heart!

2. To fill the left side of the heart with blood to remove air trapped in the left heart, the child is briefly ventilated, a few puffs to the lungs. This increases pulmonary venous return to the left heart and thereby removing any remaining air. This manoeuvre is referred to as Valsalva.

3. Rewarming is achieved by warming the blood from the heart-lung machine, by irrigating the heart topically with warm saline, and/or the use of heating blankets.

4. The venous cannula(e) are removed prior removal of the aortic cannula for the perfusionist to transfuse blood to the child to maintain an adequate systolic pressure, if required.

5. Perioperative nurses should be familiar with the departmental policies and procedures on surgical counts of the health care institution they work at.

6. Temporary pacing wires are almost always routinely inserted and are sutured to the right ventricle. Some surgeons may routinely attach pacing wires to the right atrium as well.

7. The scrub nurse must ensure, that no blood be returned to the heart-lung machine, once half dose protamine has been administered.

8. The third and final count is to be performed at skin closure.

---

**SURGEON'S COMMENT**

*Do not push instruments into the hands of the surgeon or the assistant surgeon during cannulation and decannulation. Have them ready in a rhythmic sequence based on daily routine of a surgical team.*

---

## EFFECTS OF CARDIOPULMONARY BYPASS ON NEONATES AND INFANTS

For the perioperative nurse to fully appreciate the trauma a neonate or infant encounters having surgical repair for heart lesions, is also to have some knowledge and an understanding of the effects of cardiopulmonary bypass (CPB), necessary to perform surgical repair. Only the development of mechanical cardiopulmonary bypass circuits in the late 1950s, made advanced congenital cardiac surgery possible. Early pioneers in cardiac surgery were motivated by the predicament of older children with *crippling* congenital heart defects, in addition to the results of good scientific investigation and the belief that application of these results to such children was practical and possible. Since then, open heart surgery and CPB circuits, have undergone much refinement, in particular, for the younger population.

---

**NURSING OBSERVATION**

*Before the parents of a child with congenital heart disease, who needs surgical repair, consent to surgery, they are not only fully informed about the benefits and risks of the surgery but they are also informed about the effects of cardiopulmonary bypass, necessary to perform heart surgery.*

---

Today, the trend in paediatric surgery is to repair congenital heart defects as soon after birth and before the heart of a neonate and small infant adapts to the abnormal physiology. As a result, most children undergo surgical repair during the neonatal period, resulting often in excellent surgical outcomes. Today, complete repair of congenital heart disease can be performed in neonates and infants who are only a few days old and smaller than 2 kg. In this chapter, a short review is outlined on the differences between infants and adults with regards to response to and affects of CPB.

## Haemodilution

Numerous differences between infants and adults affect the response to CPB, and these must be accounted for in CPB management strategies.[34] Procedures performed in infants and children may require extremes of temperature, haemodilution, and perfusion flow rates. Certain anatomic features, such as the presence of large aortopulmonary collateral vessels or an interrupted aortic arch, require an alteration of bypass strategies and cannulation techniques. Circuit capacity cannot currently be reduced in proportion to patient size, (although advances are progressive). Therefore, significant haemodilution in neonates and small infants is unavoidable. The CPB machine or circuit needs to be primed and these priming volumes are often 200–300% greater than the tiny baby's total blood volume. A neonate or infant smaller than 10 kg has 85 ml of blood per kilogram. This means that a baby weighing 3 kg has 255 ml of blood circulating through their small body. Even with the latest technology, the minimum prime volume for circuits is 220 ml.

Haemodilution increases tissue perfusion during CPB and allows the use of hypothermia, which is needed to protect vital organs (in particular the brain, heart, and kidneys) against ischaemia during periods of low flow and circulatory arrest. Haemodilution also reduces donor blood requirements during CPB. However, haemodilution increases water loss into the extracellular compartments (leading to total body oedema) and increases postoperative blood loss as a result of clotting or coagulation disturbances. Haemodilution causes a significant dilution of clotting factors, red blood cells (RBC) and other plasma proteins, requiring the transfusion of fresh forzen plasma FFP, cryoprecipitate, platelets and RBC.

In addition to the decrease in haematocrit associated with haemodilution, significant dilution of clotting factors and plasma proteins also occurs, resulting in dilutional coagulopathy. Other organ systems in neonates and infants are not mature. For example, the production of vitamin K-dependent clotting factors by the liver is diminished. Neonates and infants require much higher flow rates per body surface area to meet metabolic demands. Neonates are often perfused at flow rates up to 200 ml/kg per minute. As the temperature is reduced, flow rates can be decreased. This has the benefit of producing less blood in a small and complicated surgical field. Thermoregulation in small children is also impaired, so that close attention to temperature monitoring is required. Furthermore, in some instances, children are cooled to profoundly hypothermic temperatures (e.g., 15 to 18°C) and the pump is then turned off (DHCA). This provides the surgeon with the opportunity to remove the cannulae from the patient and perform a precise repair in an operative field unencumbered by blood, cannulae, or other apparatus related to CPB. When CPB is resumed, children are re-warmed to their normal temperature.

## Inflammatory Response

Exposure to the foreign surface area of the CPB circuit (aortic, venous cannulae and circuit tubings) causes significant inflammatory reactions in tiny babies. Furthermore, it causes platelet counts to decrease rapidly. More significantly, the platelet function is affected. Both haemodilution and inflammatory reactions will lead to considerable water retention and oedema, including myocardial oedema, pulmonary oedema and cerebral oedema in the postoperative period. Renal immaturity in neonates and small infants, and decreased cardiac output postoperatively, further delay the return to normal body water content. Furthermore, neonates and small infants have higher metabolic demands and therefore, require a higher perfusion flow rate. However, many cardiac lesions are repaired on CPB with low perfusion flow rates, the use of deep hypothermia with circulatory arrest (for the repair of some cardiac lesions). As a result, CPB in neonates and infants has a profound physiologic effect on most organs of the body.

Excessive total body water may prolong the ventilatory support and increase morbidity and mortality. Intravenous diuretics and inotropic support are frequently necessary to counteract the effects of haemodilution.

Numerous strategies have been researched to minimize some of the complications of CPB.

One strategy to decrease the harmful effects of CPB is to minimize the amount of exposure to the CPB circuit by keeping the duration on CPB as short as possible and limiting the amount of artificial surface area to which blood must be exposed. Often, the same CPB machine used for adults is the same used for paediatric patients. To have a smaller CPB machine and reduce the circuit size, by decreasing the overall length of and diameter of the tubing used, would be one method of decreasing the exposure to artificial surface area and therefore limiting the inflammatory response. Another advantage of a smaller circuit is smaller priming volumes, and therefore, less haemodilution and less oedema in the postoperative period. Improvements in technology have reduced the morbidity associated with CPB. The safe conduct of CPB in the neonate and infant requires a comprehensive understanding of the physiologic alterations associated with CPB, in addition to the implications of circuit design, haemodilution, choice of cannulae, degree of hypothermia, acid-base strategies, and selected flow rates.

## Postoperative Bleeding

The coagulation system of a neonate undergoing CPB is profoundly affected by haemodilution. Limiting haemodilution in neonates is difficult when the cardiopulmonary bypass circuit requires priming volumes that are two to three times the blood volume of the neonate. This extreme haemodilution contributes significantly to coagulation disturbances in the postoperative period. Current research into using lower priming volumes in neonates and its effects on the coagulation factors after bypass has demonstrated reduced coagulation disturbances in the postoperative period. Neonates and infants are at higher risk of bleeding after cardiac surgery than older children and adults, due to immature clotting factors. Anticoagulation, during bypass is crucial, however, more challenging in neonates and infants as this patient group can either show a greater resistance or sensitivity to heparin than adult patients.

## Pulmonary Hypertension

Pulmonary artery hypertension is a common problem after CPB in children. The goal is to reduce pulmonary vascular resistance. One way of achieving this is by administering nitric oxide. Nitric oxide is an endothelium derived vasodilator that can be administered as an inhaled gas. Although a nonselective smooth muscle vasodilator, nitric oxide, is rapidly inactivated by haemoglobin, and therefore, when it is administered via an inhaled route, the systemic circulation is protected from its vasodilating properties. Reduction in pulmonary vascular resistance has been demonstrated in children with reactive pulmonary hypertension after congenital heart surgery.

To summarize, the worst responses to CPB are at the extremes of age, the very young and the very old. In infants and neonates, the response is characterized by post-bypass acute respiratory distress syndrome, pulmonary hypertension, total body oedema, coagulation abnormalities, myocardial dysfunction, and haemodynamic instability. These adverse sequelae translate into prolonged ventilation, prolonged inotropic support, renal dysfunction, bleeding and later thrombosis, inability to close the chest in the operating room, and potentially the need for mechanical support after open heart surgery. In particular, the pulmonary injury seems to be quite profound and is a major source of morbidity in the young patient population.

Blood and blood products that are routinely ordered from the blood bank for any heart surgery are the following:

- **Fresh frozen plasma (FFP)** is a blood product produced by centrifugation of donated whole blood, frozen within eight hours from collection, stored in frozen state and used after thawing. FFP contains adequate levels of all soluble coagulation factors, as well as albumin (blood protein, which has the ability to draw interstitial fluid, lost through haemodilution, back into the blood circulation), immunoglobulin (blood protein or antibody in the blood), and naturally occurring anticoagulants. FFP should be of the same ABO group as the child. Coagulation disturbances and inadequate heparin reversal are two important factors contributing to perioperative bleeding after paediatric CPB surgery. FFP, as well as platelets, cryoprecipitate, RBCs and antifibrinolytic drugs (blood clot promoting drugs such as aprotinin and tranexamic acid) are administered to correct the coagulopathy and stop bleeding. FFP must be stored in designated refrigerators at a temperature < −18 °C. Once thawed, it can be kept in a designated refrigerator (1–6°C) until transfused to the child. FFP should be clear with the colour varying from yellow/straw to light green to orange. If anything seems abnormal, this should be reported or checked with the blood bank.

- **Cryoprecipitate or cryo** is the part of the blood, which contains only certain clotting factors. Cryo is usually given along with FFP to help replace the clotting factors, which can be low due to the cardiopulmonary bypass.

  *Note:* Cryo is not a concentrate of FFP, in fact, a unit of cryo contains only 40%–50% of the coagulation factors found in a unit of FFP. These factors are more concentrated in the cryo (less volume) and therefore preferred over FFP to transfuse in very small infants. Each dose of cryo is given over a 10 to 30 min period. A dose must not exceed an infusion time of greater than four hours. Cryo must be stored at temperatures between 20 and 24°C (room temperature). Cryo will usually be cloudy.

- **Platelets or thrombocytes** are small blood components that help the clotting process by sticking to the lining of blood vessels. Platelets are made in the bone marrow and survive in the circulatory system for about nine days, before being removed from the body by the spleen. The platelet helps prevent massive blood loss and blood vessel leakage resulting from trauma, such as cardiopulmonary bypass. Platelets are stored at room temperature and can be kept for up to five days. Platelets cannot be frozen and must be stored at temperatures between 20 and 24°C (room temperature). The colour of platelets will usually be clear to yellow/straw to light strawberry.

- **Packed red blood cells (PRBCs)** are made from a unit of whole blood by centrifugation and removal of most of the plasma. The known benefits of PRBC transfusion include an increase in the oxygen carrying capacity of blood, improved tissue oxygenation, and improved hemostasis. Whole blood is not readily available in Saudi Arabia and usually family members donate for their child. This has implications with regards to the development of transfusion-associated graft-versus-host disease (TA-GVHD). TA-GVHD is a life-threatening complication that may occur in immunocompromised children following the transfusion of cellular blood components (red blood cells and platelet concentrates). It is a rare complication. The only way to prevent TA-GVHD is to inactivate the T lymphocytes[*] present in the blood by a process called irradiation. TA-GVHD has developed following transfusion of red cells, platelets, and granulocytes. There have been no documented cases of TA-GVHD following the use of fresh frozen plasma and cryoprecipitate and these non-cellular components do not require irradiation. Red cells, platelets and granulocytes derived from HLA[**] matched donors and first degree relatives should be irradiated, as HLA sharing can cause TA-GVHD even in immunocompetent patients. Not indicated for full-term neonates.

  PRBC should be stored at 1–6° C in designated refrigerators. PRBC left out of a monitored refrigerator for more than 30 min cannot be returned to the refrigerator. Transfusion should be completed within four hours.

---

[*]T lymphocytes are a type of white blood cells essential for immunity.
[**]HLA stands for *Human Leukocyte Antigen*. These antigens are protein molecules we inherit from our parents.

## PERITONEAL DIALYSIS CATHETER

Fluid overload is a common complication following cardiac surgery in infants. This may be caused by pre-existing cardiac dysfunction, exogenous fluid during cardiopulmonary bypass, postsurgery acute kidney injury and the strain on the heart caused by the surgical procedure (low cardiac output). Conservative management such as the use of diuretics is often insufficient to adequately manage fluid overload. The insertion of a peritoneal drain (commonly referred to as a PD catheter, or Tenckhoff catheter, Fig. 4.36) and its use to remove peritoneal fluid postoperatively is commonly used in pediatric cardiac surgery especially in newborns with complex diseases.

### ULTRAFILTRATION AND MODIFIED ULTRAFILTRATION

As neonates and infants tend to accumulate large amounts of fluid during bypass, resulting in total body oedema with pulmonary and myocardial dysfunction, several different ultrafiltration techniques have been developed to minimize fluid retention in the postoperative period. Conventional ultrafiltration removes fluids from the bypass circuit throughout the bypass period, or whenever the venous reservoir volume is sufficient to allow filtration.

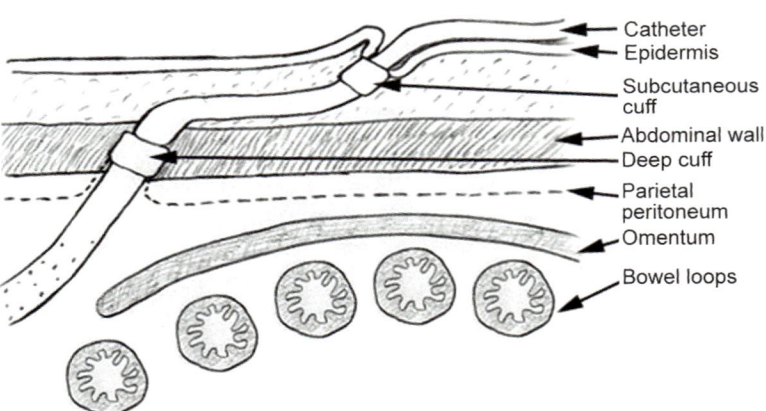

**Fig. 4.36:** The insertion of a peritoneal drain, PD or Tenckhoff catheter, is sometimes inserted to remove peritoneal fluid post-cardiac surgery

**Modified ultrafiltration (MUF)** is used after the patient is weaned off the cardiopulmonary bypass machine and before protamine is administered. Most commonly, blood is removed from the aortic cannula, passed through a hemofilter, and then returned as oxygenated, concentrated, and ultrafiltered blood to the cannula in the right atrium. Modified ultrafiltration has the advantage of filtering only the child's extracellular blood volume and not the CPB circuit, which results in greater hemoconcentration. Both conventional and modified ultrafiltration have been shown to remove inflammatory mediators from the circulation.

## CARDIOPLEGIA AND HYPOTHERMIA

Effective myocardial protection remains the key element for the success of any heart surgery. The word **cardioplegia** means *cardio* referring to the heart and **plegia** means *paralysis.* This involves stopping or arresting the heart so that intracardiac procedures can be done on a still heart. To protect the myocardium, hypothermia (cooling of the heart) is used. Hypothermia lowers the myocardial metabolism and oxygen demand during ischaemia, when the heart is arrested. There are many cardioplegic solutions available but it is the high concentration of potassium, in these solutions, that causes the heart to arrest.

Antegrade (forward flow) cardioplegia is the injection of a cardioplegic solution through the aortic root and into the left and right coronary arteries, with a cross-clamped aorta. This is the most common mode of administration. Retrograde cardioplegia is administered through the coronary sinus and flows in a retrograde fashion. Cardioplegia can be administered as a cold or warm solution.

## CIRCULATORY ARREST

Deep hypothermic circulatory arrest (DHCA) is generally reserved for neonates and infants requiring complex cardiac repairs. However, certain older children with complex cardiac disease or aortic arch anomalies may benefit from a short period of circulatory arrest. For the most part, deep hypothermia is selected to allow the surgeon to operate under conditions of low-flow (e.g., in repairing the pulmonary arteries of children with substantial aortopulmonary collateral flow) or DHCA (e.g., in repairing the aortic arch). Low pump flows improve the operating conditions for the surgeon by providing a nearly bloodless field and better visualization of critical portions of the repair at selected times during the procedure. When the strategy is to use DHCA for the intracardiac portion of the repair, venous return can be accomplished with a single atrial cannula. This has the advantage of providing optimal venous return, concomitant venting of the heart, and generally uncomplicated venous return.

During DHCA, the surgeon can remove the atrial or aortic cannula. With this technique, surgical repair is more precise because of the bloodless and cannula-free operative field. Arresting the circulation, even at deeply hypothermic temperatures, introduces the question of how well deep hypothermia preserves organ function, with the brain being of greatest concern. Prolonged deep hypothermic cardiac arrest (DHCA) is associated with brain injury, but the safe duration of circulatory arrestre mains unknown. Research suggests that neurodevelopmental outcomes for these children are not adversely affected unless the duration of DHCA exceeds a threshold of 41 min. The increased neurological morbidity associated with prolonged periods of circulatory arrest has led some cardiac surgical teams to promote continuous low-flow cardiopulmonary bypass as an alternative strategy. Low-flow cardiopulmonary bypass, maintains continuous cerebral circulation but may increase exposure to known pump-related sources of brain injury, such as embolism or inadequate cerebral perfusion. Some researches claim worse outcomes when using continuous low-flow perfusion with increased cerebral oedema, pulmonary dysfunction, and neurological injury after prolonged exposure to low-flow perfusion. Opinions are divided whether shorter periods of circulatory arrests are better tolerated than continuous perfusion.

## DEFIBRILLATION PADDLES

During open heart surgery, a pair of internal defibrillation paddles may be used to restart the infant's heart. It sends an electrical shock to the heart to either restart or to stop irregular heartbeat (referred to as atrial fibrillation) and restore a normal heartbeat. It enables the heart's natural pacemaker to regain control and establish a normal sinus rhythm. Each internal defibrillation paddle comprises a handle attached to a shaft attached to a spoon electrode. The paddle handles are held by the surgeon while the spoon electrodes are placed on the child's heart in direct contact with the myocardium. An electric discharge is passed from one spoon electrode through the infant's heart to a second spoon electrode (Fig. 4.37). The spoon electrode is of variable size depending on the size of the child's heart (Fig. 4.38).

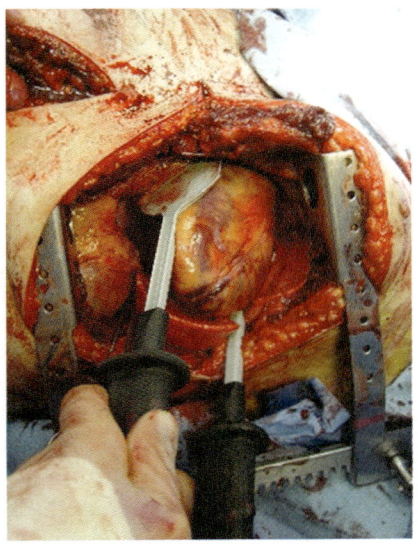

**Fig. 4.37:** During open-heart surgery, a pair of internal defibrillation paddles may be used to restart the infant's heart. (*Note:* The picture shows the heart of an adult)

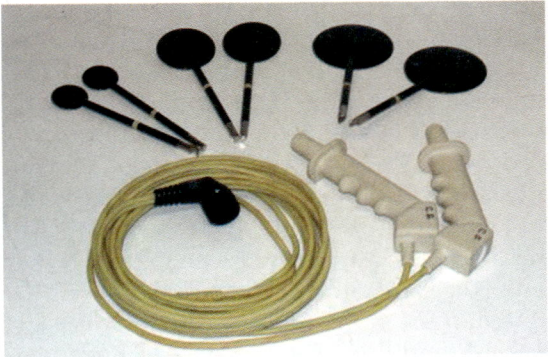

**Fig. 4.38:** The spoon electrode is of variable sizes depending on the size of the child's heart

## PACING THE HEART

Cardiac pacing is the use of a small electrical current to artificially produce a heartbeat. A pacing box creates a current and a specialised wire (atrial or ventricular pacing wire) on the outside surface of the heart delivers the electrical stimulation to the heart. Postoperative arrhythmias are a major cause of mortality and morbidity after cardiac surgery for congenital heart disease (CHD). Children with CHD are especially vulnerable to rhythm disturbances in the early postoperative period. Atrial and/or ventricular temporary pacing wires are frequently inserted at the end of a cardiac surgical procedure as a preventative measure. Their main purpose is to improve haemodynamic function in the presence of arrhythmias as well as to suppress atrial and ventricular tachyarrhythmias. Atrial/and or ventricular pacing can be started in the operating room if necessary, as well as in the cardiac intensive care unit to optimize cardiac function by maintaining an adequate heart rate and, therefore, increasing cardiac output. The most important arrhythmias necessitating pacing include bradycardia, nodal or junctional arrhythmias and atrioventricular block. Many surgeons choose to insert ventricular and/or atrial pacing wires routinely, in particular, when the right atrium is opened during the surgical repair, since the electrical conduction pathways lie across the right atrium (Fig. 4.39).

Temporary pacing wires are available in unipolar and bipolar pacing wires (Fig. 4.40). Choice is generally dictated by the surgeon's preference. Atrial pacing wires are sutured to the right atrial appendage or the body of the right atrium. The wires are usually sutured using 5-0 polypropylene sutures. The wires are passed percutaneously to the right of the midline and secured to the skin with a silk suture. Ventricular pacing wires are placed on the anterior surface of the right ventricle. They are inserted into the muscular portion of the ventricle to ensure adequate myocardial contact (Fig. 4.41).

The wires are passed through the skin to the left of the midline and secured to the skin with a silk suture (Fig. 4.42). Pacing wires are usually removed on the fourth postoperative day. If longer term pacing is required, the infant may need a permanent pacemaker insertion.

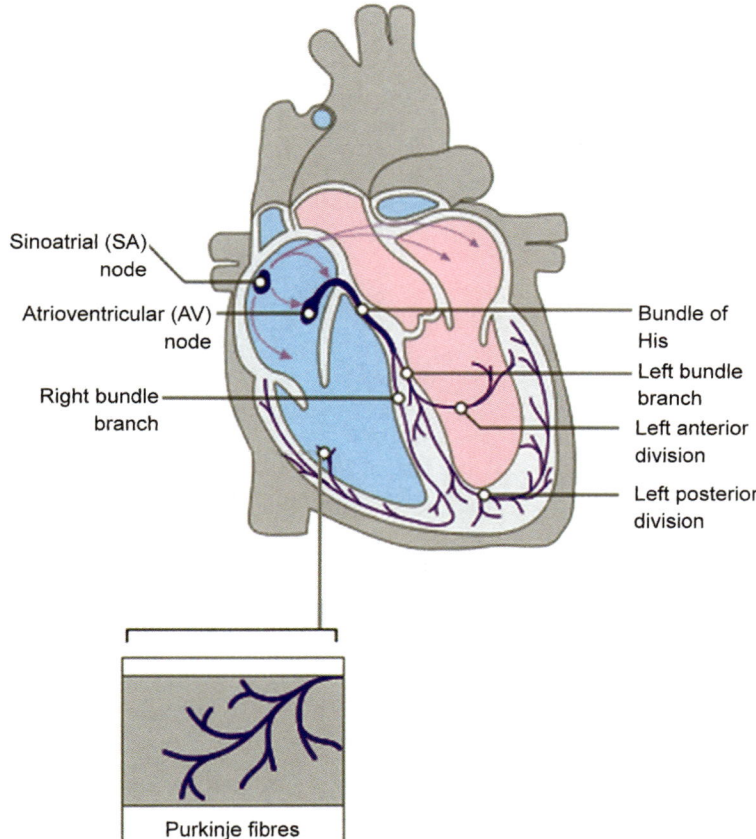

Purkinje fibres

**Fig. 4.39:** Each electrical impulse usually begins in the sinoatrial node (SA node) and travels through the right and left atria causing them to contract and push blood through to the lower sections of the heart (ventricles). Electrical impulses then reach the atrioventricular node (AV node) and pass down through the conduction fibres lying both between and around the ventricles. This causes the ventricles to contract and blood to be pushed out of the heart to the rest of the body. Many surgeons choose to insert ventricular or atrial and ventricular pacing wires routinely postoperatively, in particular, when the right atrium is opened during the surgical repair, since the SA node and conducting pathways lie across the right atrium

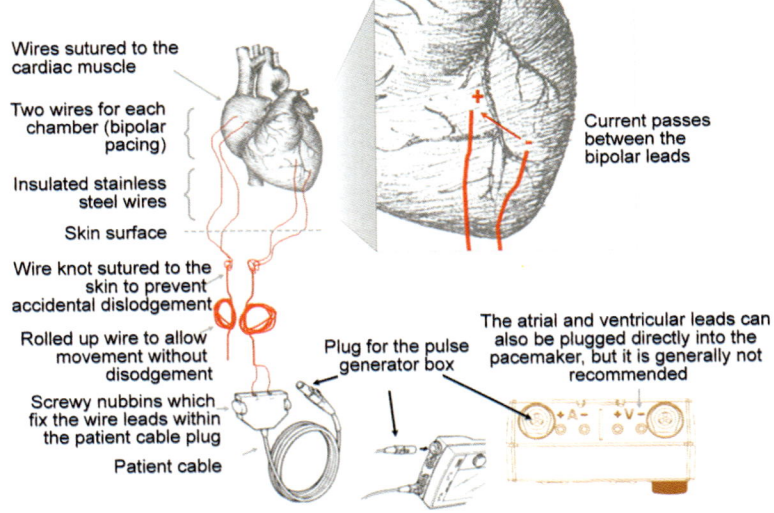

Wires sutured to the cardiac muscle

Two wires for each chamber (bipolar pacing)

Insulated stainless steel wires

Skin surface

Wire knot sutured to the skin to prevent accidental dislodgement

Rolled up wire to allow movement without disodgement

Screwy nubbins which fix the wire leads within the patient cable plug

Patient cable

Current passes between the bipolar leads

Plug for the pulse generator box

The atrial and ventricular leads can also be plugged directly into the pacemaker, but it is generally not recommended

**Fig. 4.40:** Temporary pacing wires are available in unipolar and bipolar pacing wires. They are connected to pacing cables, which are connected to a pacing box

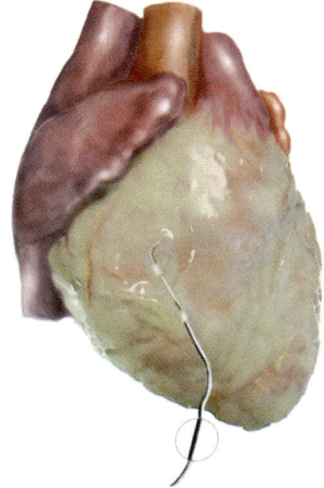

**Fig. 4.41:** Ventricular pacing wires are placed on the anterior surface of the right ventricle. They are inserted into the muscular portion of the ventricle to ensure adequate myocardial contact

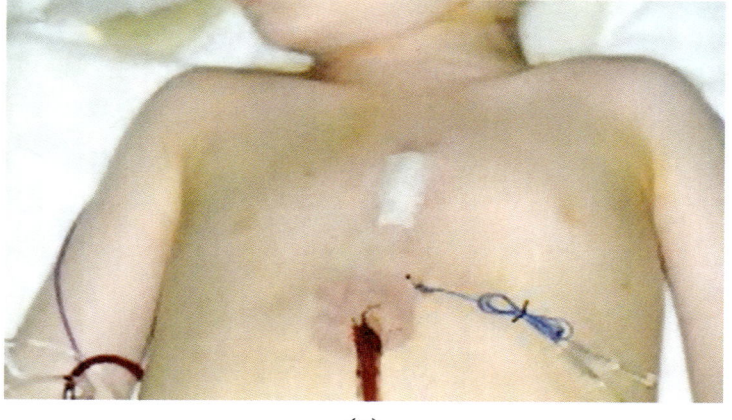

(a)

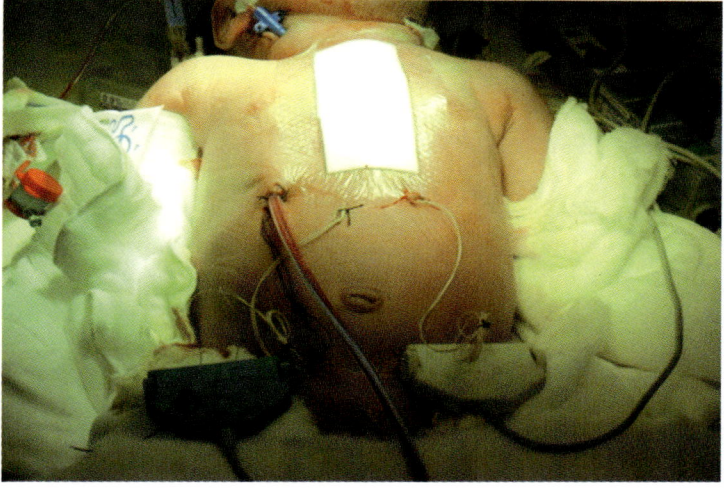

(b)

**Fig. 4.42:** Ventricular pacing wires are passed through the skin to the left of the midline and secured to the skin with a silk suture (a). When atrial pacing wires are required, these will be passed through the skin to the right of the midline (b). *(Photo (b) by EDJ, courtesy of KAMC, National Guard Hospital, Riyadh, Saudi Arabia)*

The pacing wires are connected to pacing cables, which are connected to a pacing box (Fig. 4.43).

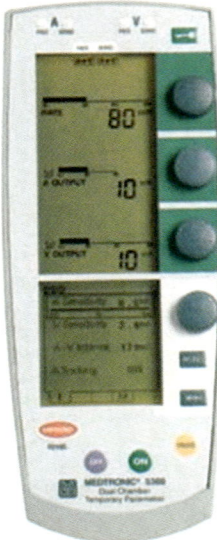

**Fig. 4.43:** Pacing box

### DELAYED CHEST CLOSURE

On occasion after an open-heart procedure, the child's haemodynamics may be unstable. Added to that, frequently there is some swelling of the heart muscle from surgery and the inflammation induced by the heart-lung machine. For that reason, at times, surgeons decide to, 'leave the chest open' only to close it a few days later. In this way, the breast bone is prevented from pushing on the heart in the most critical and early hours after an operation. Despite this, the heart itself is not exposed; a layer of soft protective material is sewn to the skin edges to provide coverage of the heart, along with sterile bandages (Fig. 4.44).

Generally, the chest is then closed in the intensive care unit under the same heavy sedation and analgesia, that is provided if the child is brought back to the operating theatres (Fig. 4.45).

### EXTRACORPOREAL MEMBRANE OXYGENATION (ECMO)

In some cases, an infant's heart is unable to resume a normal heart function and the child is unable to come off cardiopulmonary bypass. In such cases, the child is placed on ECMO (Fig. 4.46).

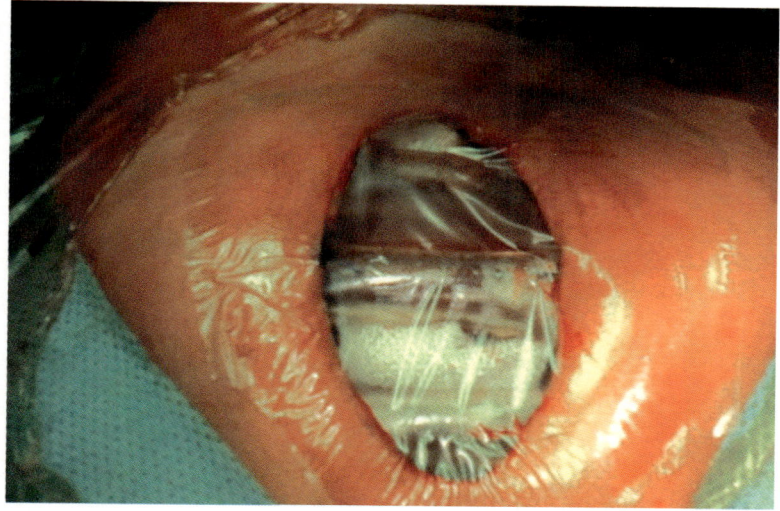

(a)

(b)

**Fig. 4.44:** Frontal view. Picture taken standing at the head of the child. The sternal edges are kept open by a 3 cm piece of tubing. The heart is further covered by a layer of transparent dressing (a) or with a patch of special designed material (b). *(Photos a, b by EDJ, courtesy of KAMC, National Guard Hospital, Riyadh, Saudi Arabia)*

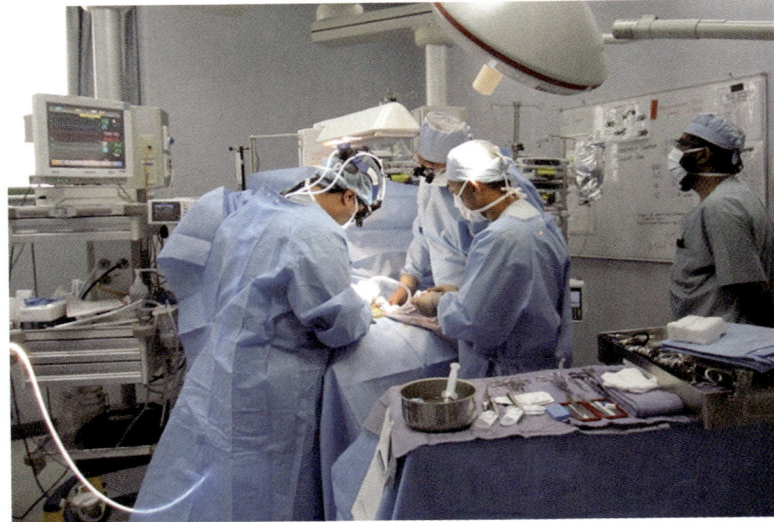

**Fig. 4.45:** Delayed chest closure in the neonatal intensive care unit. *(Photo by EDJ, courtesy of KAMC, National Guard Hospital, Riyadh, Saudi Arabia)*

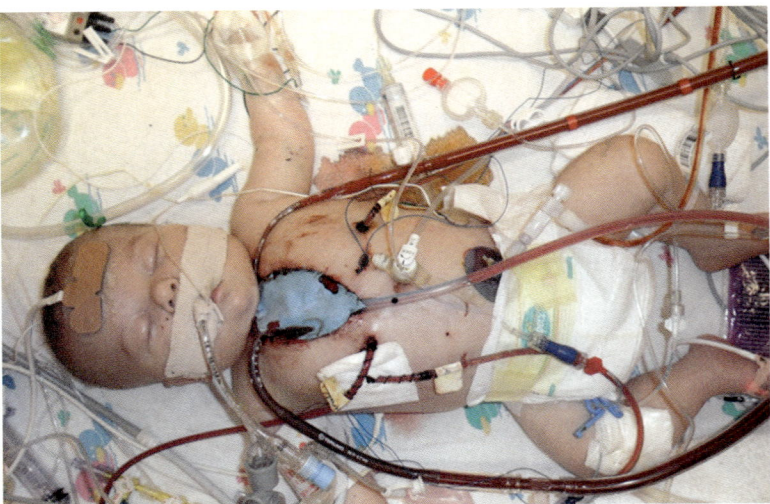

**Fig. 4.46:** In some cases, an infant's heart is unable to resume a normal heart function and the child is unable to come off cardiopulmonary bypass. In such cases, the child is placed on ECMO

ECMO stands for *extracorporeal* (outside the body) *membrane oxygenation* (artificial lung). It is similar to the heart-lung or cardiopulmonary bypass machine. However, unlike cardio-pulmonary bypass, which is used for short-term support during cardiac surgery, ECMO is used for long-term support and can be safely used from three to ten days. ECMO was first used successfully in the United State of America in 1979. It was introduced in the United Kingdom in 1989. In children, the most frequent use for ECMO is respiratory failure. ECMO is usually initiated in the operating theatre. The aortic cannula remains *in situ,* but if bicaval venous cannulae were used, these are usually replaced by a single stage cannula placed in the right atrium.

Infants placed on ECMO are critically ill and already may have a disturbed haemostasis secondary to sepsis, shock or profound hypoxia, predisposing them to intracranial haemorrhage. The continuous contact of blood with the surface of the ECMO circuit results in activation of the coagulation cascade. The use of heparin to prevent clot formation in the circuit and the decrease in platelet number and function from interaction with the circuit puts the neonate or infant at risk for bleeding. The necessity for multiple blood components for neonates on ECMO often result in high donor exposures.

## EMERGENCY CHEST REOPENING IN THE NEONATAL INTENSIVE CARE UNIT

The main indications for emergency chest reopening are bleeding, haemodynamic instability (suspicion of cardiac tamponade), or cardiac arrest. Emergency chest reopening of a postcardiac surgical neonate or infant in the intensive care unit can be a highly stressed, but infrequent procedure, which requires a high-level team response and a unique skill set. Although, the intensive care unit (ICU) does not provide a sterile environment, general operating theatre routine is followed. Curtains or blinds should be drawn to isolate the child, parents, if present, should be accompanied and leave the room. Traffic in and out the room should be kept to a minimum. All medical and nursing staff, who are present in the room during the procedure should wear a theatre hat and mask, although, policies in different institutions may vary. The re-exploration team, usually, consist of the consultant surgeon, or the surgeon's assistant, and an operating theatre nurse, all of whom scrub and dress in a sterile gown, gloves, mask, and theatre hat. If the procedure is performed after operating hours, an *on-call* team will be activated. In some institutions, cardiac theatre nurses may not be *on site* after operating hours and ICU nurses may be trained to initially assist the surgeon during the procedure till the on-call cardiac theatre nurse arrives.

The child's sternum is prepped with povidone-iodine solution and sterile drapes are used to isolate the operating site. The procedure is done under general anaesthesia with an anaesthesiologist present throughout the procedure. The sternum is opened and sternal edges are inspected for any bleeding points. Any clots within the chest cavity are evacuated and systematic inspection of all operative sites, suture lines, etc. is undertaken. Bleeding sites are controlled by sutures, stainless steel clips (*liga* clips), electrocautery, or application of thrombostatic material. The chest drains are cleared of any clotted blood. Provided, hemostasis is achieved, the sternum is closed in a standard fashion. In cases, where surgical bleeding cannot be controlled, the sternum is packed with gauze and left *open* (*see,* delayed chest closure). A main concern with regards to re-exploration in the ICU is increased incidence of sternal wound infection. Often, antibiotics are added to irrigation fluids as a preventative measure.

### NURSING OBSERVATION

*It is important for cardiac perioperative nurses to stay focussed and be able to prioritise. Assisting the surgeon in a timely manner is of paramount importance. Skin knife first followed by wire cutter to remove the sternal wires. At the same time, ensure, suction tubing is handed out and connected to a suction device and in working order!*

### SURGEON'S COMMENT

*It is important that scrub nurses or the intensive care unit nurses temporarily covering them, should be fully familiar with the contents of the re-opening set especially the skin knife, the wire-cutter, wire-holder and the appropriate-sized sternal retractor. They should be able to provide sterile gowns, sterile drapes, and gloves expeditiously and should set-up diathermy and suction systems and if required defibrillation pads as quickly as possible. A reasonable supply of fine prolene sutures should also be readily available. There should be no hesitation in asking for an extra helping hand if there is shortage of personnel. Despite the urgency of the situation, sterility should be observed as strictly as possible.*

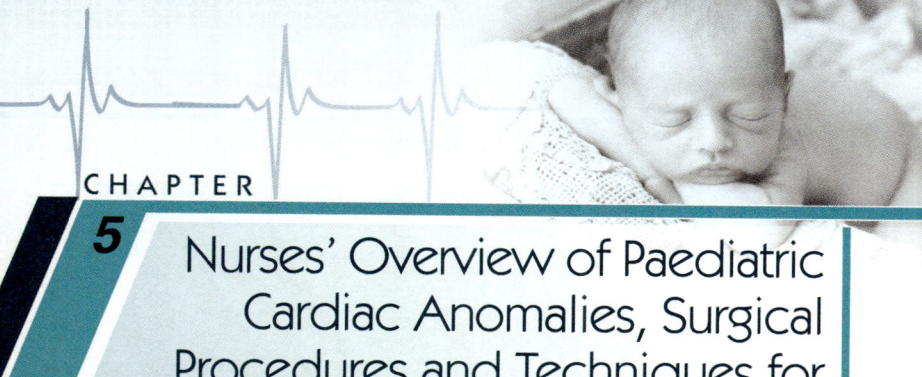

# Nurses' Overview of Paediatric Cardiac Anomalies, Surgical Procedures and Techniques for Congenital Heart Defects

## INTRODUCTION

The history of cardiac surgery is associated with great surgeons. Their pioneering surgeries and successes are recognized by having the surgery named after them (Figs 5.1 and 5.2). An overview of congenital cardiac anomalies and their subsequent surgical treatments are described in this chapter. However, it must be pointed out that surgical techniques are by no means uniform. Surgical techniques often vary, based on different (surgical) philosophies, surgeons' personal experience and their training at different hospitals worldwide. In other words, the techniques described in the following sections reflect views of individual surgeons. Other expert surgeons may perform the same surgery differently.

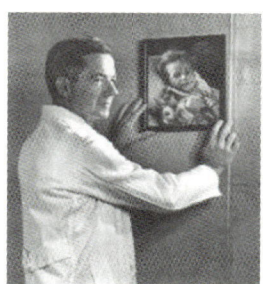 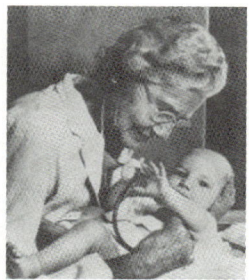 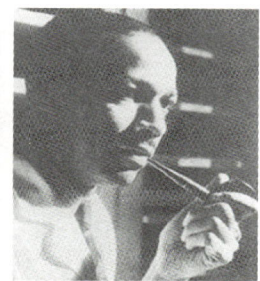

**Fig. 5.1:** Dr. Alfred Blalock (1899–1964), Helen Taussig (1898–1986), and Vivien Thomas (1910–1985). Vivien Thomas was a pioneer in the field of surgery. He worked as a lab technician for Dr. Alfred Blalock, and together they developed a procedure to alleviate a congenital heart defect, the Tetralogy of Fallot, also known as blue baby syndrome. The procedure was what became known as the Blalock–Taussig shunt. Vivien's name was not acknowledged till years later

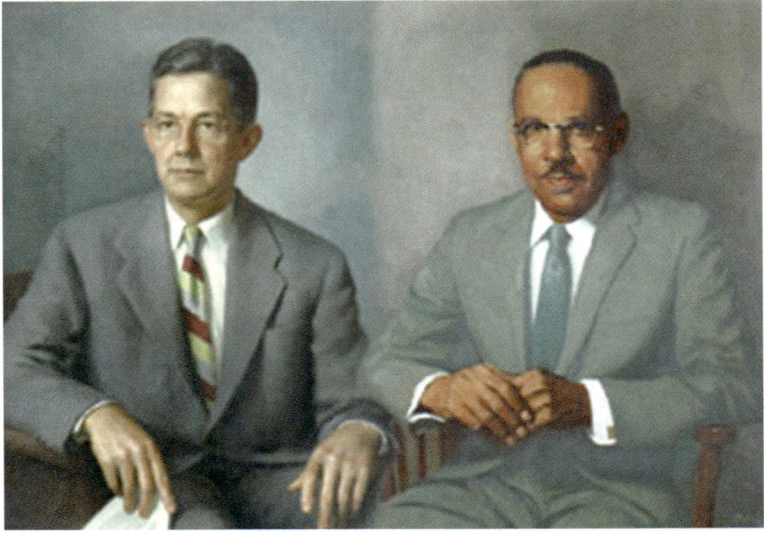

**Fig. 5.2:** At a time when racial segregation was an immutable fact of life, the two men stood together, Blalock wielding the scalpel and placing the sutures, Thomas watching every move and quietly answering the surgeon's questions. For it was Thomas, whom Blalock had relied on to work out the details of the procedure in dogs. As Blalock's surgical laboratory technician, it was Thomas who'd performed the surgery dozens of times. Blalock had been through the steps only once

## Section 1

### WHEN CHAMBERS AND VALVES ARE IN NORMAL SEQUENCE AND NORMAL POSITION AND SHUNTING IS PREDOMINANT

In the structurally normal heart, (i.e. the heart chambers and valves are in their normal sequence and normal position), the right and left side of the heart is divided, and is without communication. Shunting refers to those blood flow anomalies where, there is an abnormal communication, such as, an atrial or ventricular septal defect, patent ductus arteriosus or a patent foramen ovale that allows abnormal flow between the right and left side of the heart. Since pressures on the right side of the heart are normally lower than those on the left side, when such defects are encountered, abnormal flow is usually left-to-right resulting in an increased blood flow to the right side of the heart and consequently to the lungs. Normally, the lungs can accommodate the increased flow without significant symptoms if the degree of shunting is small or moderate. When significant shunting is present and exceeds the ability of the lungs to accept the increase, the lungs are literally flooded and symptoms of congestive heart failure result, in which the heart cannot effectively meet the oxygen demand of the body's organs. Where no congestive heart failure is clinically evident, such shunting, over time, may result in reactive changes in the pulmonary vasculature and result in pulmonary hypertension. Pulmonary hypertension causes a higher pressure within the right heart and eventually exceeds the pressure on the left side of the heart. Instead of left-to-right shunting of blood, blood flow will be shunted from right-to-left (Fig. 5.3). Depending on the clinical situation, such changes may be permanent and cause irreversible right-to-left shunting. This phenomenon is referred to as **Eisenmenger syndrome** and is associated with *clubbing* of finger and toe nailbeds (Figs 5.4 and 5.5). Eisenmenger syndrome was first described by Hippocrates (400 BC), *clubbing* of finger and

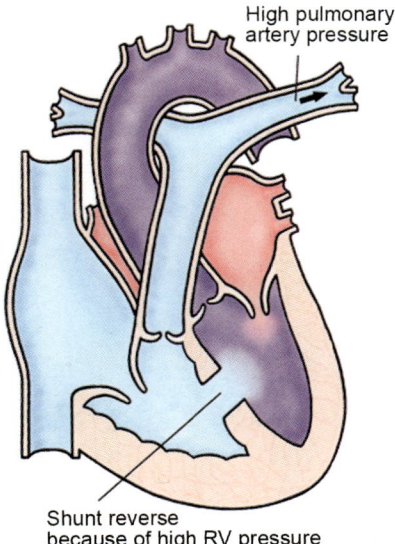

High pulmonary
artery pressure

Shunt reverse
because of high RV pressure

**Fig. 5.3:** The previous left-to-right shunt is converted into a right-to-left shunt, secondary to the elevated pulmonary artery pressure and associated pulmonary vascular disease

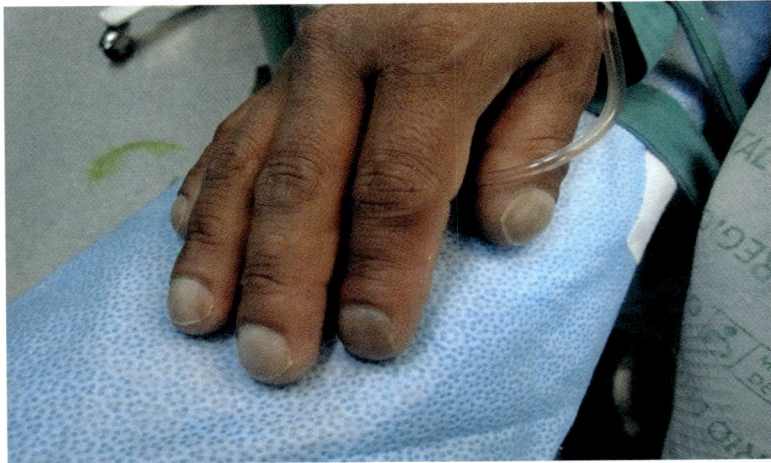

**Fig. 5.4:** Clubbing of fingers in a 33-year-old female patient with Eisenmenger syndrome. *(Photo by EDJ, courtesy of Hospital Regional Honorio Delgado in Arequipa, Peru)*

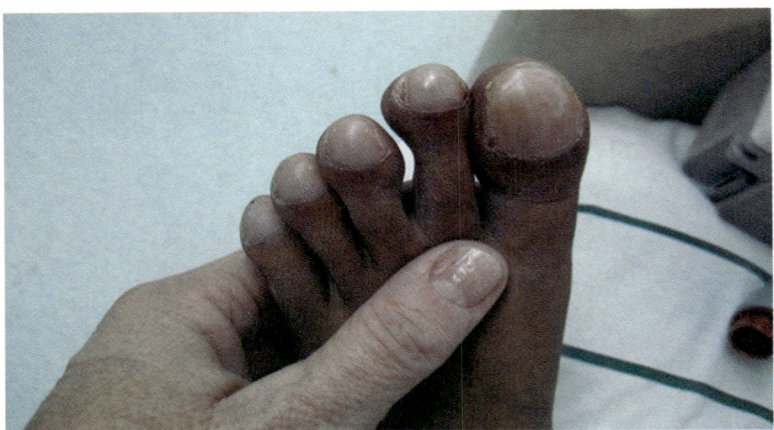

**Fig. 5.5:** Clubbing of toenails in a 4-year old child with pulmonary atresia, and MAPCA's. Hypoxia has been proposed as an explanation for clubbing in cyanotic heart disease, and pulmonary disease, and is often seen in patients with congenital heart disease resulting in hypoxia. However, the exact mechanism of clubbing remains unclear. *(Photo by EDJ, courtesy of KAMC, National Guard Hospital, Riyadh, Saudi Arabia)*

toe nailbeds is also known as **hippocratic fingers.** Eisenmenger syndrome was so named after Dr. Victor Eisenmenger, (German physician, 1864–1932), who first described the condition in 1897.[35] Without early recognition and correction, these *simple* heart problems may result in permanent, inoperative damage to the lungs. In addition, any communication between the right and the left side of the heart may allow for the possibility of venous emboli entering the arterial circulation and cause a stroke, heart infarct or necrosis of a distal extremity.

In the following section, the congenital anomalies in which shunting is predominant will be described and their surgical repair explained.

## PATENT DUCTUS ARTERIOSUS (PDA)

### Introduction

During foetal life, the ductus arteriosus is a normal structure that allows most of the blood leaving the right ventricle to bypass the pulmonary circulation, and pass into the descending aorta.[36, 37] The foetus does not breathe air, and thus blood does not need to pass through the lungs to be oxygenated. Typically, only about 10% of the right ventricular output passes through the pulmonary vascular bed. The ductus arteriosus connects the main pulmonary artery to the descending aorta distally, at the origin of the left subclavian artery. In most individuals, the ductus arteriosus is located on the left side. However, if a right aortic arch is present, the ductus arteriosus may be located on the right or the left side. The ductus arteriosus is very rarely bilateral. The structure varies in length and diameter. Histologically, the media of the ductus is composed of smooth muscle, and the intima is much thicker than that of the aorta. Contraction of this muscular media after birth causes shortening of the ductus and its functional closure. Patent (the word **patent** means *open*) ductus arteriosus is a defect in which the ductus arteriosus fails to close in an infant soon after birth. If the ductus remains patent, the condition leads to abnormal blood flow between the aorta and pulmonary artery, shunting (Fig. 5.6). Most neonates have a patent ductus arteriosus in the first 8 hours of life, with spontaneous closure occurring in 42% at 24 hours of age, in 90% at 48 hours of age, and in almost all infants at 96 hours (4 days). Permanent anatomic closure of the ductus arteriosus occurs within 3 weeks to 3 months after birth.[38]

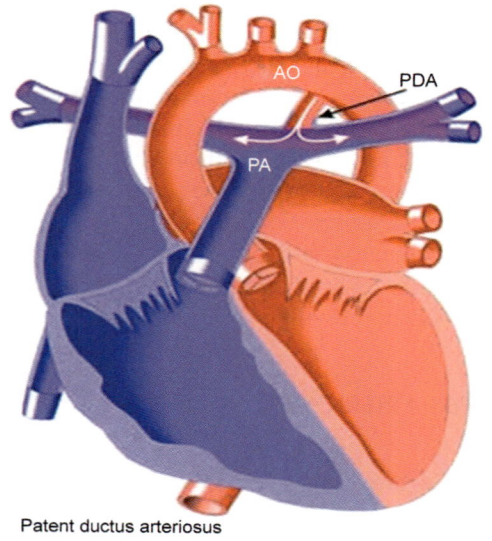

Patent ductus arteriosus

(a)

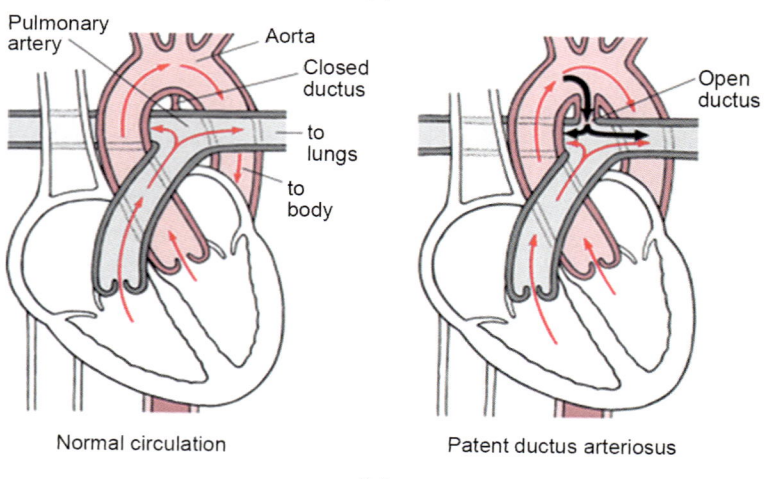

Pulmonary artery    Aorta

Closed ductus

to lungs

to body

Open ductus

Normal circulation      Patent ductus arteriosus

(b)

**Fig. 5.6:** The ductus arteriosus connects the main pulmonary artery to the descending aorta distally, at the origin of the left subclavian artery (a). If the ductus remains patent the condition leads to abnormal blood flow between the aorta and pulmonary artery. This is referred to as shunting (b)

## What Causes a Patent Ductus Arteriosus?

At birth the newborn changes from placenta to pulmonary oxygenation of the blood and the placenta is no longer part of the blood circulation. After the newborn baby takes his or her first breath the lungs expand, pulmonary vascular resistance falls, and blood flow into the lungs increases considerably. The rise in oxygen levels of the newborn blood is a potent stimulus for constriction of the ductus arteriosus within 10 to 24 hours after a full-term birth. Neonates born prematurely may lack constrictive muscle in the ductus, resulting in delay or prevention of closure of the ductus. Babies born at high altitude are also more likely to have a patent ductus arteriosus. The effect of high altitude becomes apparent at altitudes of over 3,000 m, and is most evident at altitudes of over 4,000 m.[39]

During a 2-week cardiac mission in the Andes Mountains in Peru in 2010, the majority of paediatric cases I assisted with, were surgical repairs of a patent ductus arteriosus (Fig. 5.7).

## Prevalence

Patent ductus arteriosus affects for reasons unknown, girls more often than boys. A patent ductus arteriosus is common in babies with congenital heart problems, and must be considered at the time of diagnosis, such as hypoplastic left heart syndrome, transposition of the great vessels, and pulmonary stenosis because in these cases, the diagnosis and treatment of a patent ductus arteriosus is, in fact, critical for the survival of the baby. The incidence of a patent ductus arteriosus in full-term babies is variably between 0.06 and 0.7%. In premature babies the presence of a patent ductus arteriosus is about 50%.[40]

## Symptoms

A small patent ductus arteriosus may not cause any symptoms. Although patent ductus arteriosus is often diagnosed in infants, it may not be discovered until childhood or even adulthood.[41] In isolated patent ductus arteriosus signs and symptoms are consistent with left-to-right shunting. An infant with a large patent ductus arteriosus may exhibit fast breathing, or shortness of breath, could tire very easily, have poor feeding and growth. The reason is that a patent ductus arteriosus allows a portion of the oxygenated blood from the left heart (the aorta) to flow back to the lungs

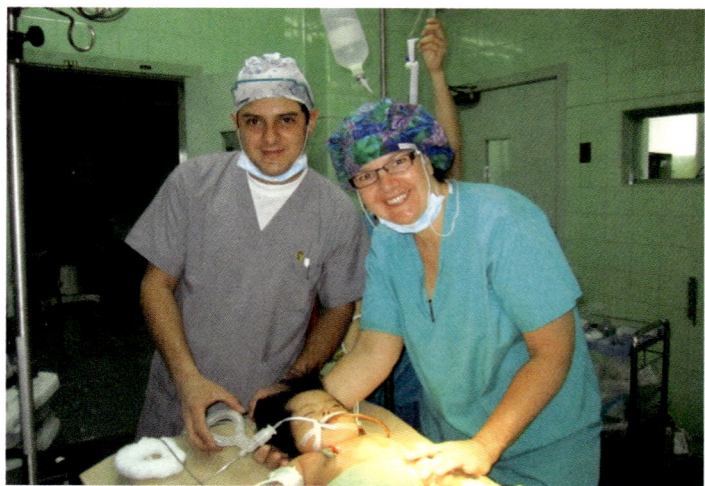

**Fig. 5.7:** A 9-month-old infant who had surgical repair of a patent ductus arteriosus (PDA) at the Hospital Regional Honorio Delgado in Arequipa, Peru. Arequipa lies in the Andes Mountains at an altitude of 2,335 metres. *(Photo by EDJ, courtesy of Hospital Regional Honorio Delgado in Arequipa, Peru)*

(left-to-right shunting Fig. 5.6). If this shunt amount is substantial, the premature neonate becomes short of breath because in addition to the normal amount of unoxygenated blood returning from the body to the lungs, more is shunted through the ductus. The neonate's work of breathing is increased, using up more calories and often interfering with feeding in infancy, and eventually, resulting in congestive heart failure. For this reason, patent ductus arteriosus is often a problem in very low birth weight infants.[42]

### Treatment

Babies with a patent ductus often have a characteristic heart murmur. The diagnosis is confirmed with an echocardiogram. Premature babies have a high rate of closure within the first two years of life. Despite this, symptomatic neonates will benefit greatly from closure of the patent ductus. In full-term infants, a patent ductus rarely closes on it's own after the first few weeks. The indications for closing a patent ductus arteriosus are several and depend on the child's age and the size of the ductus. In premature infants with poorly developed pulmonary artery smooth muscle, this lesion can cause severe congestive heart failure and chronic lung disease. In older children and adults, even an asymptomatic patent ductus arteriosus places the child at risk for subacute bacterial endocarditis. Therefore, treatment is often surgical ligation of the patent ductus, if it fails to close spontaneously or medical therapy is ineffective.[43]

## Patent Ductus Arteriosus Repair—Overview

### History

Galen initially described the ductus arteriosus in the early first century. Harvey undertook further physiologic study in foetal circulation. However, it was not until 1888 that Munro conducted the dissection and ligation of the ductus arteriosus in an infant cadaver, and it would be another 50 years before Robert E. Gross successfully ligated a patent ductus arteriosus in a 7-year-old child.[44] This was a landmark event in the history of surgery and heralded the true beginning of the field of congenital heart surgery. Catheter-based closure of the structure was first performed in 1971.

There are a number of options for surgical repair of a patent ductus arteriosus including ligation via a left thoracotomy (Fig. 5.8) or median sternotomy, video-assisted thoracoscopic surgery (VATS) and transcatheter device occlusion (Fig. 5.9). The

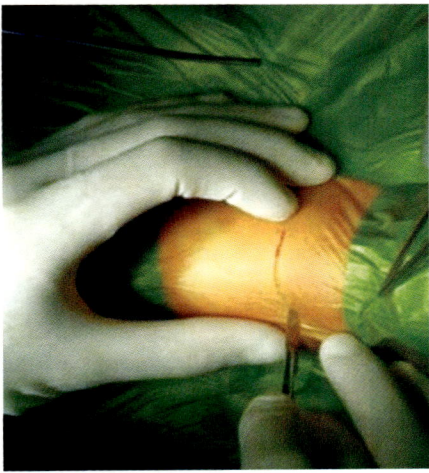

**Fig. 5.8:** There are a number of options for surgical repair of a patent ductus arteriosus including ligation via a left thoracotomy

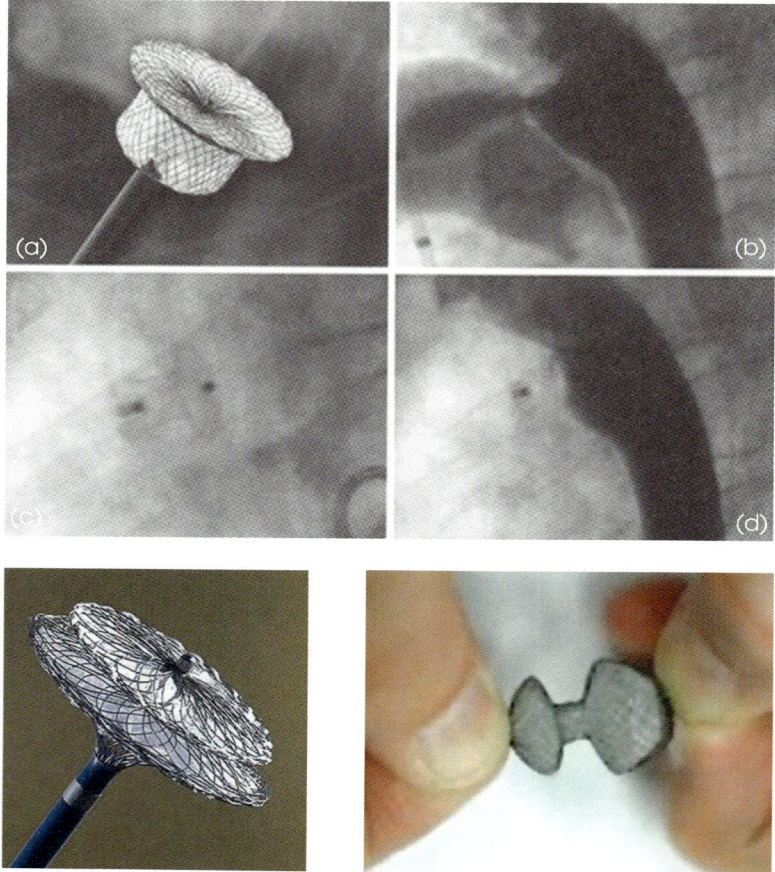

**Fig. 5.9:** Example of a patent ductus arteriosus occlusion with an Amplatzer duct occluder device. Image of an Amplatzer duct occluder device (a). Lateral angiograms demonstrating closure of the patent ductus arteriosus with the device (b through d)

latter is performed in the cardiac catheterization laboratory. Sometimes, transcatheter device occlusion fails and these infants will then be presented as an emergency to the cardiac operating room to perform surgical closure.

The following technique described for ligation of a patent ductus arteriosus is the one performed through a left thoracotomy, since this is, in most institutions, the most common approach.

## Patent Ductus Arteriosus Repair—Technique

Patent ductus arteriosus repair is a *closed heart procedure*. The terms *open* or *closed* heart surgery are used to differentiate whether or not a procedure uses the heart-lung bypass machine support.

1. General anaesthesia is established and the neonate is placed in a right lateral position. A left thoracotomy incision is made (Fig. 5.8). Individual surgeons may use a marker pen to mark the incision before prepping the baby.

2. Skin incision is made and the chest wall and intercostal muscles are divided using diathermy. The ribs are carefully retracted with a rib retractor and opened in stages to avoid rib fractures (Fig. 5.10). The lung is retracted anteriorly and the mediastinal pleura opened over the aorta and suspended with silk sutures (Fig. 5.11). The pleural incision is carried up to the subclavian take-off. (*Note:* The ductus arteriosus connects the main pulmonary artery to the descending aorta distally, at the origin of the left subclavian artery (Fig. 5.12a).

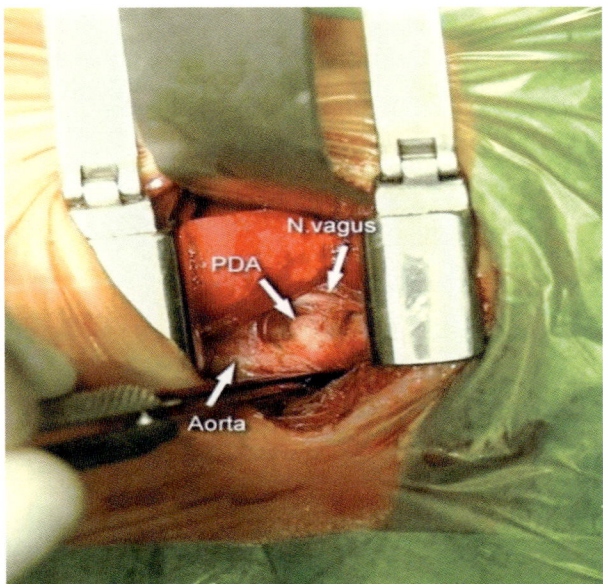

**Fig. 5.10:** The ribs are carefully retracted with a rib retractor and opened in stages to avoid rib fractures. The recurrent laryngeal nerve is a branch of the vagus nerve, N. vagus, vagus nerve

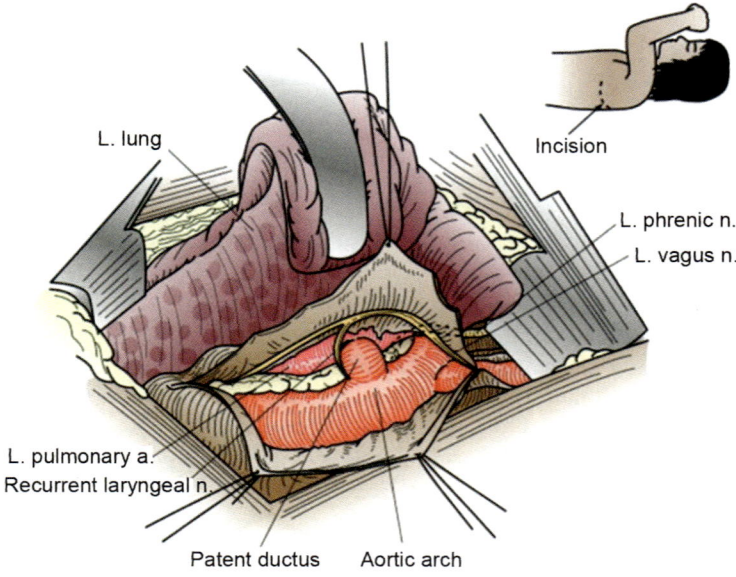

L. lung

Incision

L. phrenic n.

L. vagus n.

L. pulmonary a.
Recurrent laryngeal n.

Patent ductus    Aortic arch

**Fig. 5.11:** The anatomic relationship of a patent ductus arteriosus exposed from a left thoracotomy. The pleura is incised and retracted with silk sutures

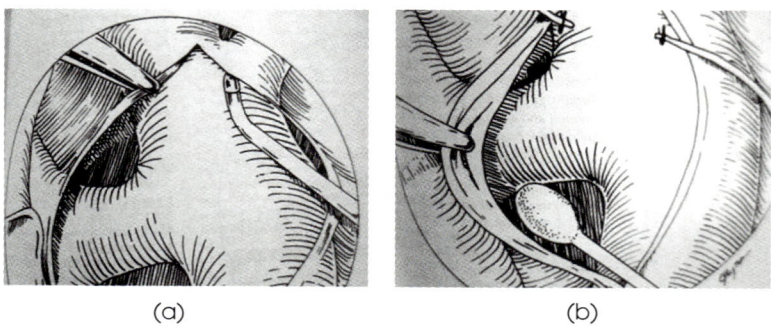

(a)                              (b)

**Fig. 5.12:** The pleural incision is carried up to the left subclavian take-off (a). (*Note:* The ductus arteriosus connects the main pulmonary artery to the descending aorta distally, at the origin of the left subclavian artery). A cotton swab may be used to bluntly dissect the ductal attachments, avoiding injury to the recurrent laryngeal nerve, which lies close to the ductus (b)

3. A cotton swab may be used to bluntly dissect the ductal attachments, avoiding injury to the recurrent laryngeal nerve, which lies close to the ductus (Figs 5.10–5.12).

4. Individual surgeons may use malleable retractors, covered with a *moist* raytec gauze, to carefully retract the left lung.

5. The ductus is identified, divided and over sewn with a non-absorbable polypropylene suture or a clip of appropriate size is placed around it and closed by applying gentle pressure on the clip holder (Fig. 5.13). A second clip can be placed to ensure the ductus is completely closed. Some surgeons may prefer to use a silk suture for ligation of the PDA (Fig. 5.15). A large PDA cannot be ligated with a clip and needs to be excised (Fig. 5.16).

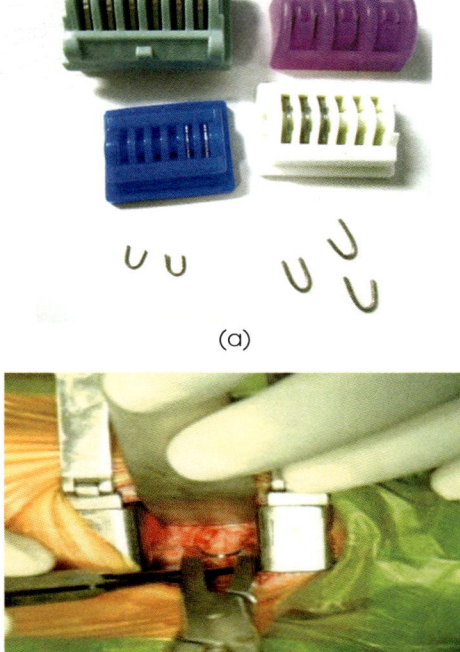

(a)

(b)

**Fig. 5.13:** A clip of appropriate size (a) is placed around the patent ductus arteriosus and closed by applying gentle pressure on the clip holder (b)

6. The rib cage is then closed with interrupted vicryl sutures. Muscle layer is closed with a vicryl suture. Skin is either closed with a subcuticular suture or skin clips depending on individual surgeon's preference.

In some institutions, the surgical repair is performed in the neonatal intensive care unit (Fig. 5.14).

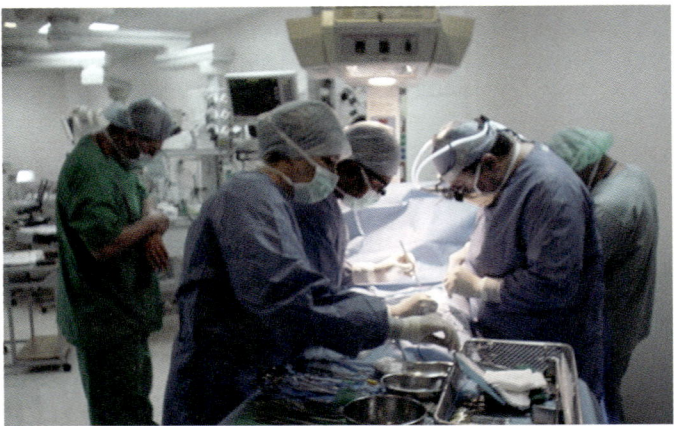

**Fig. 5.14:** Patent ductus arteriosus ligation performed in the neonatal intensive care unit. *(Photo by EDJ, courtesy of King Faisal Specialist Hospital, Jeddah, Saudi Arabia)*

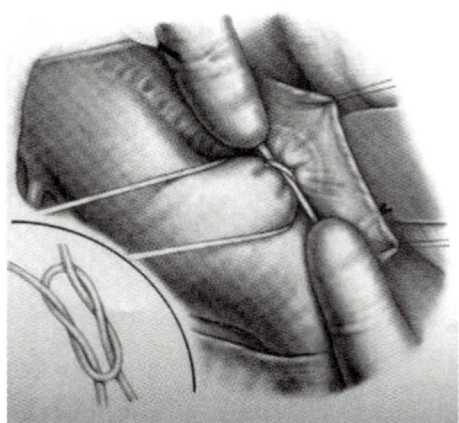

**Fig. 5.15:** Some surgeons may prefer to use a silk suture for ligation of the PDA

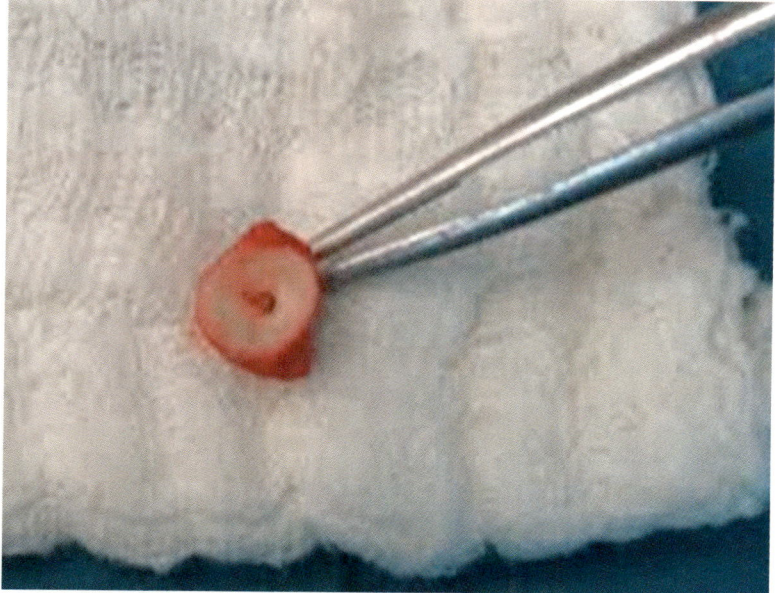

**Fig. 5.16:** PDA-tissue. A large PDA cannot be ligated with a clip and needs to be excised. This is often the case in coarctation of the aorta in which the PDA is usually large

### NURSING OBSERVATION

*It is important for nurses to know that this procedure is often performed through a left thoracotomy. Although in the rare case of a right aortic arch, the PDA may be on the right and a right thoracotomy is performed. Either way, for neonates, the procedure is, in some institutions, performed in the (neonatal) intensive care unit rather than the operating room. Surgical closure performed in the neonatal intensive care unit eliminates transport risks and is ultimately safer and easier than transporting a neonate to an operating room.*

### SURGEON'S COMMENT

*It is important that nurses ensure the correct site of surgery and are aware of surgeon's preference for technique of lung retraction and ligation of the ductus. Some surgeons do not leave a chest tube after the ductus ligation.*

## PATENT FORAMEN OVALE (PFO)

### Introduction

The patent foramen ovale (PFO) is a flaplike opening between the atrial septum primum and secundum (Fig. 5.17). In the foetus, the PFO serves as a functional connection between the right and left atria till the pulmonary circulation is established after birth. Once a baby is born, the left atrial pressure increases, which causes the PFO to close.

### What Causes a Patent Foramen Ovale?

The interatrial septum forms during the first and second months of foetal development. The Latin term **septum** means *something that encloses, a wall*, dividing a cavity or structure into smaller ones. Formation of the septum occurs in several stages. The first is the development of the septum primum, a crescent-shaped piece

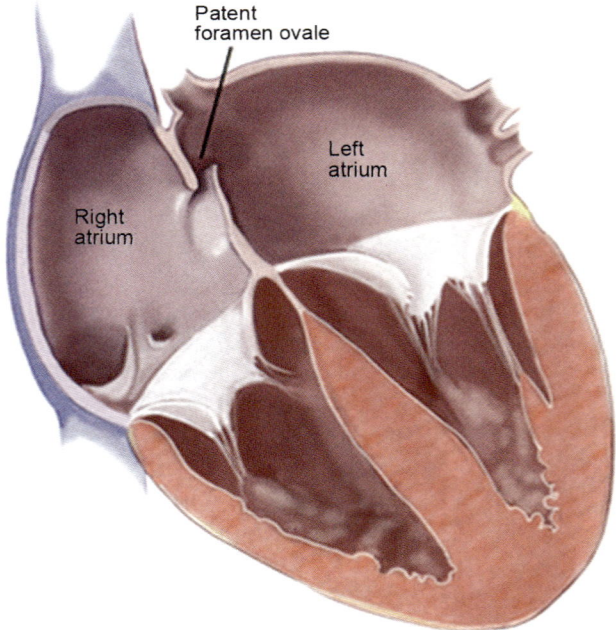

Patent
foramen ovale

Left
atrium

Right
atrium

**Fig. 5.17:** A patent foramen ovale (PFO) is a flap-like opening between the atrial septum primum and secundum

of tissue forming the initial divider between the right and left atria. Because of its crescent shape, the septum primum does not fully occlude the space between left and right atria; the opening that remains is called the ostium primum. The term **ostium** means *small opening* or *orifice*. During foetal development, this opening allows blood to be shunted from the right atrium to the left atrium. As the septum primum grows, the ostium primum progressively narrows. Before the ostium primum is completely occluded, a second opening called the ostium secundum begins to form in the septum primum. The ostium secundum allows continued shunting of blood from the right atrium to the left atrium.

This thick, muscular structure initially takes on the same crescent shape as the septum primum, except that it originates anteriorly, whereas the septum primum originates posteriorly. As the septum secundum grows, it leaves a small opening called the foramen ovale. The foramen ovale is continuous with the ostium secundum, again providing for continued shunting of blood.

The ostium secundum progressively enlarges, and the size of the septum primum diminishes (Fig. 5.18). Eventually, the septum primum is nothing more than a small flap that covers the foramen ovale on its left side. This flap of tissue is called the valve of the foramen ovale and opens and closes in response to pressure gradients between the left and right atria. When the pressure is greater in the right atrium, the valve opens; when the pressure is greater in the left atrium, the valve closes. Because the lungs are nonfunctional in foetal life, pressure in the pulmonary circulation is greater than that of the systemic circulation. Consequently, the right atrium is generally under higher pressures than the left atrium, and the valve of the foramen ovale is normally open.

At birth, there is a reversal in the pressure gradient between the atria, resulting in functional closure of the valve of the foramen ovale. Permanent anatomical closure of the foramen ovale occurs with time in normal infants. Inappropriate closure of the foramen ovale results from incomplete adhesion between the original flap of the valve of the foramen ovale and the septum secundum after birth.

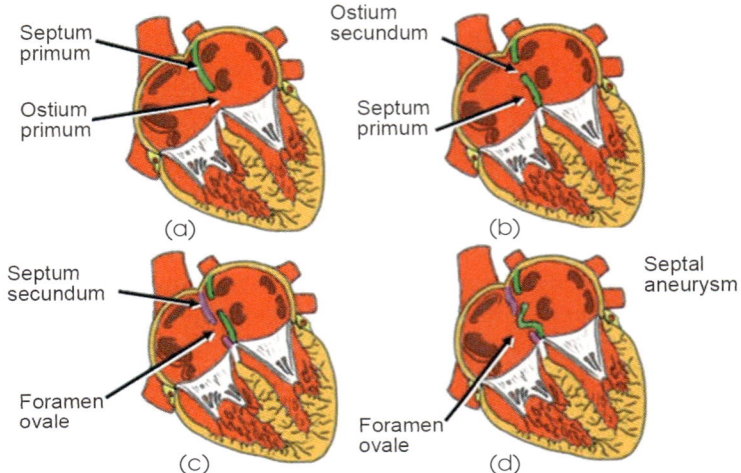

**Fig. 5.18:** Formation of atrial septum. Understanding the formation of the atrial septum explains the various types of atrial septal defects

## Prevalence

The prevalence of a patent foramen ovale is similar for males and females. It is a common congenital defect and detected in 10–15% of the general population.[45]

## Symptoms

Most neonates, infants and children with isolated patent foramen ovale are asymptomatic. Some studies in the past suggest a strong relationship between a PFO and cerebral embolism (i.e. a stroke is caused by paradoxical embolism which is carried from the venous side of the circulation to the arterial side through the PFO), particularly in young adults.[46–48]

## Treatment

Surgical closure is rarely necessary. Anatomic closure of the PFO occurs later in infancy in the majority of cases, but studies have demonstrated that anatomic closure is incomplete in approximately 1 in every 4 adults.[49] Sometimes the PFO is closed through transcatheter device closure the same method as is used for PDA closure (Fig. 5.19). This is performed in the catherization laboratory.

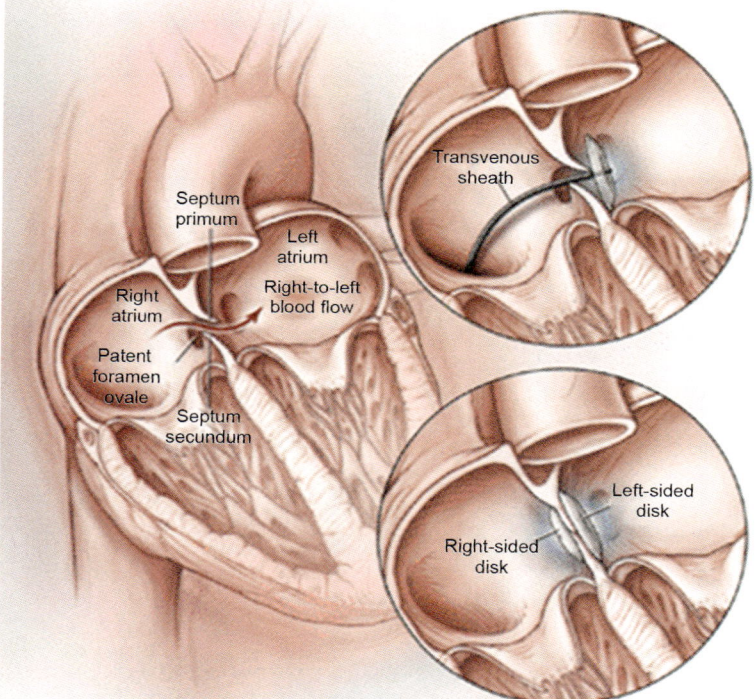

**Fig. 5.19:** Example of a patent foramen ovale occlusion with an Amplatzer duct occluder device

## ATRIAL SEPTAL DEFECT (ASD)

### Introduction

An atrial septal defect is an unwanted communication between the left and right atria (Fig. 5.20). In this condition, blood shunts from the left atrium to the right atrium through the hole because left atrial pressure normally is slightly higher than right atrial pressure. Depending on the size of the defect this pressure difference or pressure gradient forces small to large amounts of blood through the defect. The left-to-right shunt results in right heart volume overload, affecting the right atrium, right ventricle, and the pulmonary arteries. Eventually, the right atrium enlarges, and the right ventricle dilates to accommodate the increased blood volume. As a result, pulmonary hypertension may develop as a complication of the increased pulmonary blood flow.[50]

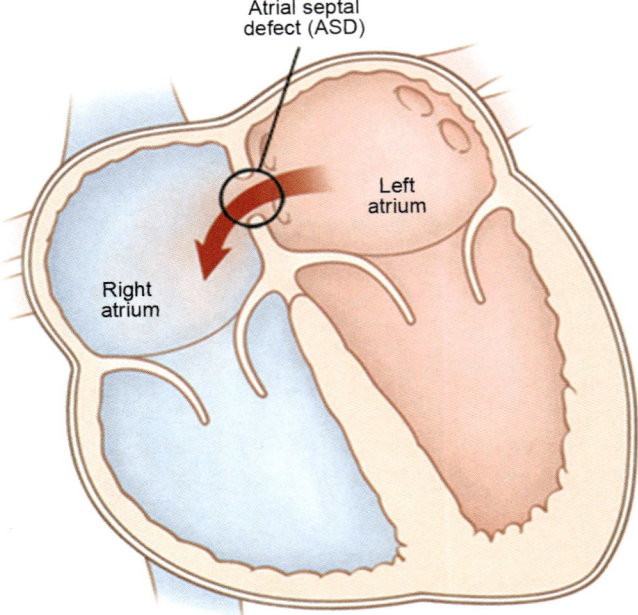

**Fig. 5.20:** An atrial septal defect (ASD) is a hole in the wall (septum) between the two upper collecting chambers of the heart. These holes may be of varying size and may be in any of several positions on the septum. The size of the defect and its location are factors which determine how serious the defect is with respect to the amount of strain on the heart and the degree to which blood crosses from one side of the heart to the other, causing a flooding of the lungs. Children with this lesion often have no symptoms, though they may have an increased incidence of lung problems. With time, however, the increased flow of blood to the lungs will cause irreversible damage. The operation for ASD involves closing the hole, either by sewing its edges together or by placing a patch in the defect

### What Causes an Atrial Septal Defect?

Atrial septal defect is caused by a spontaneous malformation of the interatrial septum.

### Prevalence

The defect occurs in 5 to 10% of all children born with congenital heart disease. For unknown reasons, an atrial septal defect is more common in females with a female-to-male ratio of approximately 2:1.[51]

## Symptoms

The size of the defect and the degree of shunting largely determine the symptoms. Symptoms become more common with advancing age. By the age of forty years, 90% of untreated patients have symptoms of exertional dyspnoea, fatique, palpitation, sustained arrthythmia, or even evidence of heart failure.

In childhood, the diagnosis is often considered after a heart murmer is detected on routine physical examination or after an abnormal finding is observed on routine chest radiographs or electrocardiogram (ECG). Unlike babies with a patent ductus where a murmur may be detected, ASD in infants exhibits few if any noticeable symptoms. In adults, one of the most common symptoms is the development of palpitations related to atrial arrhythmias.

## Common Types of Atrial Septal Defects

The most common types of ASD include the following:[52]

1. **Ostium secundum:** This defect is in the central part of the atrial septum (Figs 5.21 and 5.22). It is the most common type of atrial septal defect, representing approximately 7% of all congenital cardiac defects and 30–40% of all congenital heart disease in patients older than 40 years. In ostium secundum atrial septal defect, most affected children are free of any major symptoms, if the defect is small. However, the risk of heart failure with pulmonary hypertension and atrial fibrillation developing later in life, makes closure of the defect desirable. Lack of symptoms is not a contraindication for repair. However, closure of an atrial septal defect is not recommended in children with a clinically insignificant shunt.

    Percutaneous closure of an atrial septal defect is currently only indicated for the closure of ostium secundum atrial septal defect with a sufficient rim of tissue around the septal defect, so that the closure device does not impinge upon the superior and inferior venae cavae, or the tricuspid or mitral valves (Fig. 5.23).

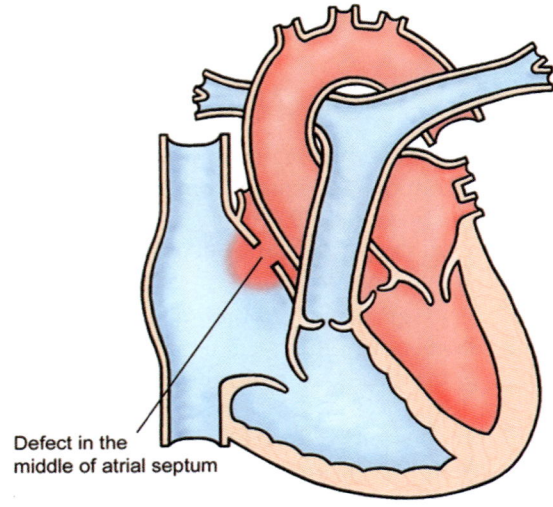

Defect in the
middle of atrial septum

**Fig. 5.21:** Ostium secundum atrial septal defect. This is the only type of ASD suitable for percutaneous closure as the defect is located in the middle of the atrial septum

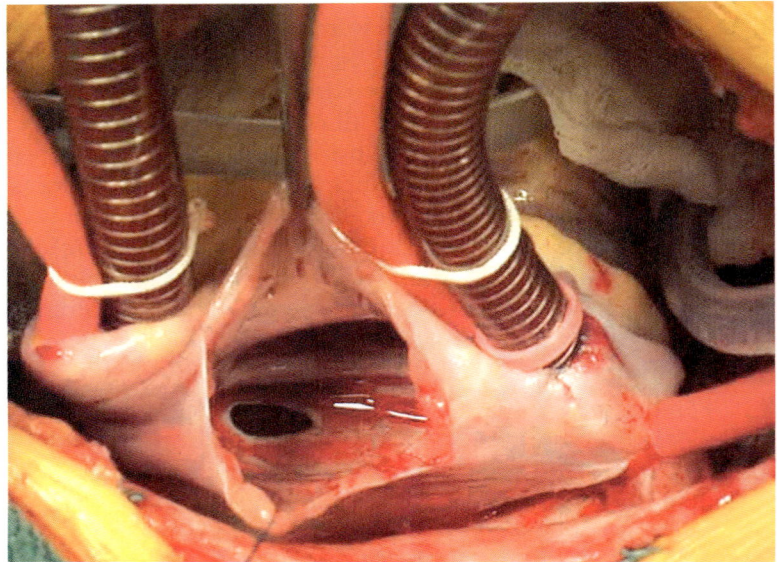

**Fig. 5.22:** Surgical view of an ostium secundum atrial septal defect

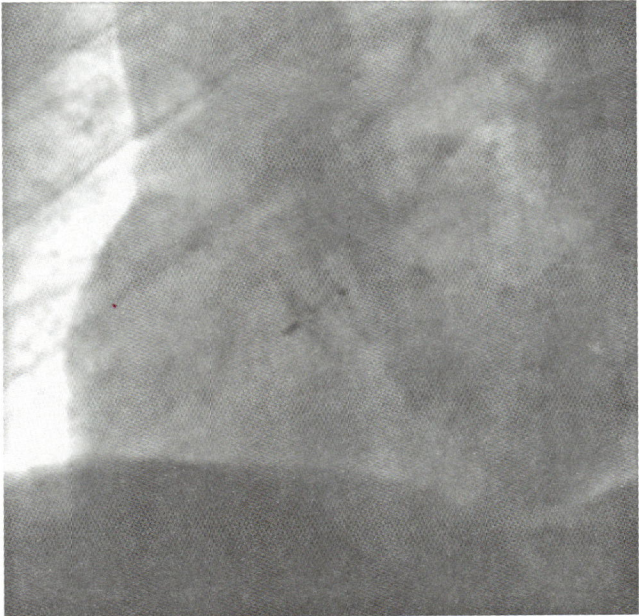

**Fig. 5.23:** Percutaneous closure of an atrial septal defect. The fluoroscopy shows the final position of the septal occluder device

2. **Ostium primum:** This is the second most common type of atrial septal defects and accounts for 15–20% of all atrial septal defects (Fig. 5.24). It is a form of atrioventricular septal defect and is commonly associated with mitral and/or tricuspid valve abnormalities. It occurs in the lower part of the atrial septum. Ostium primum atrial septal defect may lead to symptoms in infancy or childhood and needs surgical closure, mitral/ tricuspid repair and sometimes mitral valve replacement. This type of atrial septal defect is not suitable for device closure. The mitral valve is often abnormal and incompetent. If not detected in childhood, ostium primum atrial septal defect may result in clinically significant mitral regurgitation in adults. It's incidence, extent, and degree of dysfunction increases with age. Mitral valve insufficiency leads to further increase in left atrial pressure and a higher degree of left-to-right shunting. Prognosis depends on size of the defect, extent of valve involvement, time of diagnosis and surgical repair.

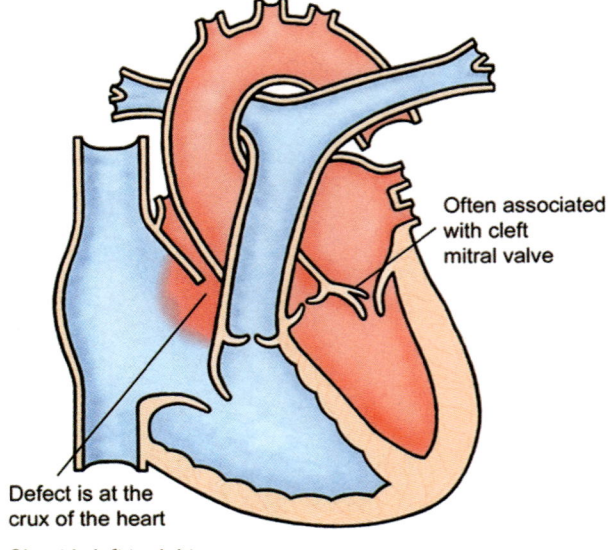

Often associated with cleft mitral valve

Defect is at the crux of the heart

Shunt is left to right

**Fig. 5.24:** Ostium primum atrial septal defect or partial atrioventricular septal defect. This defect is often associated with cleft mitral valve

3. **Sinus venosus:** Sinus venosus defects are seen in 5–10% of all atrial septal defects and are usually located along the superior (upper) aspect of the atrial septum (Fig. 5.25). Anomalous connection of the right-sided pulmonary veins is common and should be expected.

4. **Coronary sinus:** Coronary sinus atrial septal defects are located in the portion of the atrial septum that includes the coronary sinus[viii] orifice and are characterized by the absence of at least a portion of the common wall that separates the coronary sinus and the left atrium (Fig. 5.26). A dilated coronary sinus often suggests this defect. Coronary sinus defects are often associated with a persistent left superior vena cava[ix] that drains into the

---

[viii]The coronary sinus is the main drainage channel of venous blood from the myocardium. It delivers deoxygenated blood to the right atrium in conjunction with the superior and inferior venae cavae.

[ix]Persistence of the left superior vena cava (LSVC) draining into the right atrium via the coronary sinus is a variation of normal systemic venous return, occurring in 0.3% of the general population.

Defect in superior
aspect of atrial
septum

Often anomalous
PV drainage

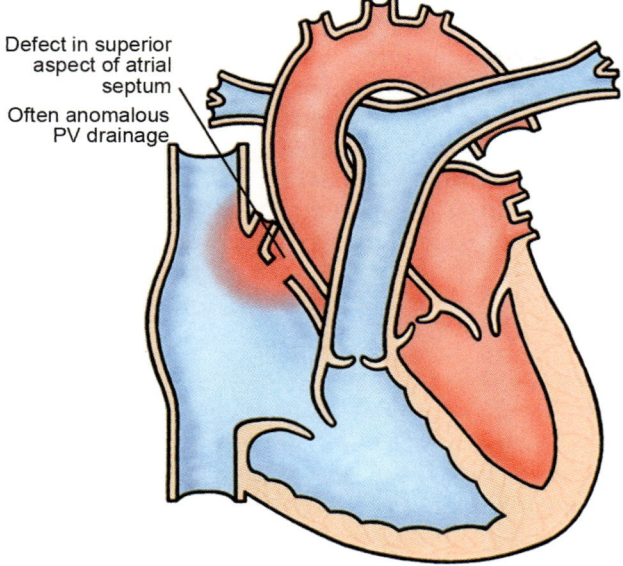

**Fig. 5.25:** Sinus venosus atrial septal defect. Anomalous connection of
the right-sided pulmonary veins is common and should be expected

Right pulmonary veins

Superior sinus
venosus defect

Secundum ASD

Inferior sinus
venosus defect

Coronary sinus defect

Primum ASD

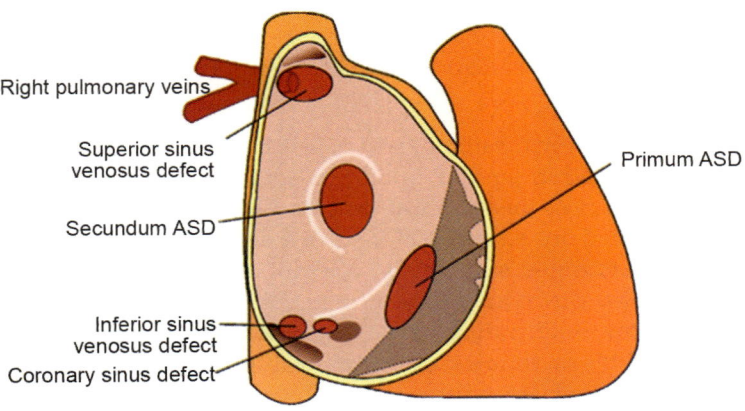

**Fig. 5.26:** Atrial Septal defects—ostium secundum, ostium primum, sinus
venosus, and coronary sinus

coronary sinus. When the wall between the coronary sinus and left atrium fails to form, the systemic venous blood (pulmonary veins) drains directly into the left atrium. This fenestration into the left atrium usually occurs between the left atrial appendage and the left upper pulmonary vein. When this fold is missing, the defect is called an **unroofed coronary sinus or unroofed coronary sinus atrial septal defect.** Coronary sinus atrial septal defects are often difficult to diagnose and may even be overlooked during surgery for complex congenital heart disease.

## Treatment

Overall, the decision to repair any kind of atrial septal defect is based on clinical and echocardiographic information, including the size and location of the atrial septal defect, the magnitude and haemodynamic impact of the left-to-right shunt, and the presence and degree of pulmonary arterial hypertension. In general, elective closure is advised for all atrial septal defects with evidence of right ventricular overload or with a clinically significant shunt. Atrial septal defect is an acyanotic lesion. Thus, the child should be normally saturated. In the rare case of severe pulmonary hypertension, atrial shunt reversal (Eisenmenger syndrome) may occur, leading to cyanosis and *clubbing* of fingers and toenails.

## Atrial Septal Defect Repair—Overview

### *History*

Rokitansky (German pathologist, 1804–1878) in 1875 first described defects of the atrial septum, but it was not until 75 years later that operations to close them were attempted. Operations to close ASDs were first tried out on artificially created defects in animals. Their success encouraged surgeons to attempt correction on humans. Some of these procedures were crude. Others were more refined, and with few modifications are in use, in some centres even today. But all of these repairs are remarkable because they were necessarily blind procedures, guided only by touch and carried out on a beating heart. In one of these attempts to close an atrial septal defect, inert lucite buttons (Fig. 5.27) were used in 1951 by Hufnagel and Gillespie.[53]

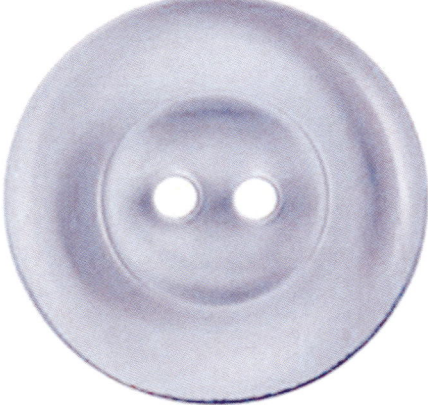

**Fig. 5.27:** To close an atrial septal defect, *inert lucite buttons* were used in 1951 by Hufnagel and Gillespie

At surgery, two opposite buttons inserted through the atrial appendage using special rod introducers were tightly screwed together on opposite sides of the atrial septum. The brilliance of this concept led to transcatheter closure of ASDs used today. Simple atrial septal defect repair was one of the first congenital heart diseases to be corrected by open heart surgery and in fact, paved the path to modern open heart surgery.

The surgical treatment options for repair of an atrial septal defect include direct suture repair, if the defect is small, or patch repair. The material used for patch repair may be the child's own pericardium (autologous), commercially available bovine or porcine pericardium, or synthetic material (Gore-tex™, Dacron).

In most cardiac centres, the surgical approach for atrial septal defect repair is through a median sternotomy, in some cases, this may be a smaller than routine skin incision and partial sternotomy (Fig. 5.28). Cardiopulmonary bypass is used with an aortic cannula placed in the ascending aorta and bicaval venous cannulation. The atrial septal defect is closed through a right atriotomy. Individual surgeons may use a left ventricular vent, which will be passed through the atrial septum, through the mitral valve into the left ventricle. In some cases, no cardioplegia is used and the child's temperature is allowed to *drift* with no active cooling.

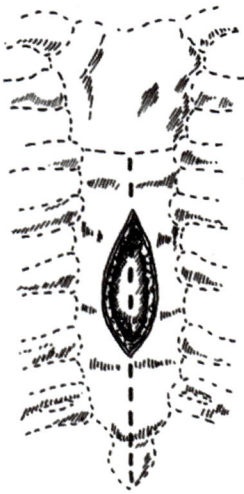

**Fig. 5.28:** A small incision across two intercostal spaces (3–8 cm) with a partial sternotomy may be used in the surgical closure of an atrial septal defect

### Atrial Septal Defect Repair—Technique

The following technique described is that of an atrial septal defect secundum repair, since this defect is the most common of atrial septal defects. However, the technique for any other atrial septal defect repair is similar to the technique described here. The majority of secundum ASDs in infants and small children with a small ASD can be closed with a single suture, whereas in older children, patch repair is almost always indicated.

1. Skin incision is made and the sternum is divided.
2. Sternal retractor is then positioned for exposure.
3. The thymus is removed to improve exposure.
4. The pericardium is opened and if used for the repair, harvested and given to the scrub nurse to prepare, either to be kept in normal saline or some surgeons prefer to treat the pericardium with glutaraldehyde because this strengthens the patch and makes it easier for the surgeon to handle (Fig. 5.30). Some surgeons prefer to leave the pericardium attached till they have inspected the size of the atrial septal defect, and then harvest appropriate size for the repair.

5. Cannulation is started by placing purse strings on the aorta, superior vena cava and inferior vena cava.
6. Once the child is cannulated, cardiopulmonary bypass is established, and the child is cooled, by cooling the blood. Mild hypothermia (32–34°C) is used in most cases. In direct atrial septal defect repair, the surgeon may prefer to *stay warm* (no active cooling).
7. A cardioplegia purse string followed by a cardioplegia needle is inserted into the aortic root.
8. The aortic crosslamp is applied and cardioplegia is delivered to stop the heart.
9. Caval tapes are placed around the superior vena cava and the inferior vena cava, as a routine before opening the right atrium.
10. The right atrium is opened and suspended with silk sutures and small vein retractors are used to facilitate exposure (Fig. 5.29).

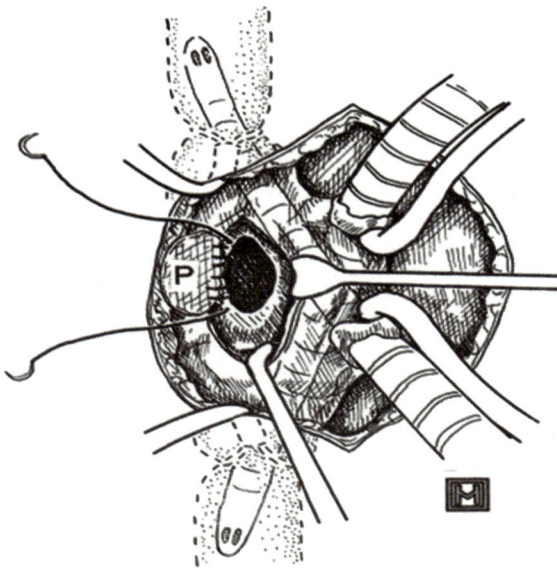

**Fig. 5.29:** A vein retractor is placed for retraction, and a cardiotomy suction catheter is placed in the coronary sinus. An autologous pericardial patch (P) is used to close the defect with a continuous suture technique

11. The atrial septal defect is inspected and it is ensured that the pulmonary and systemic venous return is normally directed to the left and right atria respectively. The defect is then repaired with either a single non-absorbable 5-0 or 6-0 polypropylene suture or in the case of patch repair, the same suture material is used to suture the patch to the edges of the defect.

12. Just before the final closure of the defect, most surgeons will ask for the left side of the heart to be filled with blood by way of hyper-inflating the lungs to increase pulmonary venous return and thereby removing any air remaining in the left heart (left atrium). This is referred to as *Valsalva*.

13. The child is positioned in a head-down position and the cross clamp is then removed.

14. Once the defect is closed, the right atrium is closed, while the child is slowly rewarmed (in case active cooling was used). The child is then weaned off cardiopulmonary bypass.

15. A single mediastinal chest drain is placed. Individual surgeons may place a right ventricular pacing wire. The sternum is rewired and the chest is closed in a standard fashion.

## PREPARATION OF AUTOLOGOUS PERICARDIUM

Prepare a small trolley, metal bowls × 3, Petri dish, glutaraldehyde 0.6%, normal saline 1 litre, carton paper (from gown), mayo and tenotomy scissors, forceps, micromosquito and extra medium size liga clip applier and clip.

## Role of the Scrub Nurse

1. Extra scrub nurse needed to prepare the pericardium (Fig. 5.30a).
2. After pericardium is harvested, place the pericardium on the carton paper (from gown), rough side of pericardium facing up (Fig. 5.30b)).
3. Take a forceps and smooth out the pericardium.
4. Cut any excess pericardium and paper ((Fig. 5.30c).
5. Staple the pericardium carefully to the paper using only few medium size liga clips ((Fig. 5.30d).
6. Immerse the pericardium in 0.6% glutaraldehyde: 10 minutes for ASD, 20 minutes for VSD ((Fig. 5.30e).
7. Then rinse in normal saline in 2 separate bowls.
8. Carefully remove the pericardium from the carton and carefully remove any white debris from the pericardium.

9. Cut a small piece from the pericardium and prepare 5–0 poly-propylene 10 mm pledgeted sutures × 3 to use for reinforcement suture if required (this depends on individual surgeons preference).

10. Immerse the pericardium in third bowl with normal saline till surgeon is ready to use it. Inform the surgeon, that the patch is ready ((Fig. 5.30f).

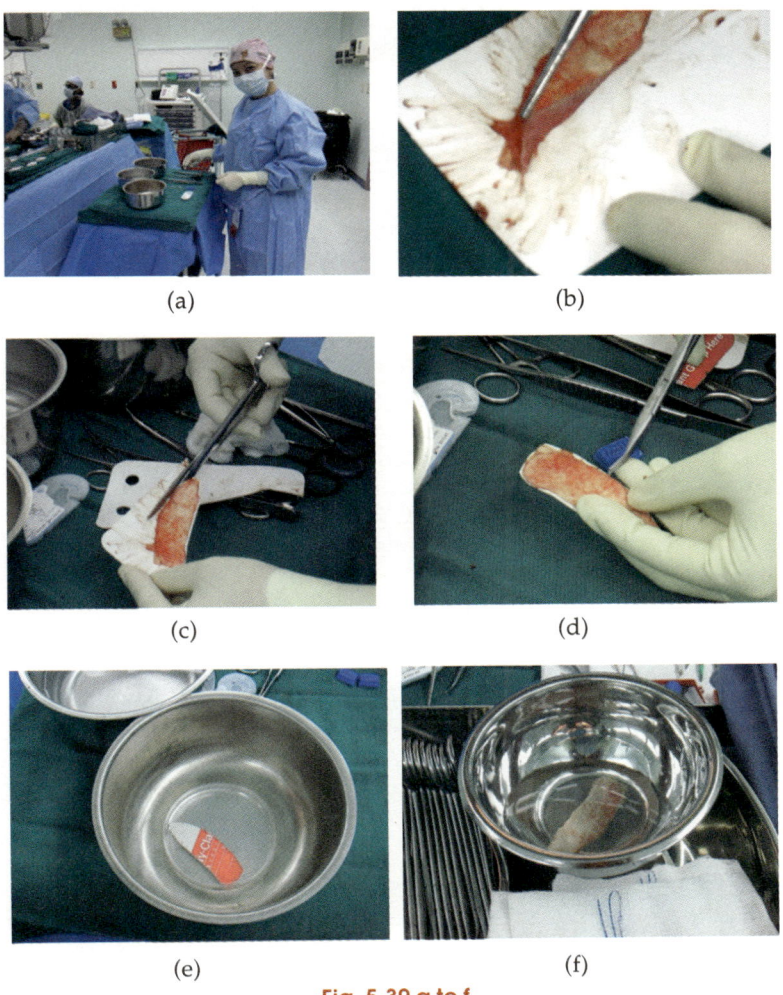

(a)

(b)

(c)

(d)

(e)

(f)

**Fig. 5.30 a to f**

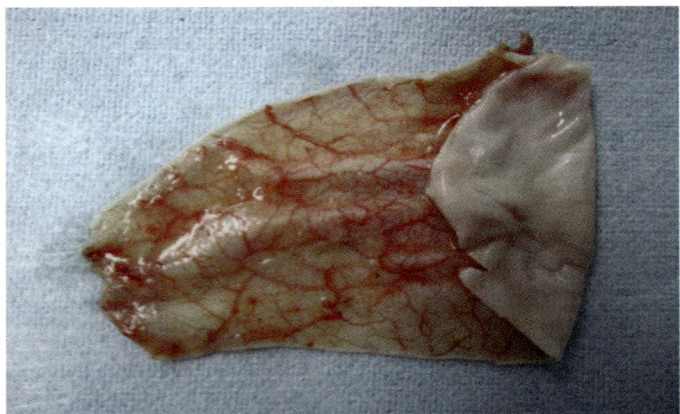

**Fig. 5.30A:** A piece of autologous pericardium is cut and refashioned to the right size and regardless of the way it will be prepared, placed into position with the smooth side towards the left atrium. *(Photos a to f by EDJ, courtesy of KAMC, National Guard Hospital, Riyadh, Saudi Arabia)*

### NURSING OBSERVATION

*This procedure is a relatively straight forward open heart procedure and a great opportunity for the orientating perioperative nurse for first time exposure in assisting the surgeon, and to become familiar with the steps of cannulation and placing a child on the cardiopulmonary bypass machine. Be familiar with the patch material, if any, used for the repair, the way it is treated, which sutures are used and which suture technique is used.*

### SURGEON'S COMMENT

*It is important that nurses follow the standard technique of cannulation of a child's heart for standard cardiopulmonary bypass with isolation of the right heart with caval snares. It is strictly observed that there is no air left in the venous cannulae because if this air goes to the right atrium, it can travel to the left heart through the ASD and lead to systemic air embolism.*

## Outcome of Surgical Repair

The results of surgical atrial septal defect (ASD) repairs are excellent. Repair of an ASD is a curative procedure that restores a normal life expectancy. Surgical mortality is less than 1% and average hospital stay is 4 days.[54]

## VENTRICULAR SEPTAL DEFECT (VSD)

### Introduction

A ventricular septal defect is a defect in the wall between the right and left ventricles of the heart (Figs 5.31–5.33). An abnormal opening in the ventricular septum allows communication of blood between the left and right ventricles. Blood flow across the defect is typically left to right and depends on the size of the defect and the pulmonary vascular resistance (PVR).

These defects can occur as an isolated lesion or in combination with other congenital cardiac anomalies, e.g. tetralogy of Fallot, complete atrioventricular canal defects or transposition of the great arteries.

### What Causes a Ventricular Septal Defect?

A ventricular septal defect is caused by embryologic malformations of the ventricular septum.

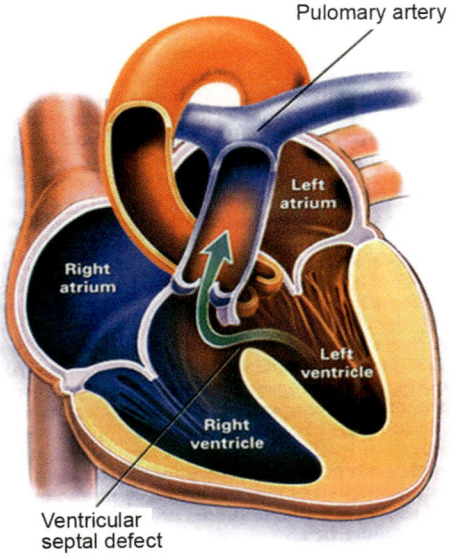

**Fig. 5.31:** Ventricular septal defect—blood flow across the defect is typically left to right and depends on the size of the defect and the pulmonary vascular resistance (PVR)

## Prevalence

VSDs are among the most common congenital heart disease. Isolated VSDs represent about 25% of all congenital heart disease (1 to 2 per 1,000 live births).[55, 56]

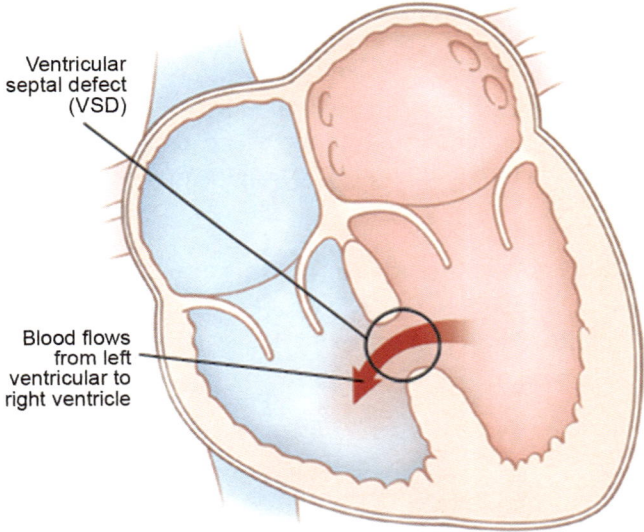

Ventricular septal defect (VSD)

Blood flows from left ventricular to right ventricle

**Fig. 5.32:** The wall dividing the two lower pumping chambers of the heart (right and left ventricles) is known as the **ventricular septum.** Abnormal development of this structure may result in a *hole*, usually located at the upper portion of the septum. Because the pressure on the left side of the heart is higher than the right, blood crosses the *hole* (VSD) and causes *flooding* of the lung vessels. The amount of overcirculation to the lungs is dependent upon the size and location of the defect. If not corrected, the increased circulation to the right side of the heart and lungs may cause an overload on the muscle and permanent damage to the lung vessels. A VSD may occur as an isolated defect, or may be one of several congenital heart malformations. The operation for VSD involves closing the defect. In some cases where the defect is small and the tissues firm, the edges may be brought together with stitches. More frequently a patch of synthetic material is sewn into place to close the defect

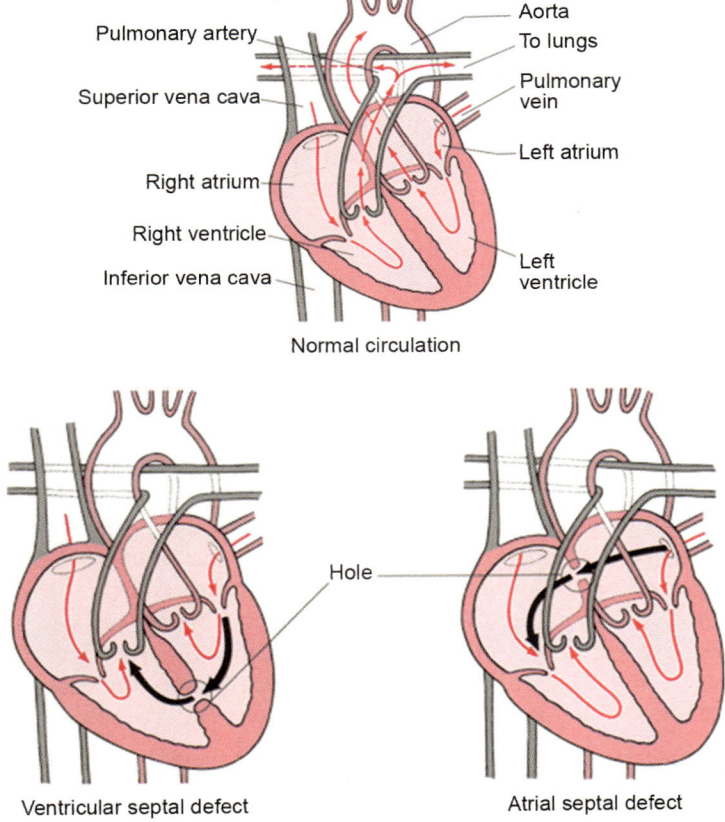

**Fig. 5.33:** Normal ciculation, ventricular septal defect and atrial septal defect

## Symptoms

These defects have a very characteristic murmur, and a cardiologist may be able to pinpoint the location and estimate the size of a ventricular septal defect just by how it sounds.

A small ventricular septal defect may never cause any problems. Large ventricular septal defects can cause problems, often developing gradually in the first few months of life. This is because before birth, the pressure on the right side of the heart is equal to the pressure on the left side of the heart. As soon as the baby takes its first breath, the pressure in the lungs and the right side of the heart starts to decrease (PVR). This process is slow and usually takes about 2 to 4 weeks for the pressure in the lungs to reach normal level. In the first 1 to 2 weeks of life, babies with large ventricular septal defects may do very well. But as the pressure in the right side of the heart decreases, blood will start to flow to the path of least resistance (i.e., from the left ventricle, where the pressure is higher, through the ventricular septal defect to the right ventricle, where the pressure is lower, and into the lungs, Fig. 5.31). This will gradually lead to symptoms of congestive heart failure (the lungs become literally flooded) and must be treated. Babies who have significant congestive heart failure will fail to thrive and will have difficulty maintaining a normal weight gain in the first few months of life. In the initial stages, the pulmonary vasculature reacts to increased flow by increasing vascular resistance and causing pulmonary hypertension, which is reversible. However, with the passage of time, irreversible and progressive changes take place in the walls of the pulmonary arteries. Once pulmonary vascular resistance has developed, and exceeds the systemic vascular resistance (the force with which the right ventricle pumps blood to the lungs), blood begins to flow from the right ventricle to the left ventricle. Once this has developed (Eisenmenger syndrome) the pulmonary vascular disease is irreversible and progressive, and the defect is irreparable.

## Common Types of Ventricular Septal Defects

Ventricular septal defects are classified by their location in the ventricular septum. The septum is divided into four components: the membranous septum, the inlet, the trabecular (muscular), and the outlet parts of the muscular septum. Therefore, there are four types of VSDs (Fig. 5.34).[57] Symptoms depend on the size of the defect and to a lesser extend to their location.

1. **Infracristal:** Ventricular septal defects can be divided into infracristal and supracristal, in relation to the crista supraventricularis, a muscular ridge in the outflow region of the right ventricle. Infracristal VSD is the most common ventricular septal defect involving the membranous septum (80% of all VSDs). The defect is also referred to as peri-membranous ventricular septal defect.

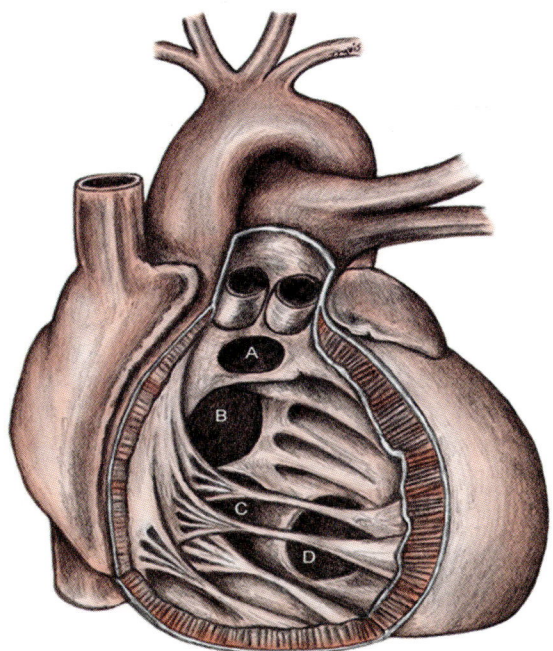

**Fig. 5.34:** Schematic representation of the location of various types of ventricular septal defects from the right ventricular aspect. A: Doubly committed subarterial or supracristal ventricular septal defect. B: Perimembranous or infracristal ventricular septal defect. C: Inlet or atrioventricular canal. D: Muscular ventricular septal defect

2. **Supracristal:** Supracristal or doubly committed VSD is the least common type of VSD, accounting for 5–8% of isolated VSDs. The location of the supracristal VSD is close to the aortic root and therefore this type of VSD commonly causes aortic valve insufficiency or regurgitation. Left-to-right shunting of blood through the defect is believed to progressively pull on the aortic valve tissue causing damage to the aortic leaflet. Supracristal is also referred to as outlet VSD (near the outflow region of the ventricles below the pulmonary and aortic valve). Morbidity and mortality in supracristal VSD is often caused by the development of aortic insufficiency. Aortic insufficiency generally begins in children between 6 and 10 years. Delayed diagnosis of this defect may lead to severe distortion of the aortic

leaflet, and aortic insufficiency, making eventual valve replacement more likely.

3. **Muscular VSD:** These types of VSDs are entirely bounded by the muscular septum and are often multiple. The term Swiss-cheese septum has been used to describe multiple muscular ventricular septal defects. These ventricular septal defects account for 5–20% of all VSD defects. About 50–70% of large muscular ventricular septal defects diagnosed during the neonatal period will become smaller or even close spontaneously within 6 to 12 months.

4. **Canal type VSD:** These ventricular septal defects lie posterior to the septal leaflet of the tricuspid valve, and are also called **inlet ventricular septal defects.** Although locations of posterior ventricular septal defects are similar to those of ventricular septal defect associated with atrioventricular valve (AV) septal defects, the AV valves are not defected or malformed. About 8 to 10% of ventricular septal defects are of this type.

## Ventricular Septal Defect Repair—Overview

Definite indications for surgery are, if an infant, regardless of age, with a large VSD, has developed congestive heart failure (due to large volumes of blood being shunted from left-to-right and flooding the lungs) and fails to grow.

In the past, pulmonary artery banding was frequently used as an initial palliative surgical intervention for infants born with a large VSD with significant left-to-right shunting and overcirculation to the pulmonary artery and lungs. The pulmonary artery band decreases the flow through the pulmonary artery, preventing overcirculation of the lungs and therefore congestive heart failure, and at the same time, allowing the child to grow. Then the band will be removed at a later stage when the infant is big enough to tolerate definite repair. Within the last 15 to 20 years, as methods of myocardial protection advanced, and surgical skills and postoperative nursing care of small infants improved, early definite repair has become more favourable. However, pulmonary artery banding still remains an initial surgical intervention in some children with left-to-right lesions. Pulmonary artery banding is a palliative but not a curative surgical procedure.

The primary goal for performing pulmonary artery banding is:

1. To reduce excessive pulmonary blood flow and protect the lungs from becoming flooded leading to pulmonary hypertension and congestive heart failure,
2. To prevent irreversible right-to-left shunting (Eisenmenger syndrome);
3. More recently, pulmonary artery banding, is used for training of the left ventricle in children with d-transposition of the great arteries;
4. Also, in certain cases of l-transposition of the great arteries, where an arterial switch operation is amendable, pulmonary artery banding, may be the initial surgical intervention, before definite repair.

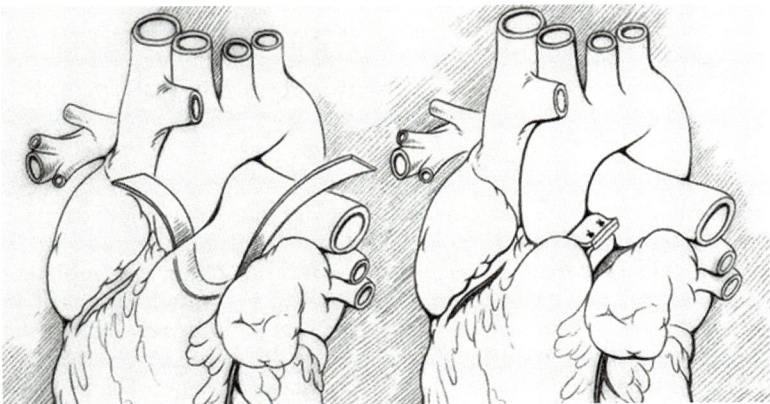

**Fig. 5.35:** Pulmonary artery banding—the pulmonary artery band decreases the flow through the pulmonary artery, preventing overcirculation of the lungs and therefore congestive heart failure

Children younger than two to three months of age (or less than 3.5 kg) may undergo ventricular septal defect repair with the technique of deep hypothermic circulatory arrest (DHCA)[x], although nowadays with advanced techniques in myocardial protection and, cardiopulmonary bypass in neonates, this is rarely necessary. Since this technique may be used, the perioperative nurse should be familiar with this.

One method of achieving deep hypothermic circulatory arrest is described below:

1. The ascending aorta is cannulated.
2. The right atrial appendage is cannulated with a small venous cannula.
3. Cardioplegia needle is inserted in the aortic root.
4. Bypass is commenced and the ductus arteriosus is ligated while the child is being cooled. (The ductus is always closed before the circulation is arrested to prevent air in the opened heart to escape through the ductus into the aorta.)
5. Once adequate cooling of the child has been reached, the aorta is clamped and a single dose of cold cardioplegia is given.
6. The circulation is then stopped, the venous cannula removed and the VSD repaired.

### NURSING OBSERVATION

*It is of paramount importance for the scrub nurse to become familiar with procedures in which circulatory arrest is used to perform a surgical repair. To operate effectively, the surgeon needs not only the expertise of his surgical assistant, the anaesthesia team and the perfusionist but needs a prepared, professional scrub nurse, ready to assist him in a timely manner.*

---

[x]Deep hypothermic circulatory arrest (DHCA) is a technique used in very small infants in which definite repair is favourable over palliative repair, for which the infant has to come back for a second and definite repair. The technique, during which the circulation of blood is completely stopped, provides the surgeon more room in very small infants with tiny hearts, to perform, e.g. a ventricular septal defect repair since the cannulae are removed during the time of circulatory arrest. The majority of infants tolerate 30 minutes of circulatory arrest at 18°C, which allows the surgeon adequate time to perform the surgery. Hypothermia is the main method of cerebral protection. Surgical techniques such as, selective antegrade cerebral perfusion may be used to prolong the safe duration of DHCA.

Nowadays, primary early repair of a VSD has been the accepted standard of practice in most cardiac centres as opposed to staged pulmonary artery banding and subsequent VSD repair. Also, the need for circulatory arrest in the very young infants is hardly necessary with advancement in cardiopulmonary bypass and myocardial protection in these neonates. Most VSDs are repaired with aortic and bicaval cannulation, aortic cross clamping, cardioplegia, hypothermia, and a left ventricular vent. This not only provides myocardial protection and a relatively bloodless intracardiac surgical field, but also relaxes the heart muscle to optimize exposure.

## Ventricular Septal Defect Repair—Technique

1. The heart is accessed through a median sternotomy.
2. In small or unstable infants, some surgeons may prefer to connect both venous cannulae to the venous line of the bypass machine and then to first cannulate, the right atrial appendage with the smaller of the two cannulae and commence cardiopulmonary bypass.
3. When on bypass, with the lungs deflated and the heart decompressed it will be easier for the surgeon to cannulate the inferior vena cava.
4. Once this has been done, the first venous cannula can be clamped and removed from the right atrial appendage, and inserted directly into the superior vena cava through a new purse string suture.
5. The ductus is ligated next, and the infant cooled to the appropriate temperature.
6. The aorta is then clamped and cold cardioplegia given to cool and arrest the heart.
7. The right atrium is opened and suspended with a silk suture.
8. A pump sucker or vent is placed in the left atrium through a natural defect (patent foramen ovale), or stab incision in the interatrial septum to keep the field blood free.
9. Alternatively, a pump sucker or vent can be placed in the left atrium via the right superior pulmonary vein. Some surgeons may use a purse string suture to keep the pump sucker or vent in place.

10. The defect is visualised by placing small vein retractors to retract the tricuspid valve.
11. In small infants the VSD may be closed with interrupted non-absorbable 5-0 or 6-0 polypropylene sutures supported with small felt pledgets (Fig. 5.36 and 5.37).[xi]
12. Mostly, patch material is needed for the repair, child's own pericardium, commercially available bovine or porcine pericardium, or synthetic material (Gore-tex™, Dacron, Fig. 5.38).
13. Standard routines are observed to remove air from the left heart before removing the cross clamp. The child is warmed, right atrium is closed and weaning from CP bypass is done as a routine. Pacing wires are placed as a routine as heart rhythm problems may be encountered at this stage or later in the intensive care unit.

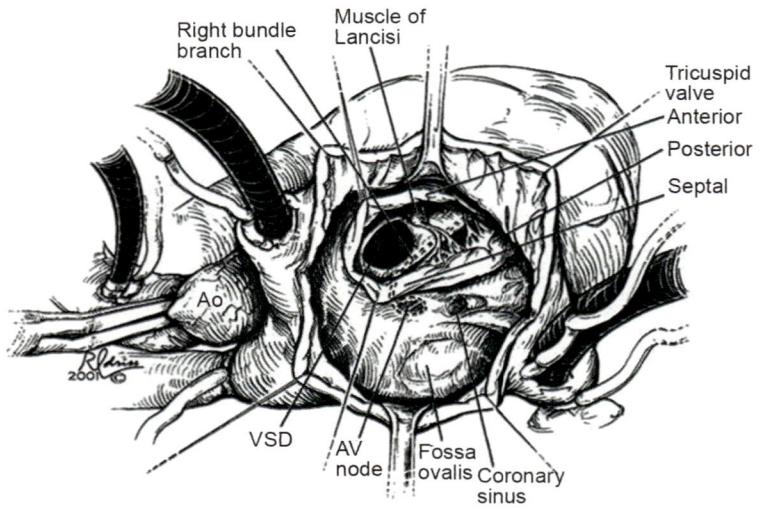

**Fig. 5.36:** Surgical exposure of a VSD. Note the AV node close to the defect

---

[xi]Felt pledgets are used as buttresses under sutures when there is a possibility of sutures tearing through tissue. These pledgets are used in various surgical suturing procedures, such as vascular closure, septal repair (ASD, VSD: Fig. 5.37), myocardial closure and valvular suturing.

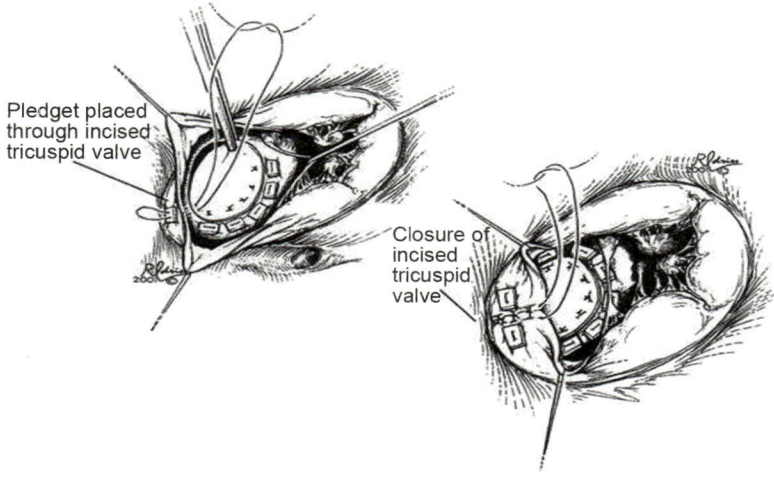

**Fig. 5.37:** Surgical repair of a VSD with a patch and pledgeted sutures

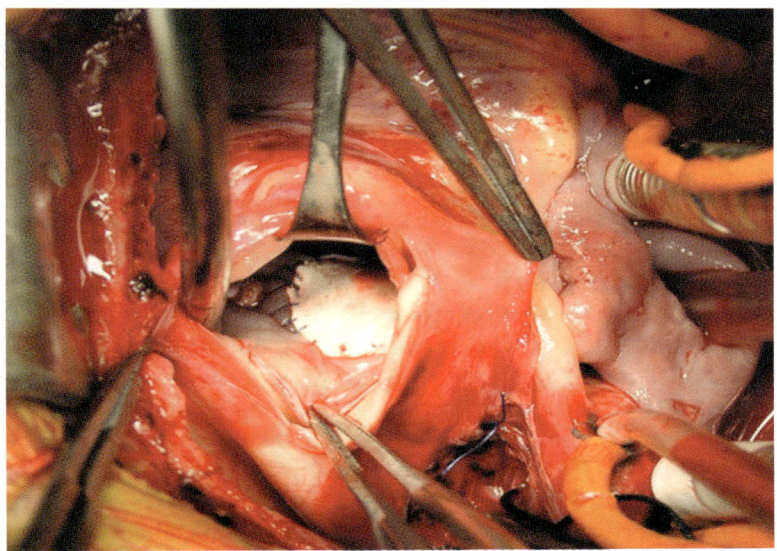

**Fig. 5.38:** Surgical closure of a VSD with a Gore-tex™ patch

**NURSING OBSERVATION**

*Both ASD and VSD repair surgeries provides the orientating perioperative scrub nurse with an excellent opportunity for first time assisting the surgeon unless circulatory arrest is used for a VSD repair which, requires advanced experience. The scrub nurse should have knowledge of what patch material is used for the VSD repair, the method in which the patch is treated and what kind of suture material is used for suturing the patch. Also different surgeons use different techniques in suturing the patch for the VSD repair. In addition, be aware that some surgeons prefer to use pledgeted sutures and it has to be prepared well in advance by the scrub nurse.*

**SURGEON'S COMMENT**

*It is important that nurses observe the standard routine for bicaval cannulation of the child's heart with caval snares. The perimembranous VSD (infracristal) is the most common VSD, which is usually closed through the right atrial incision after retracting the tricuspid valve with small vein retractors. The inlet type (canal type) and muscular VSD can also be closed through the right atrium. However, the outlet VSD (supracristal) is more easily approached by opening the main pulmonary artery and retracting the pulmonary valve with small vein retractors. The conduction tissue of the heart runs very near the edge of the VSD in most cases and a heart block may occur, if care is not taken to avoid injury to the conduction bundle.*

## Outcome of Surgical Repair

Outcome and prognosis is variable depending on the size of the VSD, associated pulmonary hypertension, and if the VSD is part of a complex congenital anomaly. For uncomplicated VSD repair, the mortality rate of surgery should come close to zero percent. The overall risk for VSD repair is less than 5%. Mortality and morbidity rates increase with multiple VSDs, pulmonary hypertension, and complex associated anomalies. The severity of these complications, if a VSD is left untreated, depends on the magnitude of the shunt, which in turn, depends on the size of the VSD, and the pulmonary vascular resistance. When surgical repair is performed before the age of two years, the long-term outlook is excellent, and the child will have the best chance of leading a normal life.[59]

## ATRIOVENTRICULAR SEPTAL DEFECTS (AVSDs)

## Introduction

Many terms are used to describe this complex defect. They include atrioventricular canal, complete atrioventricular canal, complete common atrioventricular canal, and endocardial cushion defect. Essentially, they all describe a similar heart problem. Atrioventricular septal defect is currently the preferred terminology. It is a combination of defects, involving malformations of the tricuspid and mitral valves and the atrial and ventricular septa (Figs 5.39 and 5.41). In some cases, the mitral and tricuspid valves are connected, forming a single opening. In addition to valvular defects, defects often occur in both the ventricular septum and the atrial septum. Atrioventricular septal defects can also occur with other types of congenital heart disease such as coarctation of the aorta or tetralogy of Fallot.

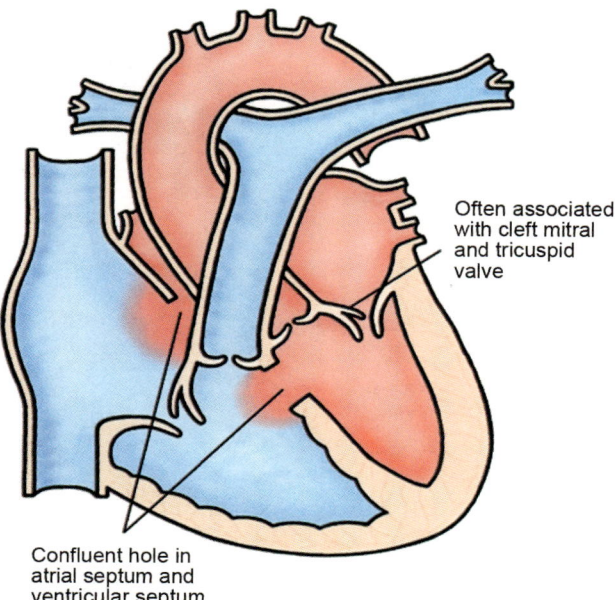

Often associated with cleft mitral and tricuspid valve

Confluent hole in atrial septum and ventricular septum

**Fig. 5.39:** Atrioventricular septal defect (AVSD). It is a combination of defects, involving malformations of the tricuspid and mitral valves and the atrial and ventricular septa

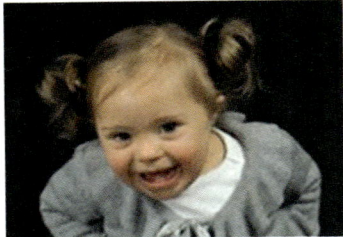 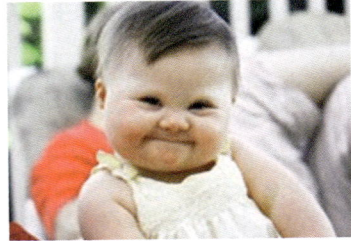

**Fig. 5.40:** Children with Down's syndrome. Atrioventricular septal defects are present in 45% of infants with Down's syndrome

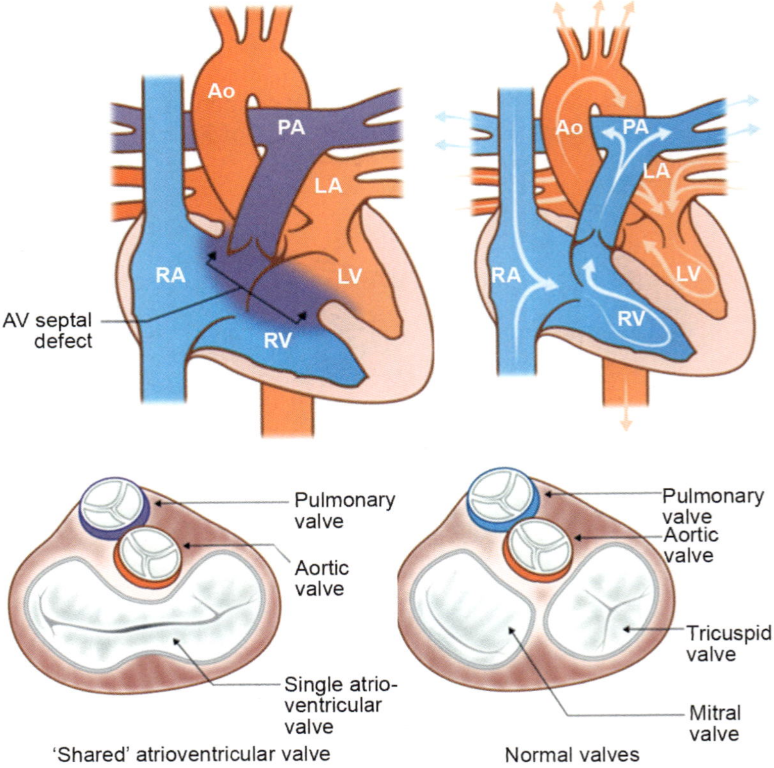

'Shared' atrioventricular valve

Normal valves

**Fig. 5.41:** Atrioventricular septal defect (AVSD). It is a combination of defects, involving malformations of the tricuspid and mitral valves, atrial and ventricular septa. In some cases, the mitral and tricuspid valves are connected, forming a single opening

## What Causes an Atrioventricular Septal Defect?

The primary defect is the failure of formation of the part of the heart that arises from an **embryonic structure** called the *endocardial cushions* (hence the name; endocardial cushion defect). The endocardial cushions are responsible for separating the central parts of the heart near the tricuspid and mitral valves, and dividing the atria from the ventricles. The structures that develop from the endocardial cushions include the lower part of the atrial septum and the ventricular septum, just below the tricuspid and mitral valves. The endocardial cushions also complete the separation of the mitral and tricuspid valves by dividing the single valve between the embryonic atria and ventricles. An atrioventricular septal defect may involve failure of formation of any or all of these structures.

## Prevalence

Atrioventricular septal defects account for 3–5% of congenital heart disease.[60] It is as common in females as in males.[61] Atrioventricular septal defects are present in 45% of infants with Down's syndrome[xii] (Fig. 5.40). Similarly, one-third of all children born with AVSD have also Down's syndrome.[62]

---

[xii]Down's syndrome, also known as **Trisomy 21,** is the single most common genetic pattern of malformation in the human race. In 1866, John Langdon Haydon Down described the physical features and associated medical problems that have come to be known as **Down's syndrome.** In the 1930s, physicians established a relationship between advanced maternal age and Down's syndrome. The chromosomal, or genetic, basis of Down's syndrome was not established until 1959. A normal human cell contains 23 pairs of chromosomes, which carry all of a person's genetic information. Due to several possible abnormal mechanisms of cell reproduction, children with Down's syndrome have an extra (third) copy of the 21st chromosome. Thus, Down's syndrome is also called **Trisomy 21.** Advanced maternal age is associated with a high incidence of Trisomy 21, but even women of typical child bearing age can have affected babies. While the diagnosis may be strongly suggested by characteristic physical findings, the final diagnosis is often made only after chromosome analysis, which includes a complete count and visualization under a microscope of the chromosomes taken from cells in the blood.

## Symptoms

Atrioventricular septal defects allow blood to move freely between the four chambers of the heart. In some infants the pulmonary vascular resistance, which usually decreases after birth, remains high and these infants may show few or no symptoms. In other infants in whom the pulmonary vascular resistance does decrease after birth, excessive blood flow will pass to the lungs and cause congestive heart failure. Children with complete atrioventricular septal defect typically develop tachypnea, repeated respiratory infections and failure to thrive. These symptoms are usually present by 6 to 8 weeks and due to blood flow through the large interventricular septal defect (left-to-right shunting). Children may survive past the first few years of life without surgical intervention if the pulmonary vascular resistance remains high, although those children may develop irreversible pulmonary vascular obstructive disease (Eisenmenger syndrome).

## COMMON TYPES OF ATRIOVENTRICULAR SEPTAL DEFECTS

Atrioventricular septal defects are classified into 5 categories:

1. **Complete atrioventricular septal defect:** A complete atrioventricular septal defect is one in which there are defects in all structures formed by the endocardial cushions. Therefore, there are defects in the atrial and ventricular septa, and the atrioventricular valve (AV valve) remains undivided or common.

2. **Partial or incomplete atrioventricular septal defect:** A partial or incomplete atrioventricular septal defect is one in which the part of the ventricular septum formed by the endocardial cushions has filled in, either by tissue from the AV valves or directly from the endocardial cushion tissue, and the tricuspid

and mitral valves are divided into two distinct valves. The defect is, therefore, primarily in the atrial septum and mitral valve. This type of atrial septal defect is also referred to as an ostium primum atrial septal defect, and is usually associated with a cleft in the mitral valve that may cause the valve to leak. Partial AVSD, as opposed to complete AVSD, of the ostium primum type is more common in children without Down's syndrome.

3. **Transitional or intermediate atrioventricular septal defect:** The transitional, also called **intermediate type of defect** looks similar to the complete form of atrioventricular septal defect, but the leaflets of the common AV valve are stuck to the ventricular septum thereby effectively dividing the valve into two valves and closing most of the *hole* between the ventricles.

4. **Balanced**, and

5. **Unbalanced atrioventricular septal defects:** In balanced atrioventricular septal defect (AVSD), the common atrioventricular valve (AVV) has a single inlet directed equally towards both ventricular chambers. Both ventricles are thus equally developed. When this common AVV opens predominantly toward one ventricle or the other an unbalanced AVSD forms. Consequently, the ventricle, which, receives most blood will be more developed than the other ventricle resulting in hypoplasia of either the right or left ventricle. This results in essentially single ventricle physiology. Importantly, the ventricles, not the common AVV, are unbalanced, thus the development of the ventricles is unbalanced with hypoplasia of the ventricle, which receives the least blood flow.

## Atrioventricular Septal Defect Repair—Overview

Pulmonary artery banding is often reserved for complicated cases of atrioventricular septal defect, such as unbalanced ventricles with single ventricle physiology and pulmonary overcirculation. Atrioventricular septal defects (AVSDs) almost invariably require surgical correction within a few months of birth. Complete AVSDs should be repaired before the age of 1 year. In many centres, surgical correction is attempted as early as three to four months to prevent development of Eisenmenger syndrome, especially in infants with Down's syndrome. Irreversible pulmonary vascular disease may be present by the age of two years in these children.

The main goals for repairing a complete AVSD are to:

1. Separate the two ventricles,
2. Separate the two atria,
3. Reconstruction of the mitral and tricuspid valve.

## Atrioventricular Septal Defect Repair—Technique

1. After a median sternotomy, the pericardium is harvested and preserved (this can be done in various ways depending on the surgeons' preference) for later use for patch repair.
2. The aorta, ductus arteriosus, and vena cavae are then mobilized.
3. The aorta and both vena cavae are cannulated, and the infant is placed on cardiopulmonary bypass.
4. Ductus arteriosus is ligated once the infant is on bypass.
5. A left atrial vent is then inserted either with a purse string suture in the right superior pulmonary vein, or through the atrial septal defect, once right atriotomy is performed.
6. Nylon or silk caval tapes are passed around both vena cavae and snared.
7. Aorta is clamped, cardioplegia is given and the child is cooled to required temperature.
8. The right atrium is opened and suspended with a silk suture.
9. The AV valve is then inspected.
10. Next, the VSD is closed using the child's own pericardium, commercially available bovine or porcine pericardium, or synthetic material (Gore-tex™, Dacron).
11. Then the common valve will be repaired, separating them into a mitral and tricuspid valve, before closing the atrial septal defect with a patch.
12. After the repair is completed and the infant is weaned off the bypass machine, ventricular as well as atrial pacing wires are inserted.
13. Chest drains are inserted and the chest is closed in a standard fashion.

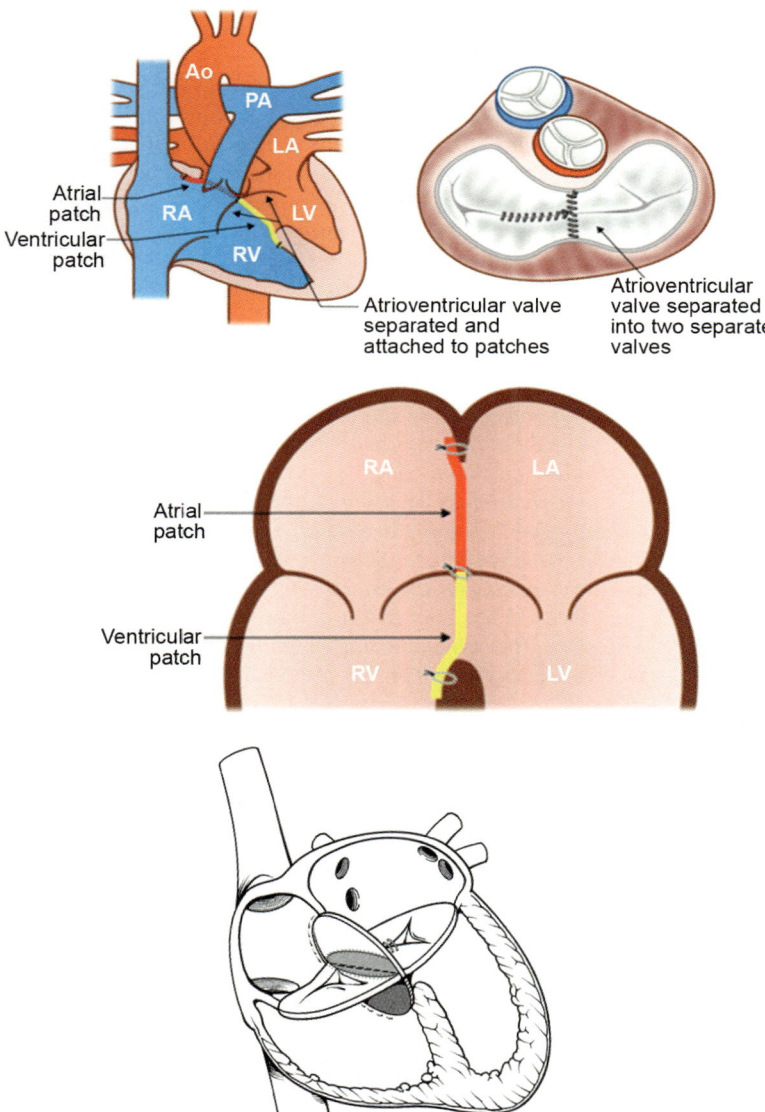

**Fig. 5.42:** Repair of atrioventricular septal defect. Both atrial and ventricular septa are closed and the single atrioventricular valve is divided into the mitral and tricuspid valves

## Outcome of Surgical Repair

Surgical morbidity and mortality rates associated with this defect have dramatically improved over the years. The surgical mortality rate should be low. In a published review of surgical outcomes of 363 patients with atrioventricular septal defects who were treated between 1982 and 1995, the early mortality rate was 10.3% and the 10-year survival rate was 83%.[63] Potential complications postsurgery include, atrioventricular block (AV block)[64], residual mitral or tricuspid regurgitation, or residual septal defects. A published study of 120 children postsurgical AVSD repair, mortality rates in-hospital were 2.5% and 6-month postsurgery were 4%. The incidence of residual septal defects and the degree of left atrioventricular valve (mitral valve) regurgitation was independent of repair type, presence of Down's syndrome, and age of operation, although younger age of operation was associated with a longer hospital stay.[65]

## WHEN CHAMBERS AND VALVES ARE IN NORMAL SEQUENCE AND NORMAL POSITION AND STENOSIS OR OBSTRUCTION IS PREDOMINANT

### Introduction

In the following section, congenital anomalies will be discussed in which the chambers and valves of the heart are in normal sequence and position but stenosis or obstruction of the heart valves causing abnormal blood flow is predominant.

It is also possible that all the cardiac chambers and most valves are in normal sequence but some valves are not well-formed, leading to absent or abnormal valvular connections. When such valves are absent, the term atresia is also used, implying that no antegrade (or forward) flow is possible across the valve. Thus, atresia of any valve may occur. Valvular atresia on the right side prevents blood from reaching the lungs; valvular atresia on the left side prevents blood from reaching the systemic circulation. For any infant with valvular atresia to survive past the first few hours of life, a shunt lesion must be present to allow blood to progress antegrade through the heart. Not all obstructive lesions prevent the total forward flow of blood. Some, such as subvalvular aortic stenosis, causes partial obstruction of the blood flow. The degree of obstruction relates to the anatomic severity of the lesion.

This section will focus on *univentricular* heart, Blalock-Taussig shunt, the Glenn and the ultimate Fontan procedure, which is the definite operation for children with valvular obstruction or atresia on the right side of the heart. This section will also concentrate on valvular obstruction or atresia on the left side of the heart (mitral and aortic valve) and surgical treatment available for this group of children.

### Univentricular Heart

Children born with a functionally univentricular heart represent a group of cardiac anomalies almost always associated with a dominant ventricle either the left or right ventricle (Fig. 5.43). Thus, a univentricular heart may be best described as a defect in which the heart has two complete atria but only one functional ventricle, either the left or the right ventricle. Most common subtypes of functionally univentricular hearts are as follows:

1. The two atrioventricular valves (tricuspid and mitral valve) drain into a dominant pumping ventricle, which is either the left or right ventricle [e.g. Double inlet left ventricle (DILV) or double inlet right ventricle (DIRV)].

2. Absence or severe stenosis of either the tricuspid or the mitral valve almost, always associated with severe hypoplasia of the corresponding ventricle (e.g. tricuspid or mitral atresia, hypoplastic left heart syndrome, or pulmonary atresia with hypoplastic right ventricle).

3. Bilateral atrioventricular connection (tricuspid and mitral valve) with either marked hypoplasia of the right or left ventricle or abnormal atrioventricular connection (unbalanced atrioventricular septal defect) or abnormal ventriculoarterial connection (complex forms of transposition of the great arteries, and double outlet right ventricle).

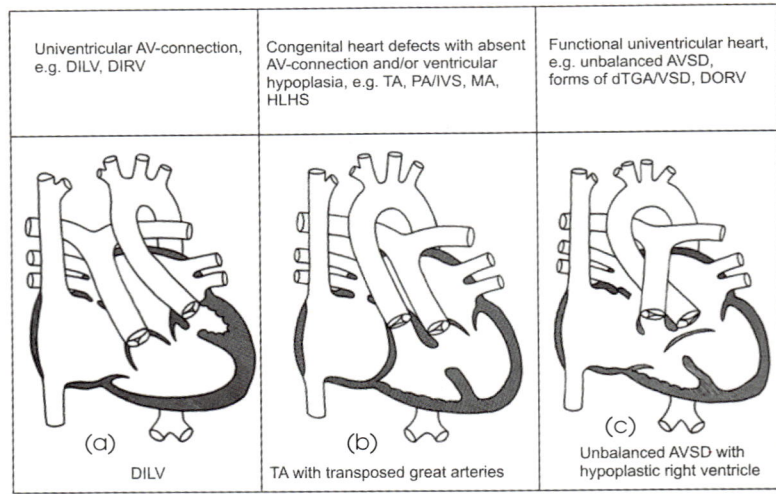

| Univentricular AV-connection, e.g. DILV, DIRV | Congenital heart defects with absent AV-connection and/or ventricular hypoplasia, e.g. TA, PA/IVS, MA, HLHS | Functional univentricular heart, e.g. unbalanced AVSD, forms of dTGA/VSD, DORV |
|---|---|---|
| (a) DILV | (b) TA with transposed great arteries | (c) Unbalanced AVSD with hypoplastic right ventricle |

**Fig. 5.43:** Functional univentricular hearts requiring palliation by Fontan-type procedures as functional correction. (DILV, double inlet left ventricle; DIRV, double inlet right ventricle; TA, tricuspid atresie; PA/IVS, pulmonary atresie with intact ventricular septum; MA, mitral atriesia; HLHS, hypoplastic left heart syndrome; AVSD, atrioventricular septal defect; TGA, transposition of the great arteries; DORV, double outlet right ventricle.) (*Note:* In Fig. 5.43a, the ventricles are reversed with the left ventricle to the right instead of the left.)

The majority of children born with a single functional ventricle or univentricular heart have to undergo various forms of surgical procedures to balance and optimise pulmonary and systemic blood flow. Initial palliations to increase pulmonary blood flow in the presence of severely reduced pulmonary blood flow include aortopulmonary shunt procedures (Blalock-Taussig) to avoid life-threatening cyanosis due to inadequate pulmonary blood flow. For children with systemic outflow obstruction or hypoplastic left heart syndrome the Damus-Kaye-Stansel anastomosis and Norwood type procedures will augment the systemic blood flow while pulmonary blood flow is controlled by an aortopulmonary shunt procedure or a right ventricular–pulmonary artery conduit.

In infants with functionally univentricular hearts who have no obstruction to pulmonary outflow, excessive pulmonary blood flow might develop as pulmonary resistance falls in the first few weeks of life. In this situation restriction of pulmonary blood flow can be achieved by surgical pulmonary artery banding to prevent *flooding* of the lungs and congestive heart failure.

### Blalock-Taussig Shunt, Glenn and Fontan Procedure

#### History

The surgical management for neonates born with cyanotic heart disease is to improve blood flow to the lungs. This can be accomplished by creating a connection between a systemic artery and the pulmonary artery. Helen Taussig (1898–1986), a paediatric cardiologist at the John Hopkins Hospital in Baltimore, USA, revolutionized the field of paediatric cardiac surgery, with her idea of creating a connection between a systemic artery and the pulmonary artery. She had noticed that children born with tetralogy of Fallot, with severe pulmonary stenosis, became severely cyanosed once the patent ductus arteriosus closed. Taussig approached Alfred Blalock (1899–1964), a paediatric cardiac surgeon at the John Hopkins Hospital and together with Vivien Thomas (1910–1985)—a laboratory technician, they decided to use the subclavian artery-to-pulmonary artery connection to improve blood flow to the lungs. Thomas experimented in the animal laboratory before Blalock performed the procedure on a 15-month old child with tetralogy of Fallot with severe cyanosis. Thomas was standing behind him on a platform and guiding him

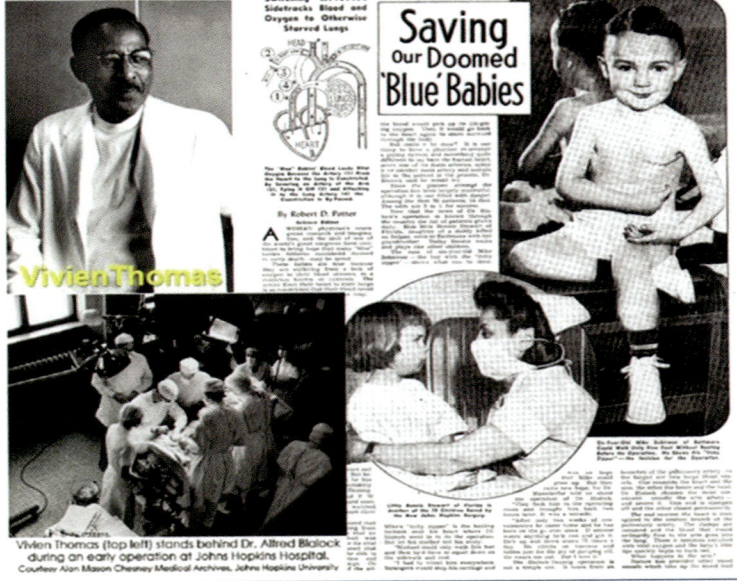

**Fig. 5.44:** Vivien T. Thomas experimented in the animal laboratory before Blalock performed the procedure on a 15-month-old child with severe cyanosis, with Thomas standing behind him on a platform and guiding him through the entire operation. Thomas was a key player in pioneering the anastomosis of the subclavian artery to the pulmonary artery. The surgical work he performed with Alfred Blalock paved the way for the successful outcome of the Blalock-Taussig shunt

through the entire operation (Fig. 5.44). The team published their results in a medical journal in 1945 to worldwide acclaim.[66]

Since its initial use in tetralogy of Fallot, many surgeons have modified the systemic-to-pulmonary shunt in terms of location of the shunt and material used. Other shunts which, proved less favourable are the in 1946, reported Potts shunt[67] (an anastomosis between the descending thoracic aorta and the left pulmonary artery) and the in 1962, reported Waterston/Cooley shunt (an aortopulmonary shunt between the posterior ascending aorta and the anterior right pulmonary artery, Fig. 5.46).

The Blalock-Taussig procedure is also used as an initial treatment for children born with other cyanotic cardiac anomalies associated with right-sided obstructed lesions, and children born

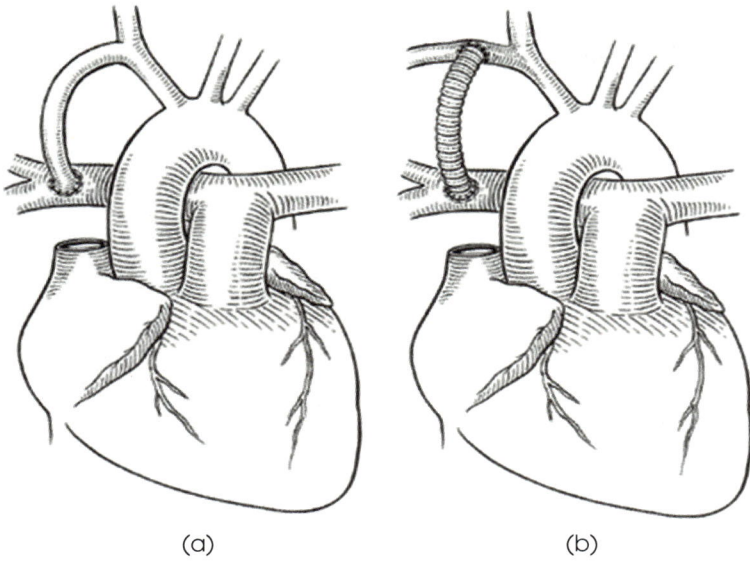

(a)  (b)

**Fig. 5.45:** Diagram (a) shows the classic BT-shunt in which the subclavian artery is divided and one end is anastomosed to the right pulmonary artery (PA). Diagram (b) shows the modified BT-shunt in which a Gore-tex™ graft is sewn between the subclavian and the right PA

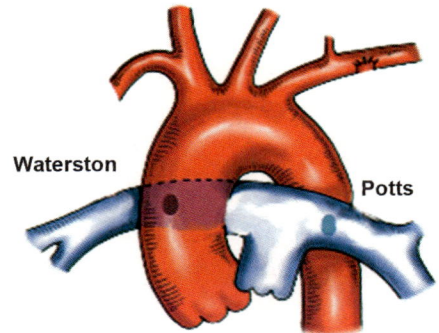

**Fig. 5.46:** Potts shunt—an anastomosis between the descending thoracic aorta and the left pulmonary artery and Waterston/Cooley shunt—an aortopulmonary shunt between the posterior ascending aorta and the anterior right pulmonary artery

with a single ventricle (tricuspid/pulmonary atresia, and hypo-plastic left heart). In some children an anastomosis is created between the aorta and the confluence of the pulmonary artery. This is referred to as a central shunt (Fig. 5.47).

### Blalock-Taussig Shunt Procedure—Overview

The Blalock-Taussig shunt (BTS) is a surgically created systemic-to-pulmonary artery shunt (aortopulmonary shunt). A systemic-to-pulmonary artery shunt increases pulmonary blood flow in children with cyanotic heart disease. The original operation involved joining the subclavian artery to the pulmonary artery. This is referred to as a classic Blalock-Taussig shunt. Nowadays, any systemic-to-pulmonary artery shunt, whether the connection is between the subclavian, innominate artery or other systemic artery to the pulmonary artery is referred to as a Blalock-Taussig shunt, or modified BT shunt (Fig. 5.45 and 5.48). This procedure diverts blood from an aortic branch to the pulmonary artery allowing blood to flow to the lungs to receive oxygen.

### Blalock-Taussig Shunt Procedure—Technique

The modified Blalock-Taussig shunt can be performed through a right or left thoracotomy or a median sternotomy. Most surgeons prefer the median sternotomy approach as this facilitates the use of cardiopulmonary bypass, if the infant suffers significant oxygen desaturation during the procedure and is believed a safer method than a thoracotomy.

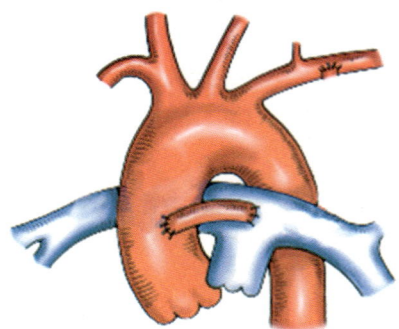

**Fig. 5.47:** An anastomosis between the aorta and the pulmonary artery confluence is referred to as a central shunt

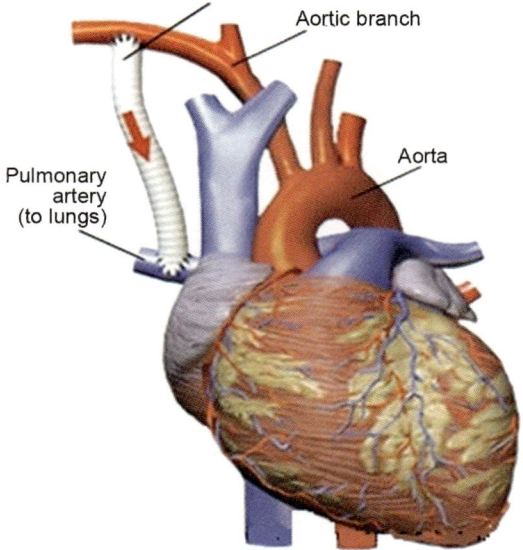

Aortic branch

Aorta

Pulmonary
artery
(to lungs)

**Fig. 5.48:** Modified Blalock-Taussig shunt—Nowadays, any systemic-to-pulmonary artery shunt, whether the connection is between the subclavian, innominate artery or other systemic artery to the pulmonary artery is referred to as a Blalock-Taussig shunt, or modified BT shunt

Cardiopulmonary bypass, if necessary, is usually with an aortic cannula and a single atrial cannula with the heart beating throughout the procedure with no active cooling of the infant.

1. The heart is accessed through a median sternotomy.
2. Mobilization of the aortic arch and head vessels is carried out and isolated with vessel loops. The left or right pulmonary artery is identified and isolated with a vessel loop. Usually, half a dose of heparin is given at this stage.
3. The systemic artery (either innominate or subclavian artery) and the left or right pulmonary artery are carefully clamped, an incision is made into the systemic artery and the graft sewn onto it with a non-absorbable polypropylene suture (Fig. 5.49).
4. Then the right or left pulmonary artery is clamped making sure that the child tolerates the clamping and does not desaturate severely. Incision is then made into the left or right

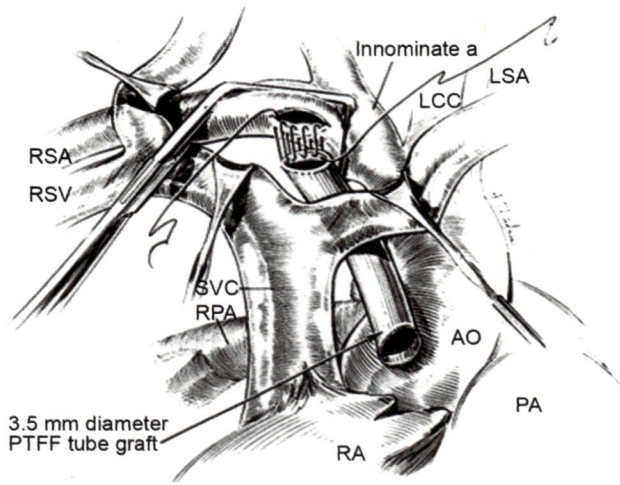

**Fig. 5.49:** Schematic diagram of right modified Blalock-Taussig shunt (RMBTS) via a sternotomy approach. RSA, right subclavian artery; RSV, right subclavian vein; SVC, superior vena cava; RPA, right pulmonary artery; RA, right atrium; PA, pulmonary artery; Ao, aorta; LCC, left common carotid artery; LSA, left subclavian artery; and Innom a., innominate artery

    pulmonary artery and other end of the graft sewn onto it with a non-absorbable polypropylene suture.

5. Vascular clamps are removed and any bleeding controlled with absorbable gelatine sponge (Gelfoam) or surgicel (Fig. 5.50).

---

**NURSING OBSERVATION**

*Most BTS surgeries are performed on a beating heart without the need for cardiopulmonary bypass. However, be prepared for going on bypass and have purse string sutures and cannulae in the room. Have a variety of shunt sizes available in the room and have knowledge of which suture material is used for the anastomoses. Some surgeons may use a finer blade such as, an ophthalmology knife or beaver blade to make the incision in the pulmonary artery and subclavian or innominate artery in very small infants. Also have a supply of haemostatic agents such as surgicel or gelfoam cut in small pieces to stop excess bleeding from the suture lines. For irrigation have small syringes with small cannulae available. Some surgeons may use heparinised saline rather than normal saline for irrigation.*

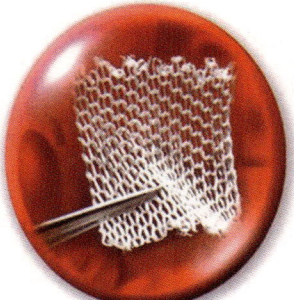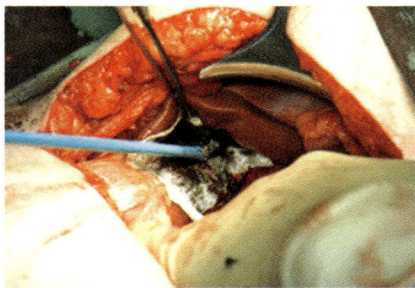

**Fig. 5.50:** Surgicel is a trademark for an absorbable knitted fabric prepared by controlled oxidation of cellulose. It is a haemostatic agent (blood-clot inducing material) used to control intraoperative haemorrhage when other conventional methods are impractical or ineffective

---

**SURGEON'S COMMENT**

*It is important that nurses are prepared for emergency conversion to cardiopulmonary bypass. The size of the shunt required should be enquired from the surgeon beforehand and its availability ensured. Appropriate types of fine vascular clamps in all sizes and shapes should be available, along with a supply of heparinized saline and fine cannulae for irrigation of the shunt.*

## Glenn Shunt Procedure—Overview

### *History*

The Glenn shunt procedure was initially performed in 1958 as a palliative procedure for tricuspid valve atresia by an American surgeon, William Glenn (1914–2003).[68] In the classic Glenn, the right pulmonary artery would be transected and ligated and the distal end would be anastomosed to the side of the superior vena cava (Fig. 5.51). When the child had a Fontan procedure, the inferior vena cava would be anastomosed to the left pulmonary artery. However, the classic Glenn would often complicate this due to necessary extensive reconstruction of the pulmonary artery (PA) at the time of the Fontan procedure. In 1966, a modification of the classic Glenn, in which the PA is not divided and the right PA is anastomosed to the superior vena cava (SVC), allowing blood to flow to the right and the left lung, hence, the term bi-directional, improved the outcome considerably.

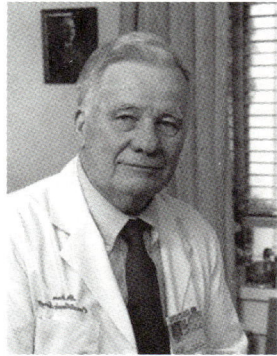 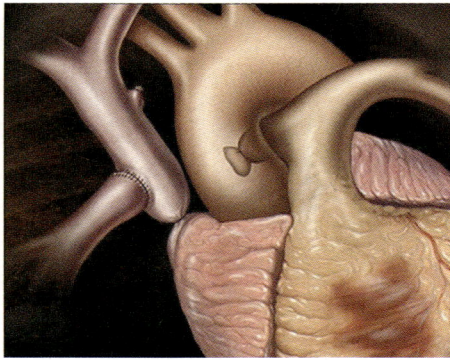

**Fig. 5.51:** Dr. William Glenn—1914–2003 who was the first to perform the classic shunt

In children with a persistent left SVC, a bilateral bi-directional Glenn shunt procedure is performed.

The Glenn shunt or bi-directional cavopulmonary shunt is usually carried out within the first four to six months of life to improve cyanosis and reduce the volume load on the single ventricle. It is a palliative procedure.

## Glenn Shunt Procedure—Technique

The concept of the Glenn procedure is to create an end-to-side anastomosis between the superior vena cava (SVC) and the pulmonary artery (Fig. 5.53 and 5.54). This will direct the venous blood return from the SVC directly to the lungs, bypassing the right ventricle and thus improving lung blood flow. The venous blood return from the inferior vena cava (IVC) will continue to flow through the right ventricle. The Glenn shunt is a low-pressure shunt as it bypasses the heart and loses out on the pump function of the heart to flow through the pulmonary artery and the lungs. Therefore, this procedure is usually performed when the pulmonary artery pressure and pulmonary vascular resistance is low, which is usually at four to twelve months of age.

The Glenn shunt procedure is normally carried out using cardio-pulmonary bypass (in some centres, the procedure may be performed without the use of cardiopulmonary bypass) and involves:

1. Aortic cannula in the ascending aorta and two venous cannulae in the innominate vein and in the right atrium.

2. All systemic-to-pulmonary artery shunts should be closed before the start of cardiopulmonary bypass to prevent blood from shunting from the systemic circulation to the pulmonary circulation and thereby compromising systemic flow (Figs 5.52 and 5.53).

3. Most commonly, vascular clamps are applied to the superior vena cava (SVC) above and below the level of transection of the SVC. The SVC is then transected and the stump or cardiac end oversewn with a continuous non-absorbable polypropylene suture (Fig. 5.53).

4. A side occlusion clamp is applied to the right pulmonary artery.

5. Then, an incision is made into the pulmonary artery and the proximal end of the SVC is anastomosed to the pulmonary artery, end-to-side anastomosis, with again a polypropylene non-absorbable suture (Figs 5.53–5.55).

6. Sometimes, when a child has a persistent left superior vena cava, a second similar anastomosis is carried out between left superior vena cava and the left pulmonary artery.

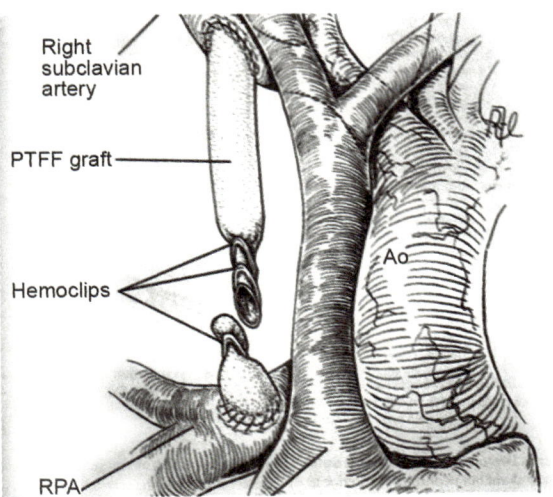

**Fig. 5.52:** Take down of BTS between the right subclavian artery and the right pulmonary artery (RPA). Some surgeons may excise all shunt material and use the same incision made in the RPA for the Glenn shunt anastomosis

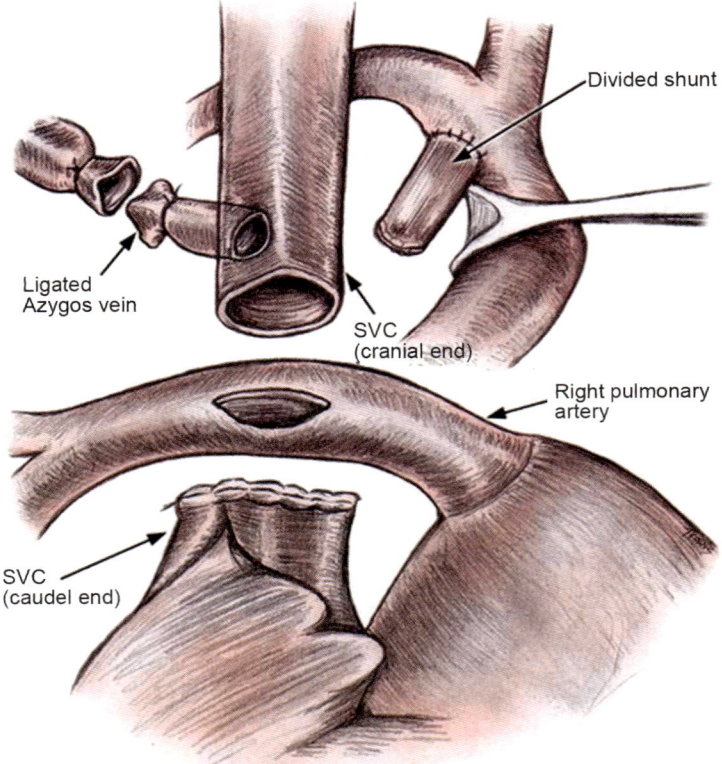

Ligated
Azygos vein

Divided shunt

SVC
(cranial end)

Right pulmonary
artery

SVC
(caudel end)

**Fig. 5.53:** The Blalock–Taussig shunt is closed, the superior vena cava (SVC) is transected and the cardiac or caudel end is oversewn

---

**NURSING OBSERVATION**

*Paediatric scrub nurses should find out if the child has had a previous Blalock-Taussig shunt (BTS), as some surgeons may prefer to excise all shunt material and use the previous incision made into the pulmonary artery for the SVC anastomosis. If the child had a previous BTS, through a median sternotomy approach, the child is prepared for redo sternotomy. In very small babies have a selection of fine vascular clamps, (e.g. titanium vascular clamps) available. For irrigation have small syringes with small cannulae available. Also have haemostatic agents such as surgicel available to stop any bleeding from anastomoses sites.*

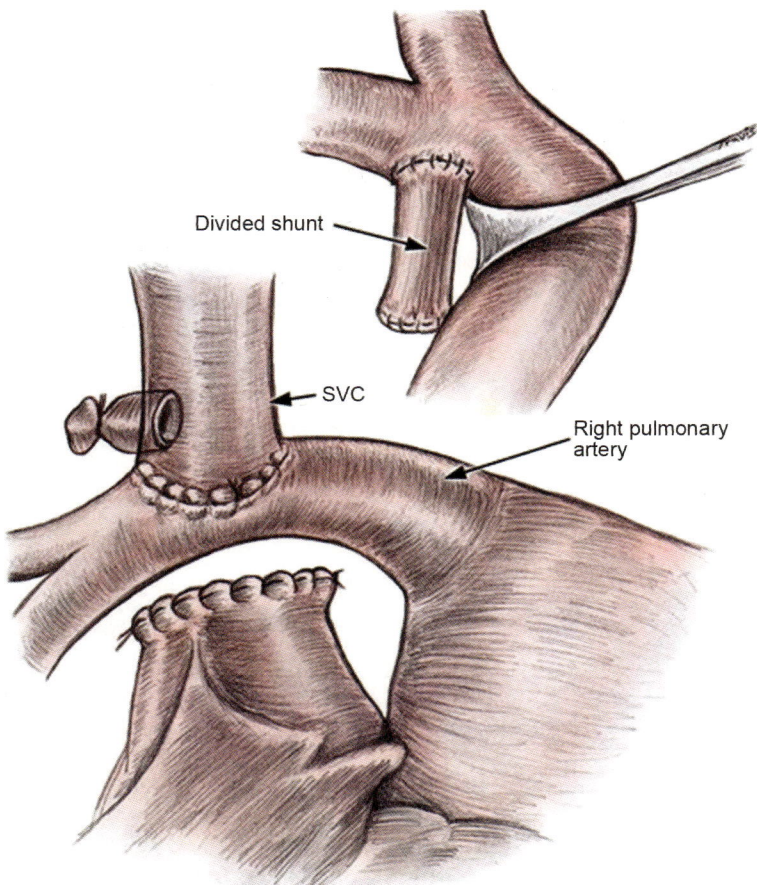

Divided shunt

SVC

Right pulmonary artery

**Fig. 5.54:** An incision is made into the pulmonary artery and the proximal end of the SVC anastomosed to the pulmonary artery-end-to-side anastomosis

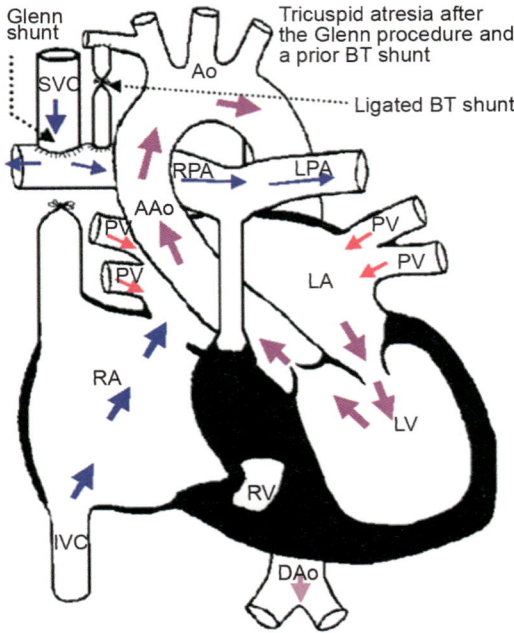

**Fig. 5.55:** Principle of the Glenn shunt procedure. The concept of the Glenn procedure is to create an end-to-side anastomosis between the superior vena cava (SVC) and the pulmonary artery

## Kawashima Procedure—Overview

### History

The Kawashima procedure is technically very similar to the bidirectional Glenn procedure (Fig. 5.56). This procedure was first performed in 1978 by a Japanese surgeon Kawashima, for children born with interrupted inferior vena cava and single ventricle physiology.[69] Interrupted inferior vena cava is a very rare congenital anomaly. It occurs in 0.6% of children with congenital heart defects. The hepatic and the prerenal segments of the inferior vena cava fail to fuse into a continuous channel. The prerenal segment of the interrupted inferior vena cava joins either the azygos vein and the right superior vena cava (azygos continuation of the inferior vena cava) or the hemiazygos vein and a persistent left superior vena cava draining into the coronary sinus (hemiazygos continuation of the inferior vena cava). Since the

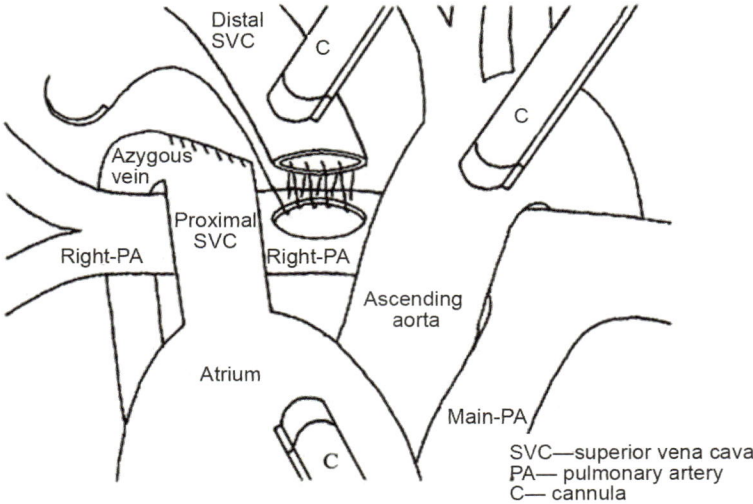

**Fig. 5.56:** The Kawashima procedure for interrupted IVC and single ventricle physiology

venous blood returns to the heart via the superior vena cava (azygos continuation of inferior vena cava to the superior vena cava), the Kawashima procedure is a final cavopulmonary anastomosis, although in some cases, a Fontan procedure may still be necessary.

## Fontan Procedure—Overview

### History

The Fontan procedure is named after Francois Fontan (1929–2018), a French cardiac surgeon, who in 1971 described this type of surgery on children with tricuspid atresia.[70] It created a separate systemic and pulmonary circulation without the right ventricle. Until then, medical opinion believed a pumping chamber was essential to move the blood through the lungs. The procedure was separately described by Guillermo Kreutzer (1934–), hence, the procedure is sometimes referred to as the Fontan/Kreutzer procedure.[71]

The Fontan procedure is to create a total cavopulmonary connection, by joining the inferior vena cava (IVC) to the pulmonary artery. This will direct the venous blood return from the IVC directly to the lungs, bypassing the right ventricle. Thus, in the Glenn procedure, venous blood return from the SVC flows directly to the lungs. In the Fontan procedure, also the venous blood return from the IVC flows directly to the lungs, thus resulting in a total venous blood return directly to the lungs, bypassing the right side of the heart completely. After the Fontan, blood must flow through the lungs without being pumped by the heart. For the same reasons as the Glenn procedure cannot be performed in the first four weeks of life, when the pulmonary artery pressure and pulmonary vascular resistance are still high, the Fontan procedure also cannot be performed in the first weeks of life. However, the age at which a Fontan procedure should be carried out remains controversial and depends on many factors.[72] The most common age at which a Fontan procedure is performed, is between two and four years of age.

Fontan connections can be achieved in a number of ways and since the first procedure it has undergone many modifications. The two most common and frequently used methods are the lateral atrial tunnel or lateral tunnel Fontan technique and the extracardiac conduit' Fontan. The lateral tunnel technique, involves placing a baffle, which is a created tunnel-like Gore-Tex™ patch (or other patch material), inside the right atrium sutured to the lateral wall of the right atrium from the IVC to the opening, or orifice of the SVC and to the undersurface of the right pulmonary artery. If required, a small hole or fenestration is punched into the baffle to offload potential pressure (Figs 5.57 and 5.58). The

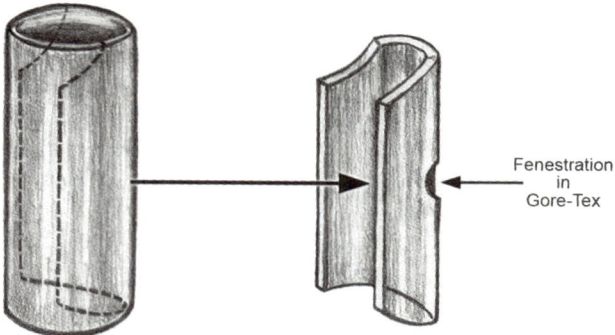

Fenestration
in
Gore-Tex

**Fig. 5.57:** Creating a tunnel-like Gore-Tex™ patch for the lateral tunnel Fontan technique

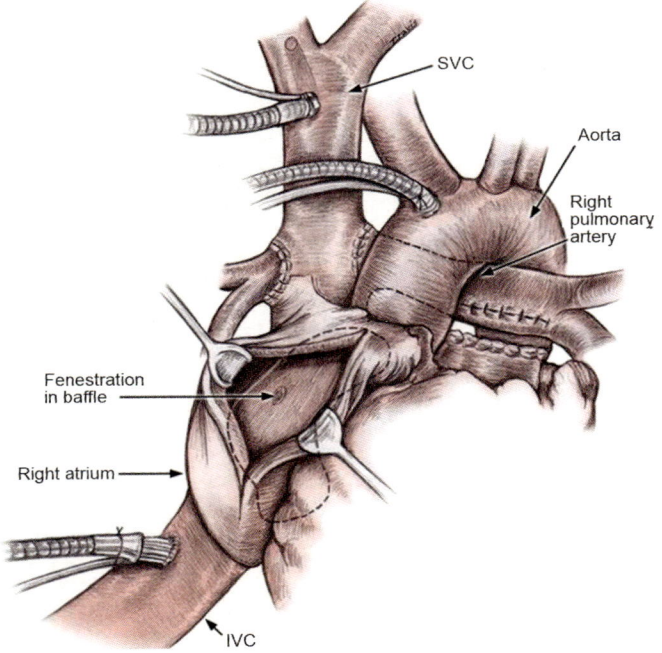

**Fig. 5.58:** Fenestrated lateral tunnel Fontan technique

lateral tunnel technique may be preferred by some surgeons in smaller infants since the remaining native atrial tissue can grow to accommodate increased systemic venous return over time when the child grows.

In the extracardiac conduit type of Fontan, one end of a synthetic tube graft is connected to the inferior vena cava and the other end to the pulmonary artery confluence. This technique has obvious size limitations since the graft cannot grow. Therefore, extracardiac Fontan operation is performed in older children in order to implant a conduit size that will be suitable into adult life (Fig. 5.59).

The extracardiac Fontan will be described in the following operative technique for Fontan procedure, since this technique is performed by the majority of cardiac surgeons.

## Extracardiac Fontan Procedure—Technique

The procedure is performed through a median sternotomy approach. If previous surgery (Blalock-Taussig shunt and Glenn

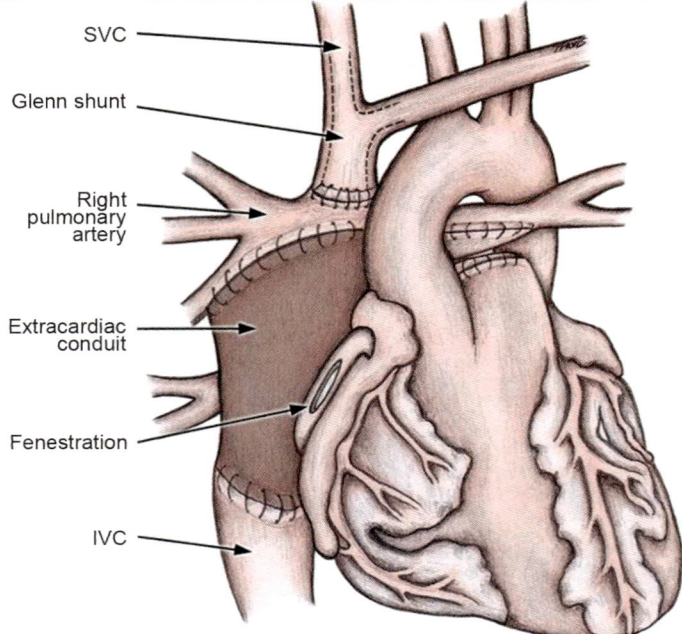

SVC

Glenn shunt

Right pulmonary artery

Extracardiac conduit

Fenestration

IVC

**Fig. 5.59:** The extracardiac Fontan technique. One end of a synthetic tube graft is connected to the inferior vena cava and the other end to the pulmonary artery (as seen in the picture) or the pulmonary confluence

procedure) was performed, this entails a re-sternotomy and external defibrillating pads must be placed on the child at the start of the procedure. The procedure is often performed using moderate hypothermia and continuous circulatory support. However, in some centres, may be performed with the use of deep hypothermic circulatory arrest. For the extracardiac conduit, different material is used, including Gore-Tex™ graft, bovine valved xenograft (Contegra®), valveless homograft or a pericardial tube.

1. A redo sternotomy and full inspection of the right heart, superior and inferior venae cavae, the previous Glenn anastomosis and the branch pulmonary arteries is carried out.
2. The child is heparinised and cannulated with an arterial cannula in the ascending aorta, and either the placement of a single venous cannula in the right atrial appendage, or venous cannulae in both the superior and inferior venae cavae.

3. Cardiopulmonary bypass is initiated and the child is cooled to target temperature.
4. The inferior vena cava (IVC) is transected from the right atrium, and right atrium is closed with a non-absorbable polypropylene suture (Fig. 5.60a).
5. One end of an extracardiac conduit is sutured to the IVC (Fig. 5.60b, c).
6. The IVC cannula is clamped next, which will fill the graft with blood. A vascular clamp is placed on the graft (Fig. 5.60d).
7. A small incision is made in the undersurface of the right pulmonary artery and the other end of the graft is sutured onto it (Fig. 5.60e). Alternatively, the surgeon may prefer to suture the distal end of the graft onto the pulmonary confluence.
8. Both clamps (IVC cannula and vascular clamp placed on the graft) are released and haemostasis is established (Fig. 5.60f)
9. The child is weaned-off cardiopulmonary bypass in the usual fashion.
10. Chest drains and pacing wires are placed according to surgeon's preference.
11. Sternum is closed in the standard fashion.

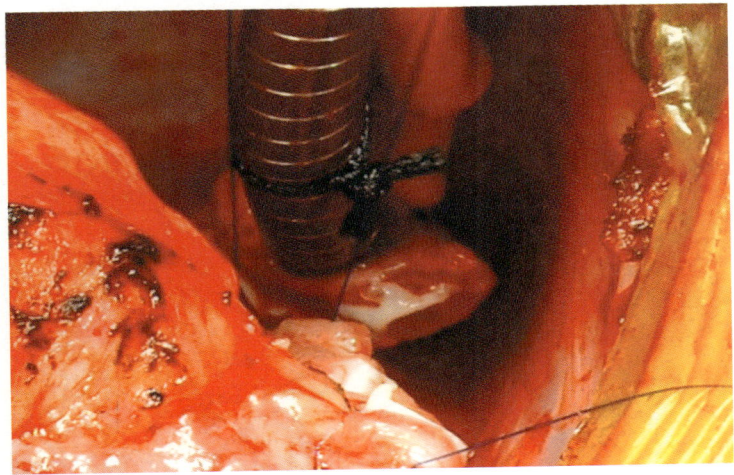

**Fig. 5.60a:** Surgical steps of the Fontan procedure. The inferior vena cava is transected from the right atrium. The defect in the right atrium is closed with a non-absorbable polypropylene suture. *(Photo by EDJ, courtesy of King Faisal Specialist Hospital, Riyadh, Saudi Arabia)*

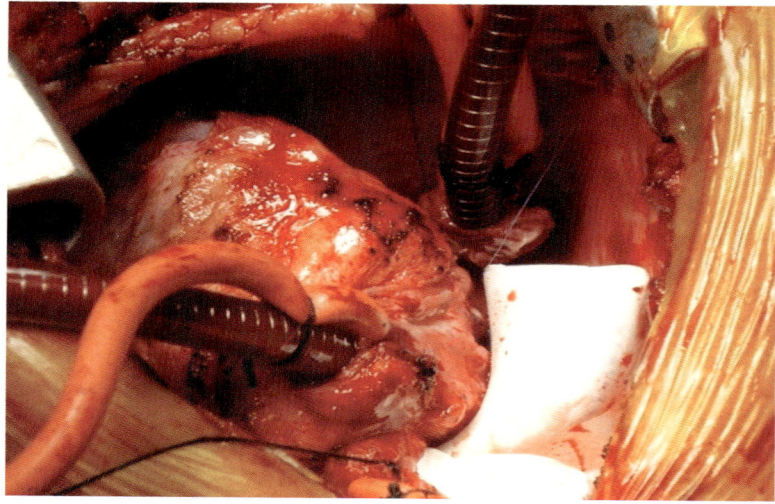

**Fig. 5.60b:** Surgical steps of the Fontan procedure. One end of a Gore-Tex™ graft is sutured onto the inferior vena cava. *(Photo by EDJ, courtesy of King Faisal Specialist Hospital, Riyadh, Saudi Arabia)*

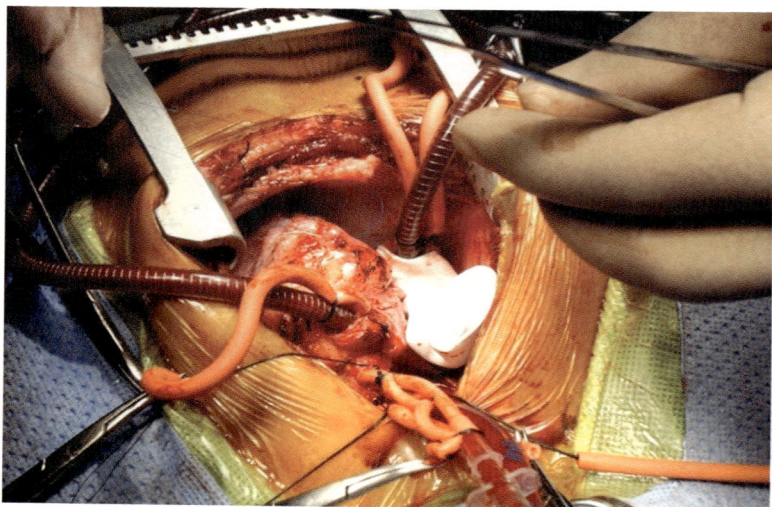

**Fig. 5.60c:** Surgical steps of the Fontan procedure. Finishing the distal anastomosis. *(Photo by EDJ, courtesy of King Faisal Specialist Hospital, Riyadh, Saudi Arabia)*

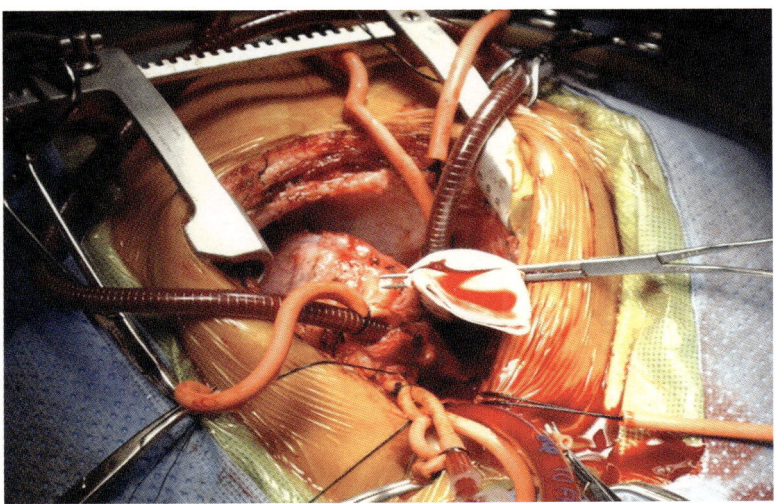

**Fig. 5.60d:** Surgical steps of the Fontan procedure. Clamp is placed on the IVC cannula (not seen) and a vascular clamp is placed on the graft. *(Photo by EDJ, courtesy of King Faisal Specialist Hospital, Riyadh, Saudi Arabia)*

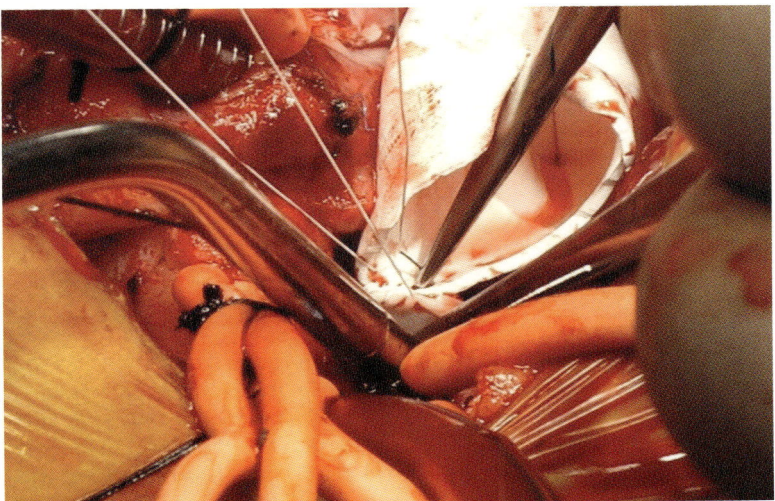

**Fig. 5.60e:** Surgical steps of the Fontan procedure. Other end of a Gore-Tex™ graft is sutured onto the pulmonary artery. *(Photo by EDJ, courtesy of King Faisal Specialist Hospital, Riyadh, Saudi Arabia)*

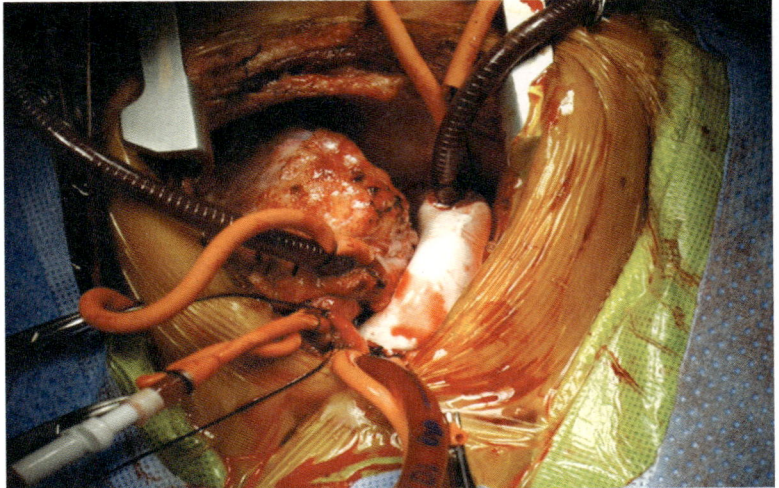

**Fig. 5.60f:** Surgical steps of the Fontan procedure. Both clamps (IVC cannula and vascular clamp placed on the graft) are released and haemostasis is established. *(Photo by EDJ, courtesy of King Faisal Specialist Hospital, Riyadh, Saudi Arabia)*

An alternative conduit is the use of a bovine valved xenograft, or Contegra®, for constructing the extracardiac Fontan connection (Figs 5.61 and 5.62). This alternative has first been reported as a successful experience by Ghassan Baslaim, a Saudi cardiac surgeon and colleagues at the King Faisal Specialist Hospital in Jeddah, Saudi Arabia in 2003.[73, 74] The advantages of using a Contegra® are easy availability, different size options, and the presence of a valve in the conduit.

---

**NURSING OBSERVATION**

*There are many variations on the Fontan procedure depending on the anatomy and age of the child and preference and expertise of individual surgeons. Plan and prepare in advance for the procedure and be familiar with the material (conduit, patch) used for the procedure and suture material used for the anastomosis. Have haemostatic agents available and a variety of fine vascular clamps. For irrigation and testing the anastomoses, have a variety of small syringes and cannulae available.*

*The Fontan procedure is performed on cardiopulmonary bypass with cardiac arrest using cardioplegia. Most of the dissection is performed before the bypass to reduce the time on bypass and cross clamp, thus improving the results of the Fontan operation. The nurses should be familiar with the conduit and the sutures used by the surgeon and ensure their availability. Fontan procedure is considered high-risk if the child's pulmonary artery pressures are higher than acceptable. In these cases, a fenestration is made between the conduit and the atrial cavity. Thus, an aortic punch may also be required. A left atrial line is also inserted at the end to monitor the left ventricular function after coming-off bypass and in the intensive care unit.*

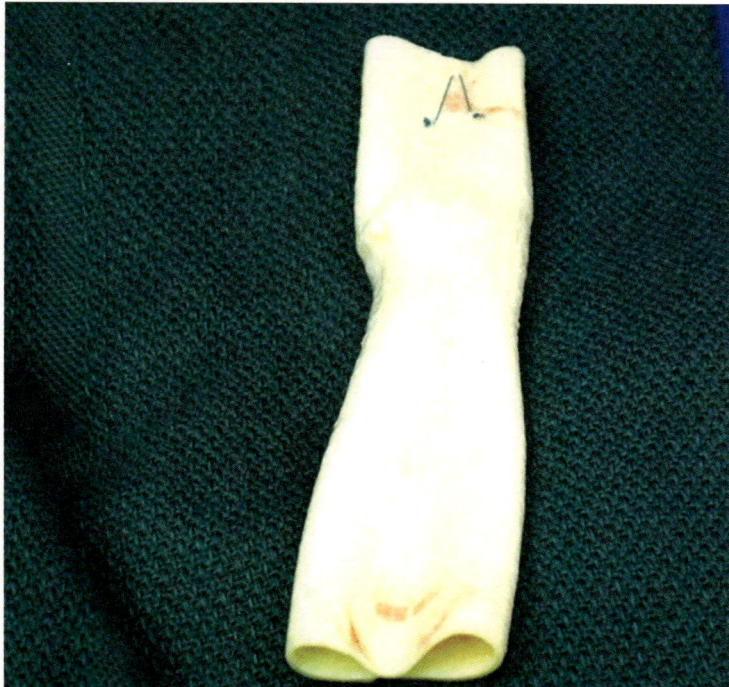

**Fig. 5.61:** An alternative extracardiac conduit is the use of a bovine valved xenograft (Contegra®). This is a bovine jugular vein with a trileaflet valve. It is preserved in glutaraldehyde solution and is available in sizes 12–22 mm. Note the arrow on the graft, which indicates the direction in which the valve opens. *(Photo by EDJ, courtesy of King Faisal Specialist Hospital, Jeddah, Saudi Arabia)*

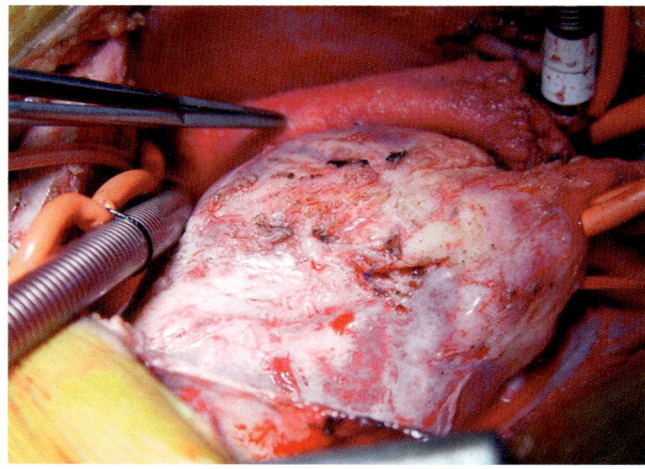

**Fig. 5.62:** Completed Fontan using a bovine valved xenograft (Contegra®). *(Photo by EDJ, courtesy of King Faisal Specialist Hospital, Jeddah, Saudi Arabia)*

## Outcome of Surgical Repair

Despite lower levels of physical health, quality of life of Fontan children is comparable with that of their healthy counterparts (Fig. 5.63).

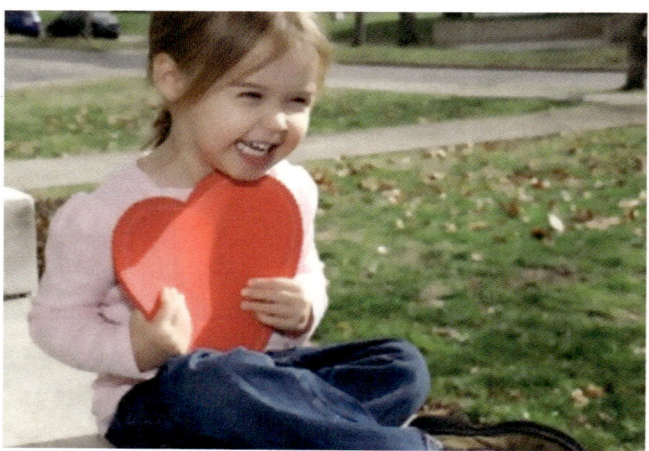

**Fig. 5.63:** A happy child after a Fontan operation

## REPAIR FOR UNIVENTRICULAR HEART IN SUMMARY

1. **Blalock-Taussig shunt:** The first operation creates a pathway for blood to reach the lungs. A connection is made usually between the aorta (right subclavian or innominate artery) and the right pulmonary artery. Some of the blood travelling through the aorta towards the body will shunt through this connection and flow into the pulmonary artery to receive oxygen. However, the child will still have some degree of cyanosis since oxygen-poor (blue) blood from the right atrium and oxygen-rich (red) blood from the left side of the heart mix and flow through the aorta to the body.

2. **Glenn shunt:** A second operation, often performed at about 4 to 12 months of age, replaces the Blalock-Taussig shunt with another connection to the pulmonary artery. In this operation, the Blalock-Taussig shunt is removed, and the superior vena cava is connected to the right pulmonary artery. Blood from the head and arms passively flows into the pulmonary artery and proceeds to the lungs to receive oxygen. However, oxygen-poor (blue) blood returning to the heart from the lower body through the inferior vena cava will still mix with oxygen-rich (red) blood in the left heart and travel to the body, so the child will remain mildly cyanotic. This operation helps to create some of the connections necessary for the final operation, the Fontan procedure.

3. **Fontan procedure:** This operation is often performed at about 18 to 36 months of age, and allows all the oxygen-poor (blue) blood returning to the heart to flow into the pulmonary artery, greatly improving the oxygenation of the blood. The Glenn shunt, connecting the superior vena cava to the right atrium, is left in place. A second connection is made directing blood from the inferior vena cava to the right pulmonary artery. This connection can be created in slightly different variations, depending on the method the surgeon prefers, and what is best for the child.

## TRICUSPID VALVE STENOSIS OR ATRESIA (OBSTRUCTED OR ABSENT ATRIOVENTRICULAR CONNECTION)

### Introduction

Tricuspid atresia is a congenital heart disease in which the tricuspid valve is missing or abnormally developed (Fig. 5.64). The defect blocks blood flow from the right atrium to the right ventricle and consequently blood flow to the lungs. If the tricuspid valve is completely absent, venous blood returning to the right atrium can only continue to flow if there is a communication between the right and left atrium, by either an atrial septal defect or patent

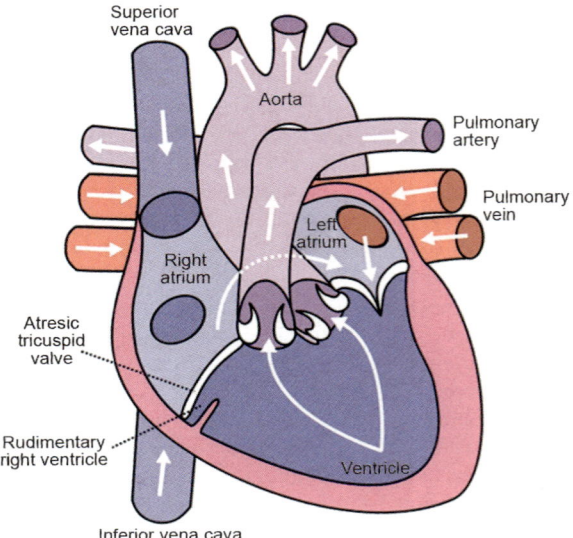

**Fig. 5.64:** Tricuspid atresia in tricuspid atresia, the right ventricle is often small (hypoplastic) or absent. This is known as univentricular heart, which means, an infant born with tricuspid atresia has only one single functional ventricle

foramen ovale. In order to sustain life, there has to be a patent ductus arteriosus that will take some of the blood back to the lungs, or a ventricular septal defect with a normal pulmonary valve to allow adequate blood flow to the lungs. Tricuspid atresia is often associated with other congenital heart diseases. Three types of tricuspid atresia are described in the literature, depending on the associated relationship of the great vessels. In type I, the great arteries are related normally; in type II, the great arteries are d-transposed; and in type III, the great arteries are l-transposed. The types are further subclassified according to the presence or absence of a ventricular septal defect and pulmonary valve pathology.[75,76]

## Prevalence

Tricuspid atresia is the third most common form of cyanotic congenital heart disease, with a prevalence of 0.3–3.7%.[77] The other two frequently observed cyanotic congenital cardiac anomalies are transposition of the great arteries and tetralogy of Fallot.

## Symptoms

Cyanosis is the most common clinical feature. The clinical features largely depend on the amount of pulmonary blood flow. The lower the pulmonary blood flow the earlier, the infant becomes cyanotic.

## Treatment

Depending on the degree of obstruction and associated cardiac anomalies, a baby born with this defect will not survive unless treated soon after birth. Common treatment for tricuspid atresia is multistage surgery to redirect blood to the lungs. This management frequently involves one or more palliative surgical interventions during the first few years of life (Blalock–Taussig shunt and Glenn shunt, see univentricular heart). These early interventions are necessary and will prepare the child for a *repair* based on the Fontan principle. The Fontan operation was first performed in children born with tricuspid atresia.

---

**NURSING OBSERVATION**

*Tricuspid atresia prevents blood from reaching the lungs and unless the tricuspid valve can be repaired these children will need at least three surgeries to bypass the right side of the heart. Extra attention should be given to these children and their parents as both may be more or less distressed depending on previous surgery and experience with hospital admissions and treatment.*

---

### *Outcome of Surgical Repair*

Infants will remain cyanotic after the first two operations until the final operation (Fontan procedure) is performed. Children will likely grow and develop more slowly than the average child because of the lower amounts of oxygen available for the body's needs. Following the Fontan procedure, when oxygen level improves, many children will see major improvements in growth, development, and can eventually catch up to normal children.

## EBSTEIN ANOMALY

### Introduction

Another variation of a normal developed tricuspid valve is Ebstein anomaly. In this condition the opening of the tricuspid valve is displaced towards the apex of the right ventricle (Figs 5.65 and 5.66).

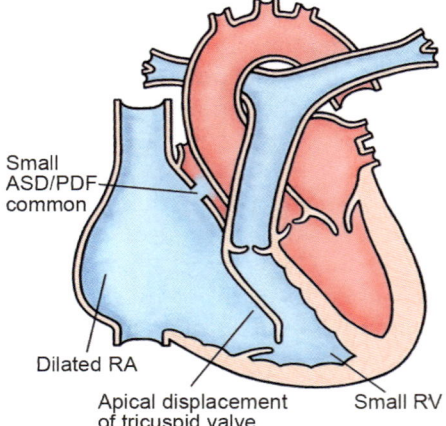

**Fig. 5.65:** Ebstein anomaly—in this condition, the opening of the tricuspid valve is displaced towards the apex of the right ventricle

The annulus of the valve is still in the normal position. The valve leaflets are to a varying degree, attached to the walls and septum of the right ventricle. Wilhelm Ebstein (1836–1912) first described a patient with cardiac defects typical of Ebstein anomaly in 1866 and the anomaly is named after him.[78] The leaflet anomaly leads to tricuspid regurgitation. The severity of regurgitation depends on the extent of leaflet displacement, ranging from mild regurgitation with minimally displaced tricuspid leaflets to severe regurgitation with extreme displacement.

## Prevalence

Ebstein anomaly probably accounts for 0.5% of cases of congenital heart diseases. True prevalence is unknown because mild forms are frequently undiagnosed.[79]

## Symptoms

This defect is characterized by remarkable morphologic variability and a broad spectrum of clinical presentations. Cyanosis is the most prominent symptom in neonates. Beyond the neonatal period, most children and adults present with dyspnea, fatigue, and some degree of cyanosis. Presenting symptoms are directly related to the severity of tricuspid valve incompetence, the presence or absence of an atrial septal defect, the degree of right

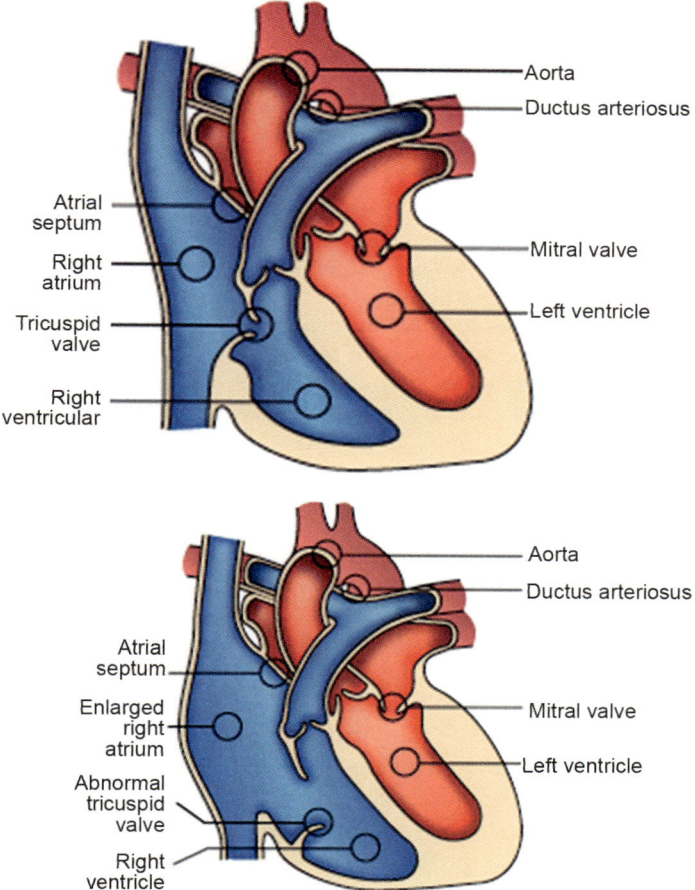

**Fig. 5.66:** The leaflets do not control the blood flow properly, resulting in a right ventricle that is too small, and a right atrium that is too large. There are varying degrees of severity of Ebstein's anomaly, and there is usually an atrial septal defect

and left ventricular dysfunctions, and the presence of arrhythmia and associated cardiac defects.

## Treatment

Early surgical attempts to treat Ebstein malformation using palliative shunts resulted in extremely high mortality rates. During the 1960s, most attempts to repair the tricuspid valve were unsuccessful, and prosthetic valve replacement became the preferred approach. Nowadays, surgeons will attempt to repair rather than replace the tricuspid valve. Overall, the treatment for Ebstein anomaly will depend on the severity of the lesion, and the expertise of the surgeon.[80]

---

**NURSING OBSERVATION**

*If the tricuspid valve cannot be repaired, a mechanical mitral valve can be used in the tricuspid position in small children. Note: There are no tricuspid prosthesis valves available on the market as in most cases the tricuspid valve is repaired rather than replaced. In bigger children and adults a tissue (mitral) valve is preferred as the blood flow through the tricuspid valve is slower due to lower pressures on the right side of the heart, making the mechanical valve more susceptible to the formation of clots.*

---

## PULMONARY VALVE STENOSIS OR ATRESIA (OBSTRUCTED OR ABSENT VENTRICULOARTERIAL CONNECTION)

### Introduction

Acquired pulmonary valve disease is very rare. Pulmonary valve disease is usually congenital. Pulmonary stenosis may be an isolated lesion or it may be associated with more complicated congenital anomalies. Tricuspid atresia in children is often associated with pulmonary stenosis. Pulmonary stenosis varies in severity from mild stenosis to complete outflow obstruction and atresia. Severe stenosis of the pulmonary valve in which the pulmonary valve is almost atretic, occurs typically in association with tetralogy of Fallot (Fig. 5.67). In true pulmonary atresia, both pulmonary arteries arise from the aorta (Fig. 5.68).

Pulmonary stenosis or atresia prevents blood flow to the lungs and results in cyanosis. The pulmonary blood flow is in most cases provided by the patent ductus arteriosus.

### Prevalence

The prevalence of isolated pulmonary stenosis has been estimated at 8 cases per 10,000 live births and this accounts for about 8% of all congenital heart disease. Tetralogy of Fallot with pulmonary atresia accounts for about 2% of congenital heart disease.[81]

## Symptoms

Symptoms of pulmonary stenosis/atresia are similar to that of tricuspid stenosis/atresia. Cyanosis is the most common clinical feature. The clinical features largely depend on the amount of pulmonary blood flow. The lower the pulmonary flow the earlier the infant becomes cyanotic.

## Treatment

Severity of the pulmonary valve stenosis determines surgical treatment. Stretching the valve with a balloon catheter, balloon

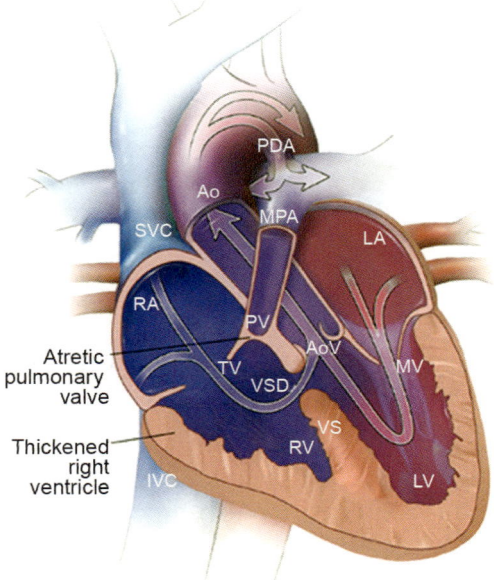

**Fig. 5.67:** Severe stenosis of the pulmonary valve in which the pulmonary valve is almost atretic, occurs typically in association with tetralogy of Fallot. RA, right atrium; RV, right ventricle; LA, left atrium; LV, left ventricle; TV, tricuspid valve; MV, mitral valve; AoV, aortic valve; PV, pulmonary valve; MPA, main pulmonary atery; Ao, aorta; SVC, superior vena cave; IVC, inferior vena cave; VS, ventricular septum; VSD, ventricular septal defect; PDA, patent ductus arteriosis

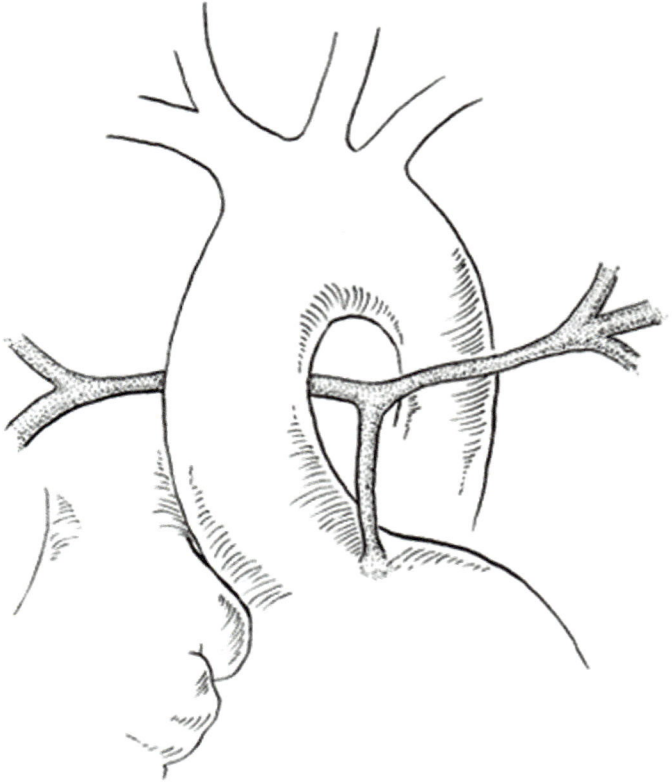

**Fig. 5.68:** In true pulmonary atresis, both pulmonary arteries arise from the aorta

valvuloplasty, may relief the symptoms (Figs 5.69 and 5.70). Usually, this produces effective long-term relief of the obstruction in isolated pulmonary valve stenosis. Some children who are unsuitable for this type of procedure, or in whom it is unsuccessful, may require surgery to correct the problem.

Surgery may include relief of right ventricular outflow tract obstruction and the placement of a transannular patch in isolated pulmonary valve stenosis (Fig. 5.71). If pulmonary valve stenosis is associated with other congenital anomalies, surgery is more complicated.

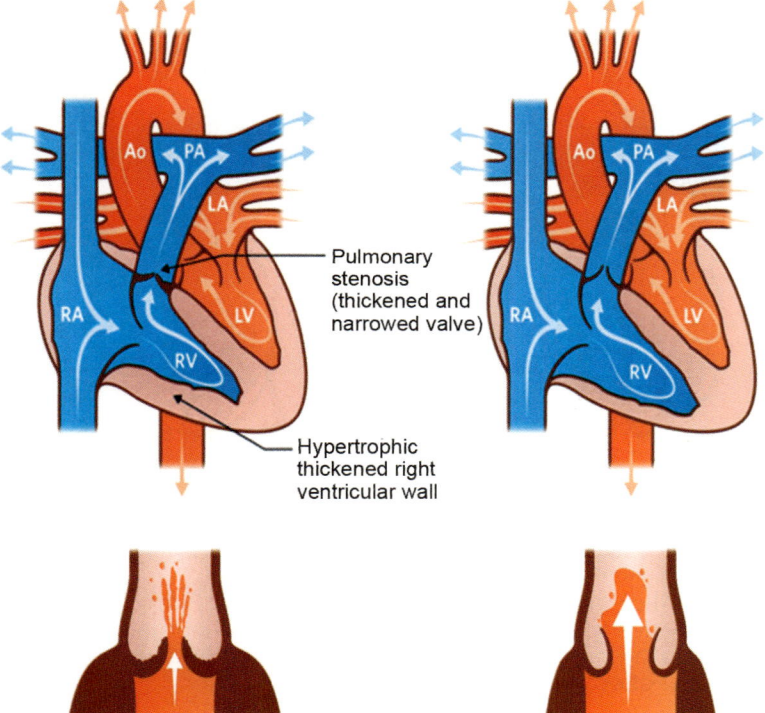

Pulmonary stenosis (thickened and narrowed valve)

Hypertrophic thickened right ventricular wall

**Fig. 5.69:** The pulmonary valve is thickened and narrowed leading to the development of abnormally high pressure in the right ventricle. The right ventricular wall becomes thickened (hypertrophied). If the problem is severe it may require treatment, which usually involves stretching the valve with a balloon catheter (balloon valvuloplasty)

---

**NURSING OBSERVATION**

*Babies born with pulmonary stenosis or atresia may present as an emergency for BT-Shunt surgery, depending on the severity of the stenosis. In isolated pulmonary stenosis, surgery would consist of the placement of a transannular patch (Fig. 5.71). Knowledge of the individual patient's anatomy presented for pulmonary stenosis repair will assist the scrub nurse in preparing for the surgery.*

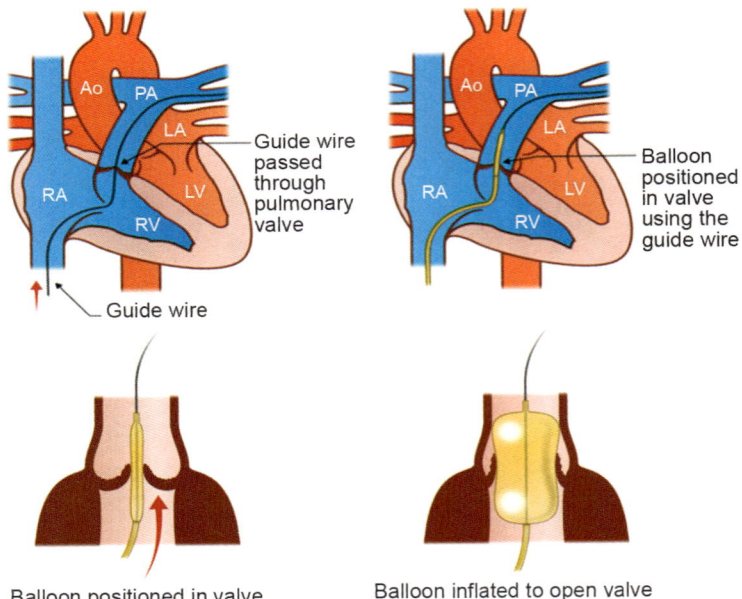

Balloon positioned in valve using a guide wire

Balloon inflated to open valve

**Fig. 5.70:** Balloon valvuloplasty—a heart catheter, with an inflatable balloon at the tip, is passed from a vein in the leg. When the tip is through the valve the balloon is inflated to stretch open the valve. Usually, this produces effective long-term relief of the obstruction

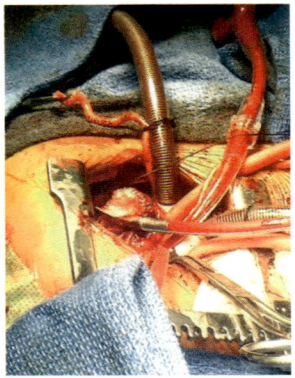

**Fig. 5.71:** Surgery may include relief of right ventricular outflow tract obstruction and the placement of a transannular patch (as shown in picture) in isolated pulmonary valve stenosis. *(Photo by EDJ, courtesy of KAMC, National Guard Hospital, Riyadh, Saudi Arabia)*

## PULMONARY STENOSIS/ATRESIA WITH A VENTRICULAR SEPTAL DEFECT

### Introduction

Pulmonary atresia with a ventricular septal defect (VSD) is associated with underdevelopment of the right ventricular outflow tract with atresia of the pulmonary valve, a large VSD, and overriding of the aorta. When a large patent ductus arteriosus (PDA) is present this lesion is managed as a severe form of tetralogy of Fallot (Fig. 5.73). When a PDA is absent or very small, pulmonary artery blood supply is provided partially or entirely by other connecting blood vessels between the aorta and the pulmonary arteries in the lungs. This is referred to as **major aortopulmonary collateral arteries or MAPCAs** (Fig. 5.72).

### Treatment

The surgical treatment for pulmonary stenosis or atresia with a VSD and MAPCAs is variable, and depends on individual anatomy and surgeon's preference. If the atresia only involves the pulmonary valve, the valve can be dilated with a balloon catheter (Fig. 5.70). Stents can be placed in stenosed aortopulmonary collateral arteries in infants with hypoplastic pulmonary arteries. Palliative systemic-to-pulmonary shunts such as the modified Blalock-Taussig shunt can be placed to promote growth of the pulmonary arteries and is connected from the subclavian or

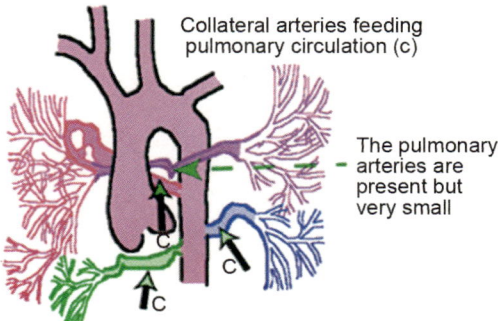

Collateral arteries feeding pulmonary circulation (c)

The pulmonary arteries are present but very small

**Fig. 5.72:** Major aortopulmonary collateral arteries (MAPCAs)—the pulmonary arteries are present but very small. The collateral vessels are usually several in number and carry blood (from the aorta) to different parts of the lung circulation

innominate artery to the pulmonary artery (when anatomy permits, Fig. 5.73). Alternatively, a direct right ventricle-to-pulmonary artery shunt may be preferred (Sano shunt) or in some cases valveless conduits or homografts may be used to connect the right ventricle (RV) to the pulmonary artery (Rastelli). This also may promote the growth of pulmonary arteries.

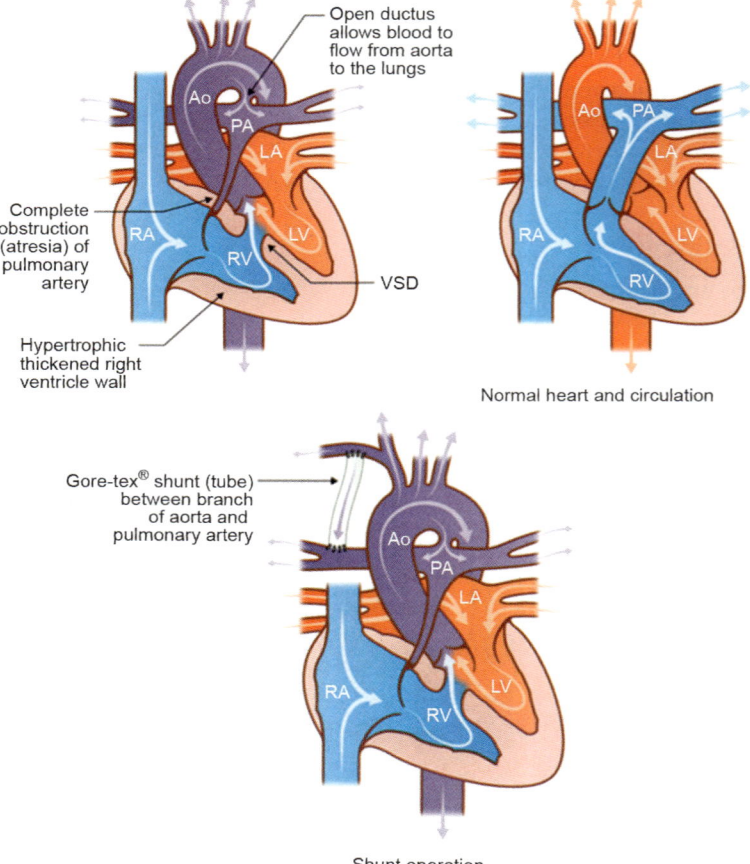

**Fig. 5.73:** When a large patent ductus arteriosus (PDA) is present, this lesion is managed as a severe form of tetralogy of Fallot. Most babies will need a shunt operation during the newborn period and complete repair is carried out at a later stage

The goal of complete repair is to create an unrestricted continuity between the RV outflow tract and the pulmonary arterial confluence using nonvalved or valved conduits (Fig. 5.74). Subsequently, all MAPCAs need to be joined to reconstruct main pulmonary arteries. This is referred to as **unifocalization**. At the time of complete repair the VSD is also closed.

When a PDA is absent or very small in children with pulmonary atresia with a VSD, pulmonary artery blood supply is provided partially or entirely by MAPCAs (Fig. 5.75). Corrective surgery is much more complicated and complexity of surgery depends on the number of collaterals (MAPCAs) and the size of the pulmonary arteries. Since the collateral circulation can be extremely complex and extremely variable, surgical correction is individualized to each child presenting with this complex anomaly.

The traditional approaches have been (1) staged unifocalization using sequential left and right thoracotomies followed ultimately by a median sternotomy with VSD closure and connection of the right ventricle to the reconstructed central pulmonary arteries (Rastelli) or (2) various surgical palliations (Blalock-Taussig shunt) to encourage growth of hypoplastic central pulmonary arteries (Fig. 5.76), followed by further unifocalization procedures, and finally intracardiac (VSD) repair. Thus, unifocalization consists of connecting as many collaterals as possible to the native pulmonary arteries. When the pulmonary arteries are hypoplastic,

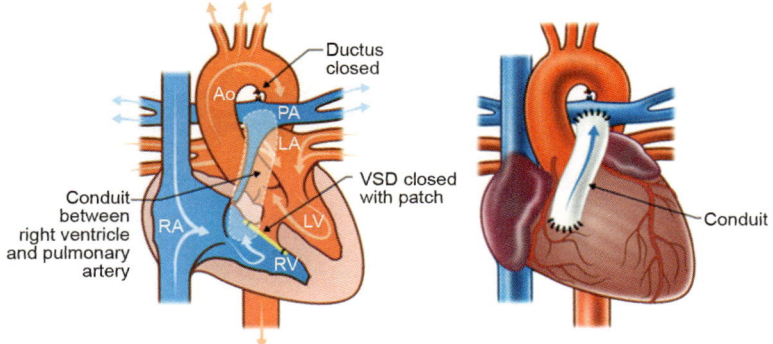

**Fig. 5.74:** Complete repair is usually postponed until the age of one to three years or sooner depending on surgeon's preference, and anatomy of the child. Repair usually, necessitates the use of a graft valve to replace the missing pulmonary valve (conduit)

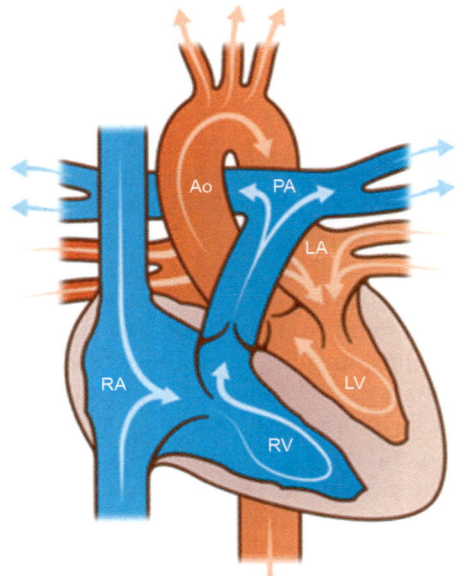

Normal heart and circulation

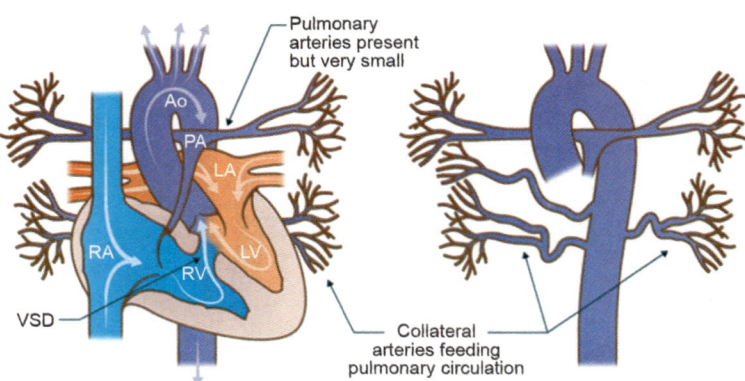

Pulmonary arteries present but very small

Collateral arteries feeding pulmonary circulation

VSD

**Fig. 5.75:** The collaterals are usually several in number and carry blood to different parts of the lung circulation. Surgery is often a matter of connecting up the multiple collaterals at different operations before performing a complete repair in suitable cases. The final repair usually involves insertion of a graft valve (conduit) to replace the absent pulmonary valve

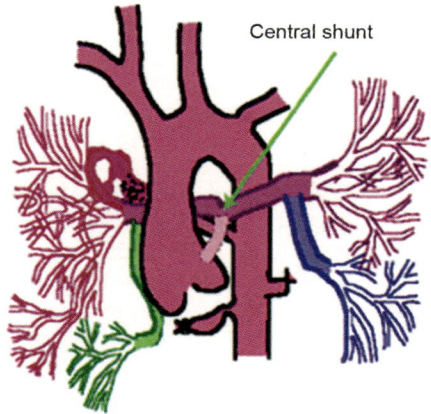

**Fig. 5.76:** Staged procedure—connecting collateral vessels, MAPCAs, to the left and right pulmonary artery with an additional central BT Shunt to allow growth of the main pulmonary artery

nonconfluent, and supplied by aortopulmonary collaterals, a multistaged repair is often required. This consists of a modified Blalock-Taussig or a central shunt to encourage enlargement and growth of these vessels so they can be successfully incorporated into the complete repair.

If the pulmonary arteries have grown after placement of the palliative shunts, unifocalization of the pulmonary arteries can be performed; this is done by incorporating the aortopulmonary collaterals and connecting them to a conduit from the right ventricle (Fig. 5.77).

---

**NURSING OBSERVATION**

*Unifocalization can be tedious for both surgeon and scrub nurse due to the complexity and extend of the surgery. The surgery is complicated and can be long and should preferably not be attempted by scrub nurses new to cardiac surgery. Since the collateral circulation can be extremely complex and extremely variable, surgical correction is individualized to each child presenting with this complex anomaly. How to prepare for this type of surgery acquires advanced experience and scrubbing skills. In most centres, few surgeons are specialized in this kind of surgery and the outcome will greatly depend on the expertise and experience of the surgeon.*

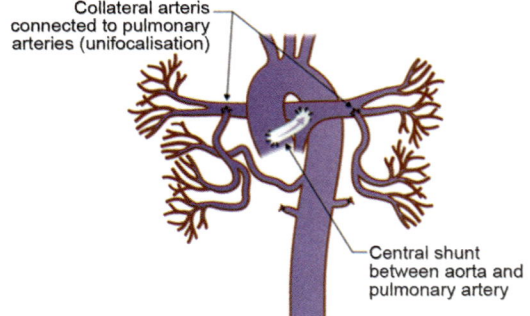

First stage of repair

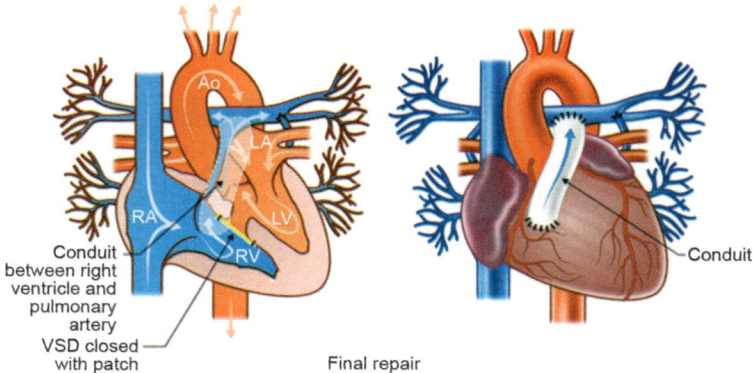

**Fig. 5.77:** Final procedure and complete repair—the VSD is closed and a conduit is placed between the right ventricle and the main pulmonary artery

## PULMONARY STENOSIS ATRESIA WITH INTACT VENTRICULAR SEPTAL DEFECT

### Introduction

As in pulmonary atresia with VSD, this defect is also associated with complete obstruction of the pulmonary artery. However, as

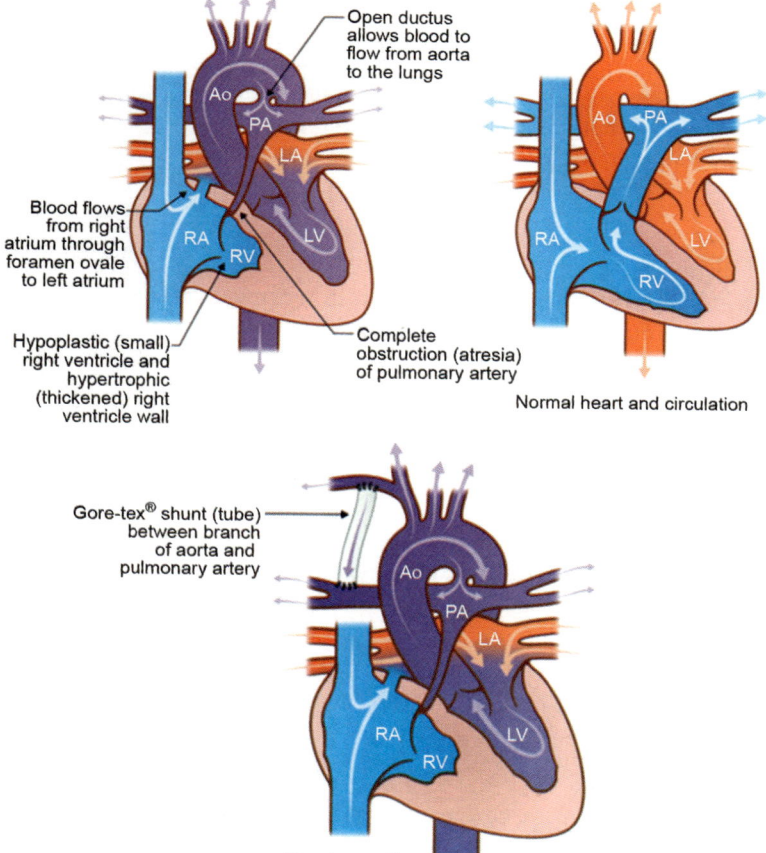

**Fig. 5.78:** Most babies will need a Blalock-Taussig shunt operation during infancy, involving insertion of a tiny piece of artificial tube (made from Gore-Tex)™ between the aorta, or a branch (usually, subclavian or innominate artery), and one of the branch pulmonary arteries (usually, the right pulmonary artery). Complete repair may be possible, but often necessitates several operations (Glenn and Fontan)

there is no associated VSD, blood is diverted from the right atrium to the left atrium via the foramen ovale. The right ventricle (RV) is usually small (hypoplastic), though its wall may be thickened (hypertrophied). Survival depends on the ductus arteriosus remaining open in the early days of life (in order for blood to reach the lungs).

---

**NURSING OBSERVATION**

*Babies born with pulmonary stenosis with intact ventricular septal defect may present as an emergency as soon as the ductus arteriosus closes, as the baby will not survive if no blood can reach the lungs. Therefore, the scrub nurse should be taught early during her training to be able to prepare and assist with cardiac surgery in a timely manner.*

### Treatment

Most babies will need a shunt operation during infancy (Blalock–Taussig shunt) (Fig. 5.78). Complete repair (Glenn and Fontan) may be possible, but often necessitates several operations.

## MITRAL VALVE STENOSIS OR ATRESIA (OBSTRUCTED OR ABSENT ATRIOVENTRICULAR CONNECTION)

### Introduction

Congenital mitral valve stenosis or atresia is rare. Mitral valve atresia is often associated with hypoplastic left heart syndrome and aortic valve atresia (*see* hypoplastic left heart syndrome).

## AORTIC VALVE STENOSIS OR ATRESIA AND SUBAORTIC MEMBRANE (OBSTRUCTED OR ABSENT VENTRICULOARTERIAL CONNECTION)

### Introduction

The most common cause of aortic stenosis in children is a congenital bicuspid valve, in which the aortic valve has two leaflets instead of the normal three leaflets (Fig. 5.79). Bicuspid valves are prone to the formation of calcium deposits and thus prone to aortic valve stenosis (Fig. 5.81). As this is a slow process, children born with a bicuspid aortic valve usually develop symptoms in their 40's and 50's. Younger children usually only have features of a leaking rather than a stenotic valve (Fig. 5.82).

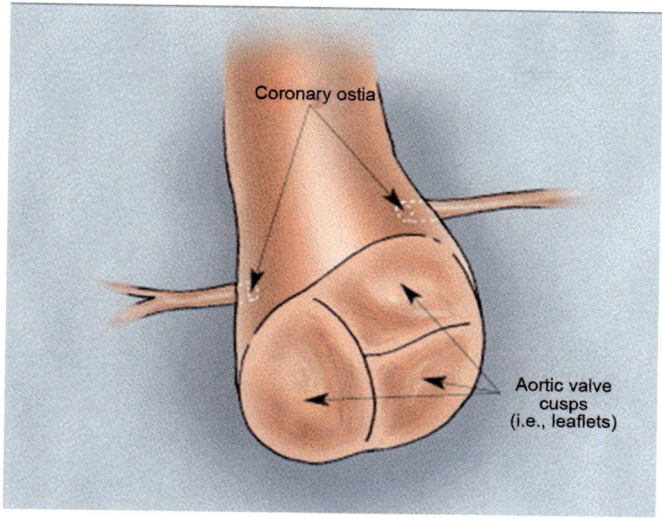

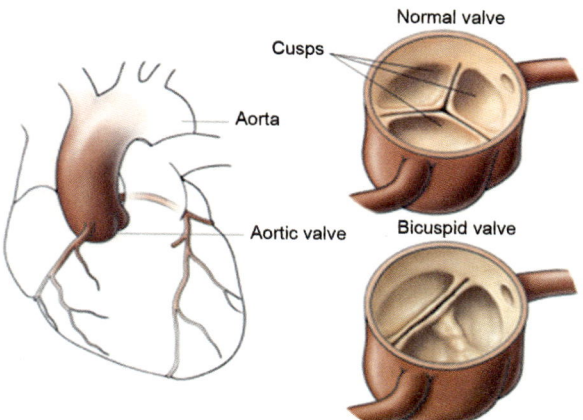

Fig. 5.79: Bicuspid aortic valve—the aortic valve has two leaflets instead of the normal three leaflets

### Treatment

Surgical treatment for bicuspid aortic valve in children is often repair (Fig. 5.80). Other non-surgical options are balloon valvuloplasty (Fig. 5.84), which is usually carried out in the catheterization laboratory. Repair can last a lifetime, but about 25% of patients will require a valve replacement within ten years.

In older children and adults, repair is performed less often and is technically more difficult than mitral valve repair. The option would then be to replace the aortic valve (Fig. 5.83).

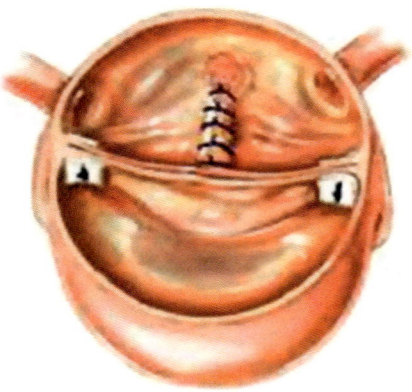

**Fig. 5.80:** Bicuspid aortic valve repair

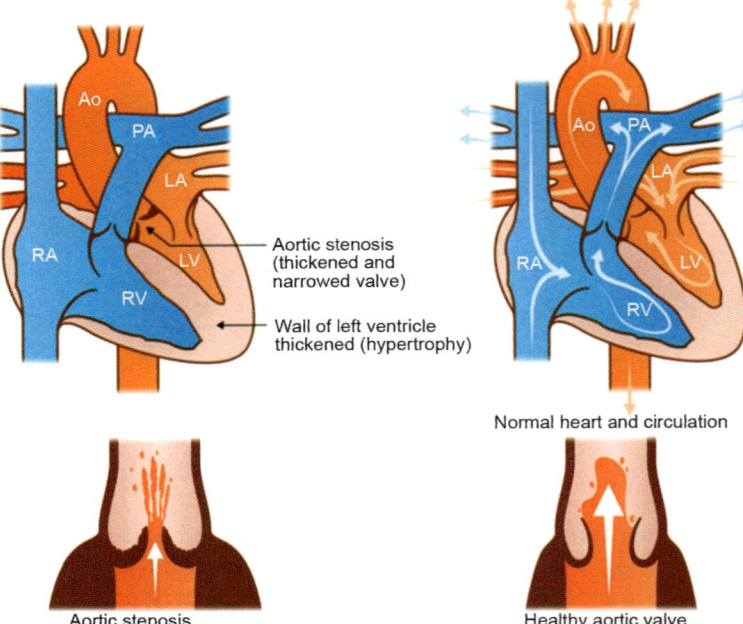

**Fig. 5.81:** Aortic valve stenosis—thickened and narrowed valve

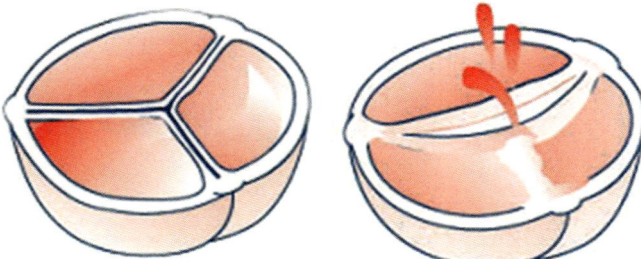

**Fig. 5.82:** Younger children usually only have features of a leaking rather than a stenotic valve

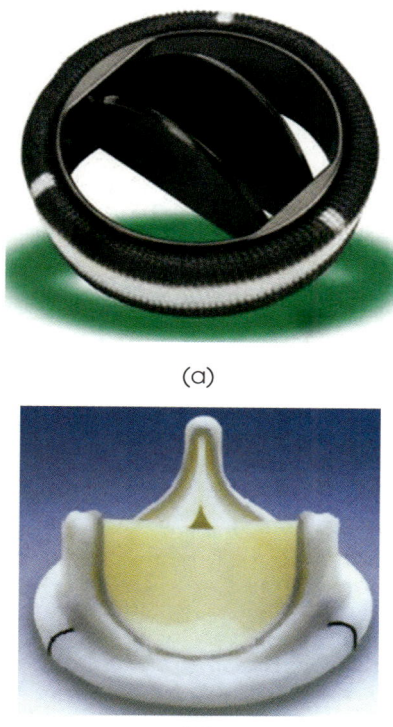

(a)

(b)

**Fig. 5.83:** In older children and adults, repair is performed less often and is technically more difficult than mitral valve repair. The option would then be to replace the aortic valve. Mechanical aortic valves are more often used in children (a). Tissue valves (b) or mechanical valves are used in adults

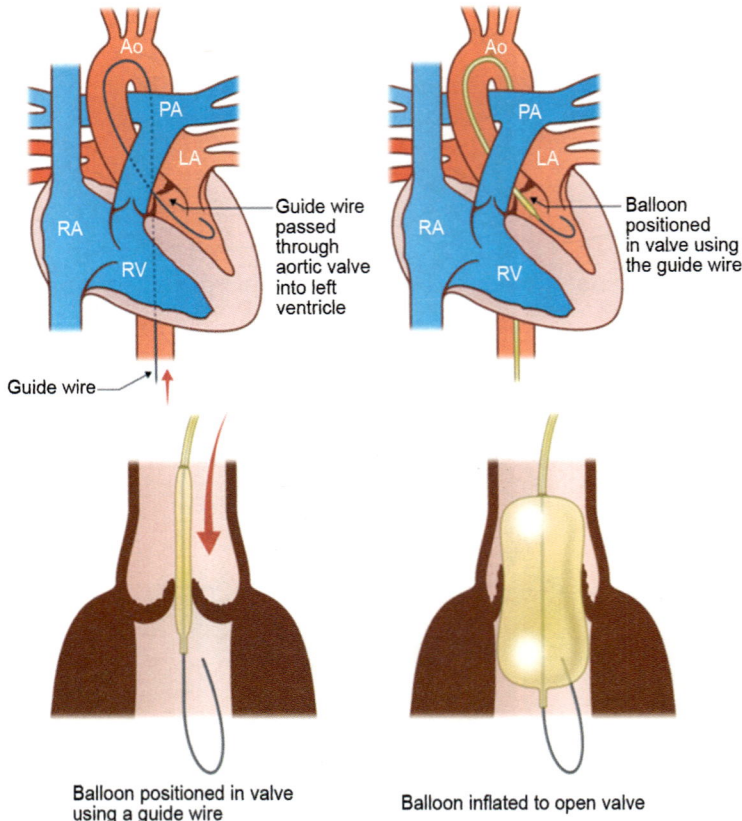

Guide wire passed through aortic valve into left ventricle

Guide wire

Balloon positioned in valve using the guide wire

Balloon positioned in valve using a guide wire

Balloon inflated to open valve

**Fig. 5.84:** The aortic valve is thickened and narrowed leading to the development of abnormally high pressure in the left ventricle. The left ventricular wall becomes thickened (hypertrophied). If the problem is severe it may require treatment, which usually involves surgery in younger children, though it may be possible to stretch the valve with a balloon catheter (balloon valvuloplasty), in older children. The catheter is passed through the femoral artery. When the tip is through the valve, the balloon is inflated to open the valve. Treatment does not completely cure the problem and the valve sometimes tends to develop further problems with time, sometimes needing reoperation or further balloon stretching. If the valve is severely abnormal a valve replacement may be required

## SUBAORTIC MEMBRANE (SAM)

### Introduction

Other congenital problems, such as malformation of the valve itself, or the formation of abnormal membranes or obstructive muscle above or below the aortic valve (subaortic membrane) may cause aortic valve stenosis (Figs 5.85 and 5.86). Because subaortic membrane interferes with the smooth flow of blood out of the left ventricle, referred to as left ventricular outflow tract obstruction, surgery is indicated to avoid elevated pressure in the left ventricle and overload. Although, subaortic membrane is classified as a congenital heart disease, it is rarely seen at birth. Its progressive course and its high rate of postoperative recurrence suggest that it may be an acquired condition.[82]

There are two kinds of subaortic stenosis.

1. **Discreet subaortic stenosis:** The more common form of subaortic stenosis occurs when the membrane made-up of fibrous tissue forms the obstruction underneath (sub-) the aortic valve.
2. **Tunnel subaortic stenosis:** Less common and more complex, occurs when the pathway between the ventricle and valve is narrow for the entire distance.

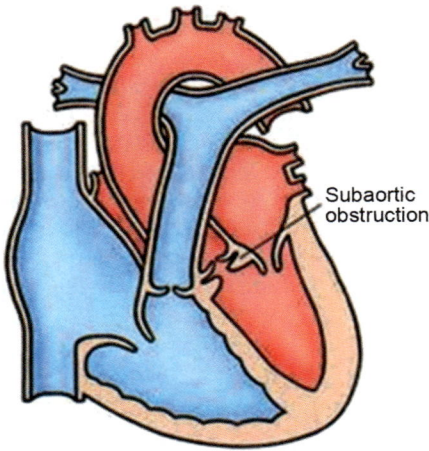

**Fig. 5.85:** The formation of abnormal membranes of obstructive muscle above or below the aortic valve (subaortic membrane) may cause aortic valve stenosis

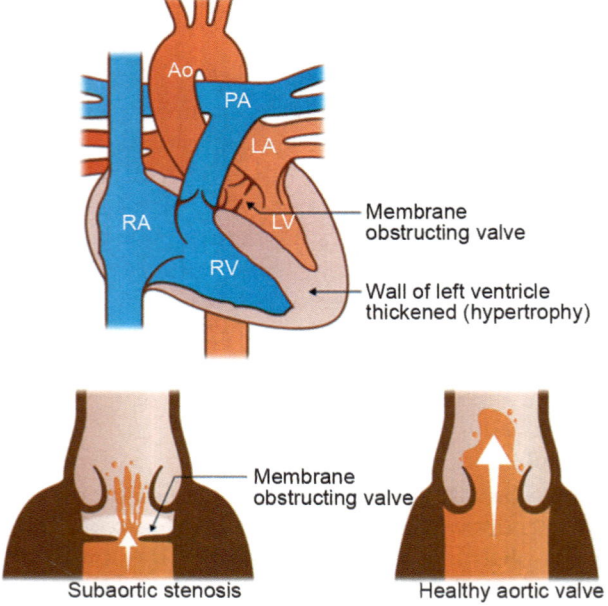

**Fig. 5.86:** Subaortic stenosis caused by subaortic membrane, which obstructs the valve

## Symptoms

Subaortic membrane causes aortic stenosis (left ventricular outflow tract obstruction) resulting in extra work for the left ventricle to pump blood through the obstruction. Turbulent blood flow created by the narrowing may damage the aortic valve, causing an otherwise normal valve to leak (aortic valve insufficiency or regurgitation).

## Treatment

Surgery involves open-heart surgery and is accomplished by carefully resecting the membrane (Fig. 5.87) and frequently may involve resection of septal muscle (myomectomy) to enlarge the left ventricular outflow tract and to reduce the likelihood of recurrence.

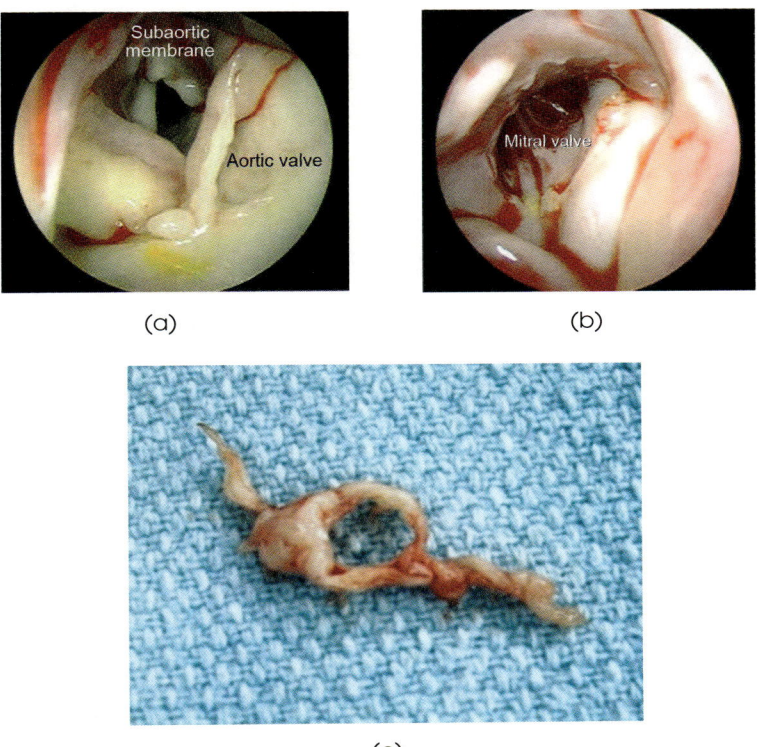

(a)                                    (b)

(c)

**Fig. 5.87:** Subaortic membrane (a), after resection (b) and resected membrane. *(Photo C by EDJ, courtesy of KAMC, National Guard Hospital, Riyadh, Saudi Arabia)*

## Subaortic Membrane Resection—Technique

1. The procedure is carried out on cardiopulmonary bypass with one venous cannula, cardioplegia, aortic cross clamping and a left atrial vent.
2. The subaortic membrane is approached by opening the aorta just above the aortic valve. The subaortic membrane can be seen through the valve.
3. Aortic stay sutures are used to carefully retract the aorta for exposure of the valve. A left atrial vent is placed to keep the operating field bloodless. Small vein retractors are placed to carefully retract the aortic valve leaflets.
4. Combination of sharp and blunt dissection is used to peel the membrane off the muscle all the way round the entire circumference of the subaortic region.
5. The child is weaned off cardiopulmonary bypass in the usual fashion. Chest drains and pacing wires are placed according to surgeon's preference. Sternum is closed in the standard fashion.

---

### NURSING OBSERVATION

*The operation is performed on cardiopulmonary bypass with mild hypothermia. One venous cannula usually provides optimal venous drainage. The scrub nurse should be familiar with the surgeon's preference to resect the membrane. The surgeon may use aorta stay sutures, which he may use to close the aorta after resection of the membrane. The scrub nurse should prepare various sizes of blunt spatulas for the membrane resection.*

---

### Outcome of Surgical Repair

Early postoperative complications such as complete heart block, as the area of conduction pathway is close to the aortic valve, may occur and is associated with too aggressive excision of the membrane and myomectomy.[83]

### Aortic Valve Replacement: Ross Procedure—Overview

Aortic valve replacement in infants and children is rarely performed. Indications for replacement in young children are hypoplasia of the aortic valve annulus in the neonate, progressive stenosis of the aortic valve in infants and children, left ventricular outflow tract obstruction, secondary to aortic valve stenosis that requires enlargement of the outflow tract, rheumatic aortic valve disease, and aortic valve disease caused by endocarditis.

Aortic valve replacement with a mechanical valve is not ideal in neonates and small children as there is no appropriate size of mechanical valve available on the market for this group of patients. Before long, replacement would be necessary as the child soon outgrows the valve. In addition, mechanical valves require life-long anticoagulants and due to potential poor compliance in children with anticoagulation protocols, would limit the child's activities such as playing sports due to higher risks for bleeding when injuries occur. For young girls difficulties with future pregnancy is often a deciding factor for not choosing a mechanical valve as a replacement for a diseased aortic valve.

Bioprosthetic and homograft valves are better options as they do not require anticoagulants. However, these prosthesis' also do not grow with the child and their durability in young children is very limited due to a higher incidence of progressive degeneration and early calcification. Also, the availability of appropriate sized bioprosthetic and homograft valves can be a problem.

If the aortic valve needs to be replaced, the best option appears to be the Ross procedure particularly, in young adults (Fig. 5.88). The Ross procedure was developed in 1967 by a South African born British surgeon, Donald Ross (1922–2014).[84] In this procedure, the diseased aortic valve is resected, and replaced with the native pulmonary valve. The pulmonary valve is then replaced with a pulmonary or aortic homograft. The main advantage of this procedure is that the child's own pulmonary valve is anatomically very similar to the aortic valve and performs better in the aortic

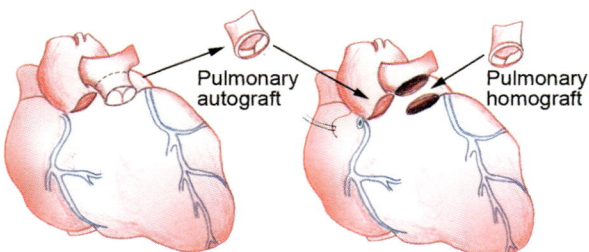

Pulmonary autograft

Pulmonary homograft

**Fig. 5.88:** The Ross procedure is a two-step procedure. First, the diseased aortic valve is replaced with the child's own pulmonary valve. Second, the pulmonic valve is replaced with a homograft

position than a replacement valve, that is, either a homograft, or prosthetic valve. The child's own pulmonary valve in the aortic valve position will grow as the child grows.

## Ross Procedure—Technique

1. The procedure is carried out on cardiopulmonary bypass with bicaval cannulation, cardioplegia, aortic cross-clamping and a left atrial vent.
2. Dissection is carried out around the aorta using forceps, diathermy and dissecting scissors to separate it from the pulmonary artery and then transected proximal (above) the ostia of the left and right coronary arteries (Fig. 5.89). The diseased aortic valve and proximal tissue is removed (Fig. 5.90), leaving the right and left coronary arteries with a button of tissue to allow for suturing to the pulmonary autograft later (Fig. 5.91).

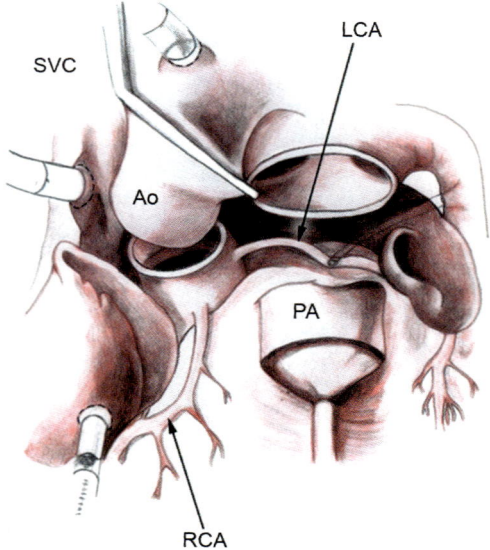

**Fig. 5.89:** The aorta is transected proximal (above) the ostia of the left and right coronary arteries. The pulmonary artery is transected near the bifurcation. SVC, superior vena cava; Ao, aorta; PA, pulmonary artery; LCA, left coronary artery; RCA, right coronary artery.

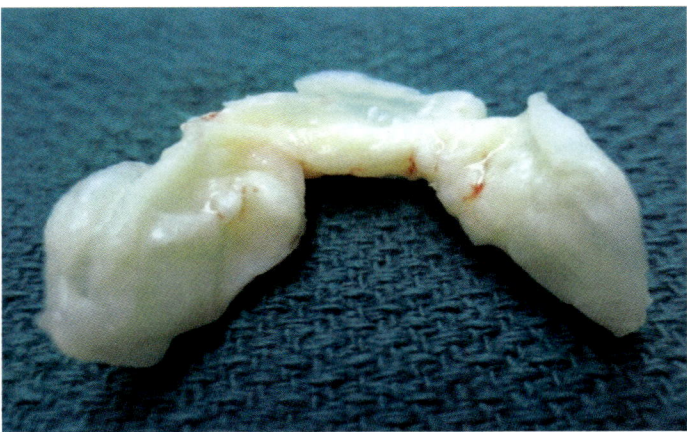

**Fig. 5.90:** The diseased aortic valve is removed

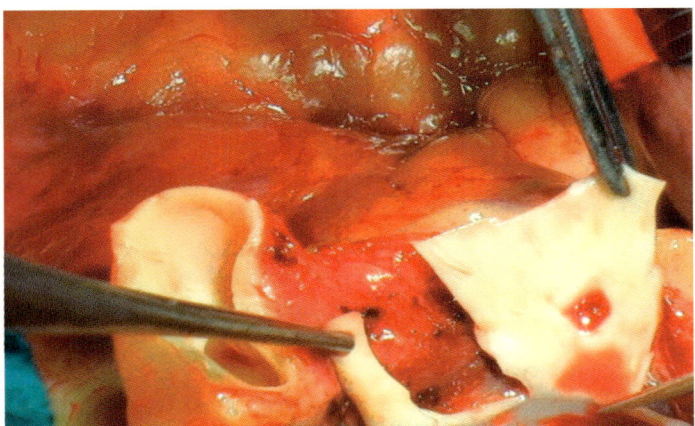

**Fig. 5.91:** The diseased aortic valve and proximal tissue is removed, leaving the right and left coronary arteries with a button of tissue to allow for suturing to the pulmonary autograft later. The right coronary button can be seen. *(Photo by EDJ, courtesy of KAMC, National Guard Hospital, Riyadh, Saudi Arabia)*

3. The pulmonary artery is transected near the bifurcation (Figs 5.89 and 5.92).
4. The pulmonary root is dissected including the pulmonary valve (Figs 5.92 and 5.93).

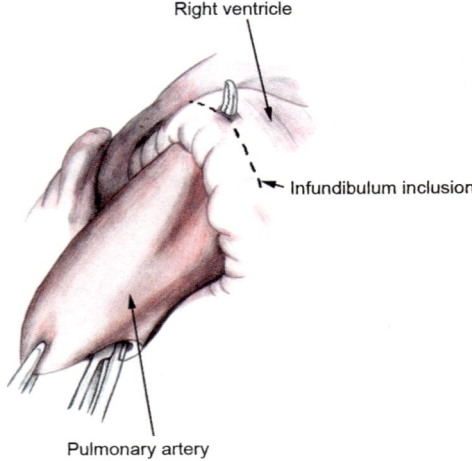

Right ventricle

Infundibulum inclusion

Pulmonary artery

**Fig. 5.92:** The pulmonary root is dissected including the pulmonary valve

5. The pulmonary autograft is then sized with standard sizers to select an appropriate size pulmonary homograft or aortic homograft depending on what is available.

6. The autograft is sutured to the aortic valve annulus using either a running or interrupted 4-0 polypropylene suture (Fig. 5.94).

7. A small opening is made in the autograft and the left coronary artery is anastomosed using a running 6-0 polypropylene suture. The distal aortic anastomosis is then constructed with a continuous 4-0 polypropylene suture.

8. The anastomosis of the right coronary artery is constructed in a similar fashion as the left coronary button. Antegrade cardioplegia can now be administered, and any bleeding from the suture line of the harvested autograft site can be checked.

9. A cryopreserved pulmonary or aortic homograft (Fig. 5.95) is then appropriately trimmed, and the distal anastomosis is performed using a continuous 4-0 polypropylene suture. The proximal anastomosis is constructed with a continuous 5-0 polypropylene suture (Fig. 5.96).

10. The patient is then placed in steep Trendelenburg position and the left ventricular vent is aspirated, the cross clamp can be removed. The remainder of the anterior portion of the

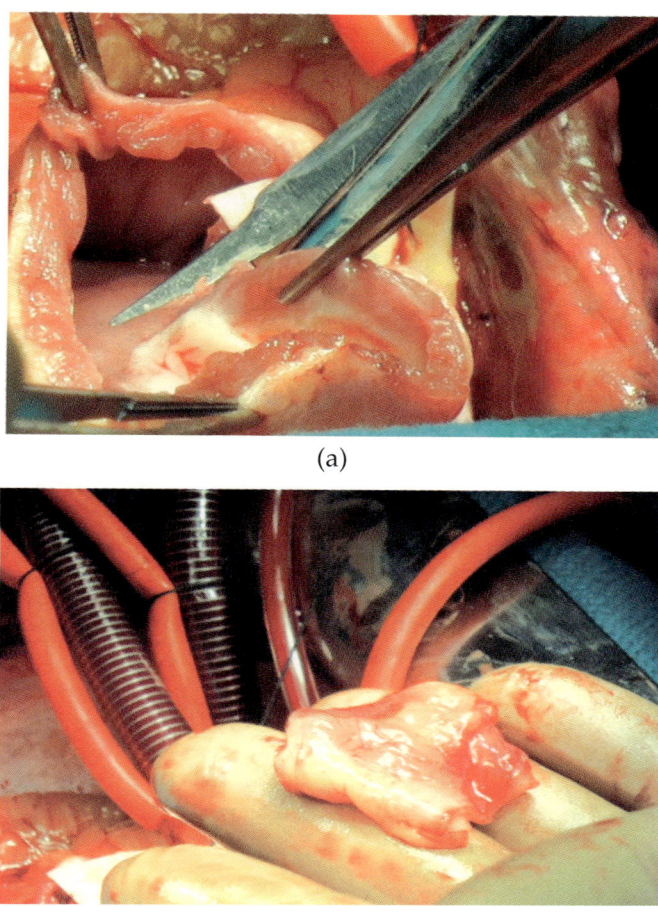

(a)

(b)

**Fig. 5.93:** The pulmonary valve and a segment of the pulmonary artery are excised (a, b). *(Photo (a), (b) by EDJ, courtesy of KAMC, National Guard Hospital, Riyadh, Saudi Arabia)*

homograft anastomosis can be completed with the heart beating (Figs 5.97 and 5.98).

11. The patient is then weaned from cardiopulmonary bypass; protamine is administered, and the patient is decannulated. Chest drains, pacing wires are inserted and chest is closed in a standard fashion.

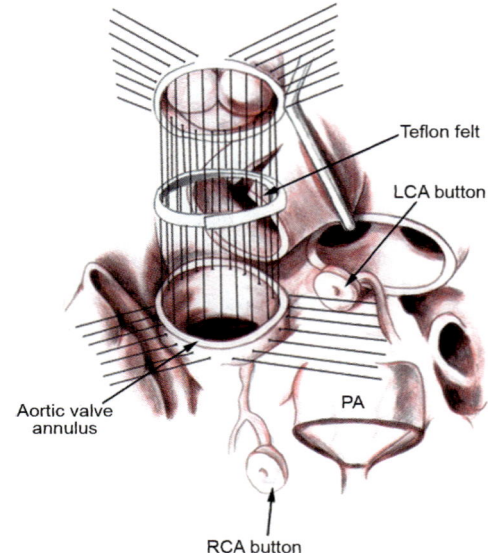

Teflon felt

LCA button

Aortic valve
annulus

PA

RCA button

**Fig. 5.94:** Placement of the pulmonary autograft into the aortic position with Teflon felt reinforcement. *Note:* The placement of a piece of teflon felt depends on the surgeon's preference

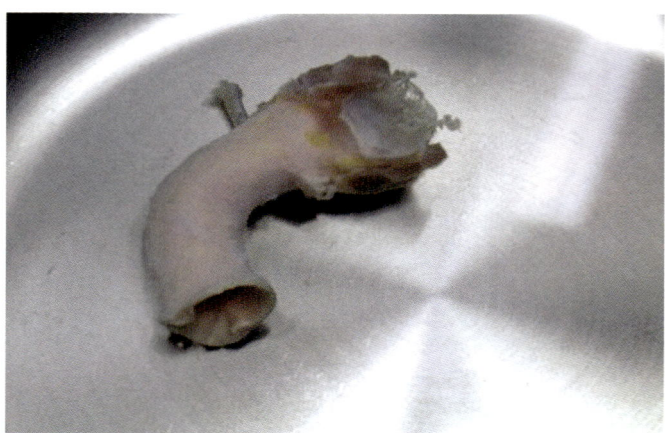

**Fig. 5.95:** Pulmonary homograft (picture shows aortic homograft; note the coronary arteries) is used for replacement of the native pulmonary valve. *(Photo by EDJ, courtesy of King Faisal Specialist Hospital, Jeddah, Saudi Arabia)*

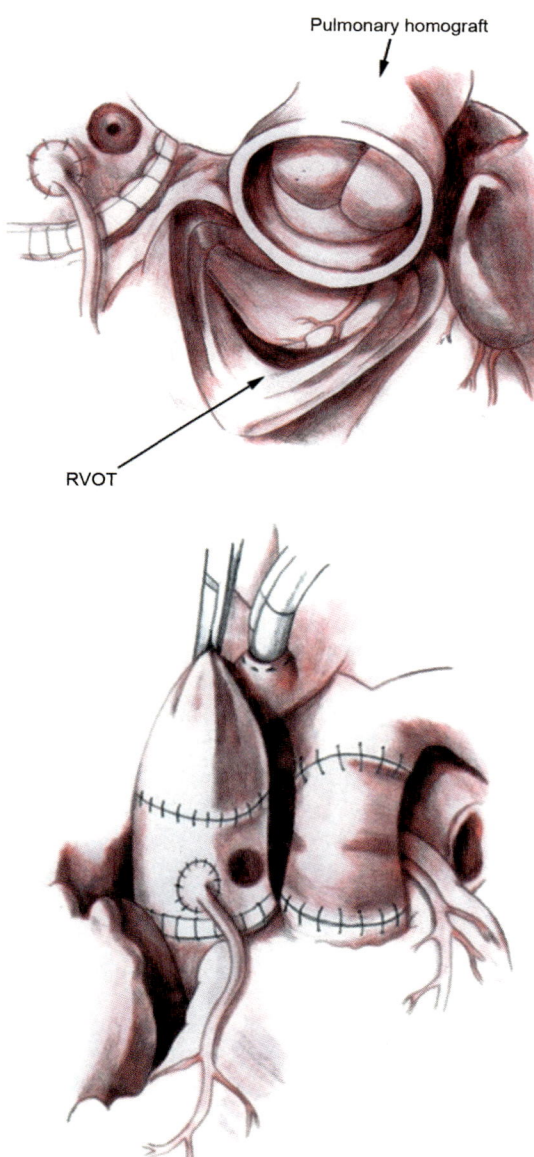

**Fig. 5.96:** Placement of the pulmonary homograft into the pulmonary position. RVOT—right ventricular outflow tract

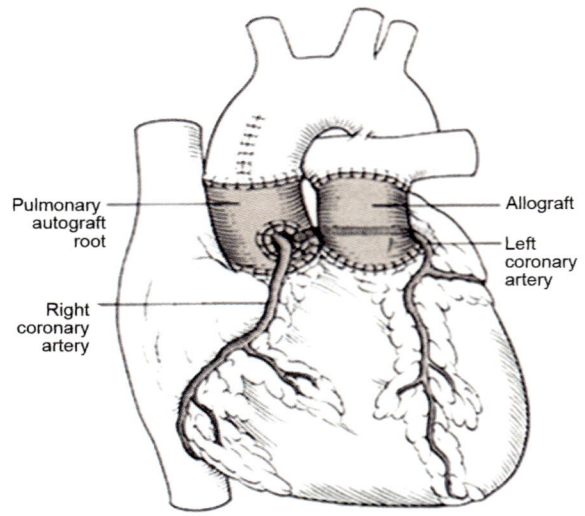

Pulmonary autograft root

Right coronary artery

Allograft

Left coronary artery

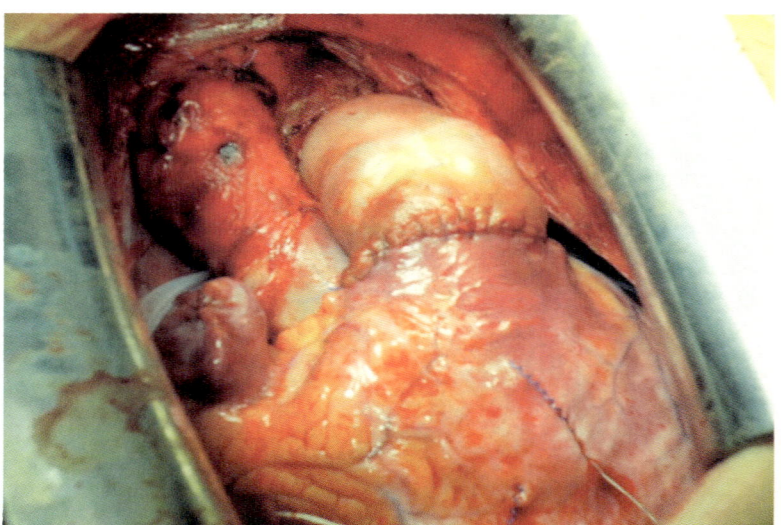

**Fig. 5.97:** Completed Ross procedure. Right ventricle can be seen with the pulmonary homograft (allograft); note the suture line. *(Photo by EDJ, courtesy of KAMC, National Guard Hospital, Riyadh, Saudi Arabia)*

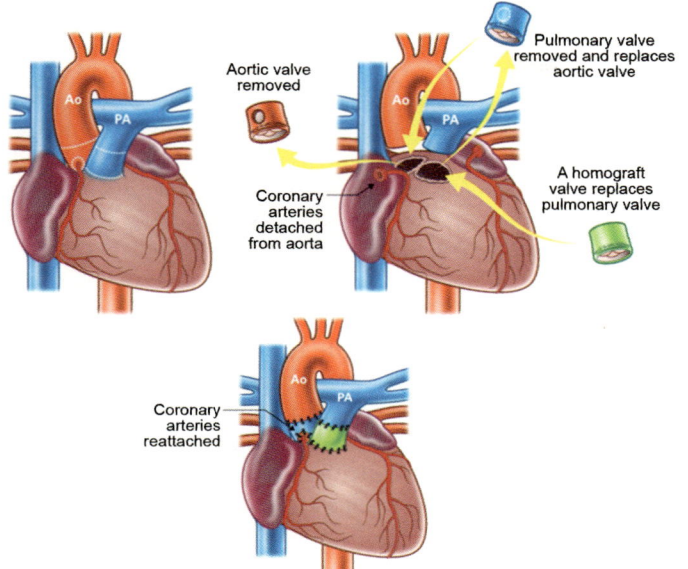

**Fig. 5.98:** The healthy pulmonary valve is removed and sewn into the position of the damaged aortic valve. The pulmonary valve itself is then replaced with a homograft valve. The advantage of this operation is that the new aortic valve will grow with the child and the homograft valve, which can be large enough to allow for growth, is not subjected to high pressure and can last much longer in the position of the low pressure pulmonary valve—though it is likely that it will eventually need to be replaced at a further operation.

---

### NURSING OBSERVATION

*The Ross procedure is technically demanding and the surgeon's experience with this operation affects the decision as well as the suitability of the patient. Have homograft/valve sizes and homograft folder on hand in the room for selecting the appropriate size and to check availability of homografts. Often an extra scrub nurse is needed to prepare the homograft. Be familiar with the guidelines and thawing process of homografts. Have sufficient supply of polypropylene sutures for the anastomoses, stay sutures, etc. In some cases, the aorta annulus may be too small to fit the pulmonary autograft. If the aortic root annulus is too small, then an aortoventriculoplasty combined with the Ross procedure (commonly known as a Ross-Konno procedure) is performed (Figs 5.99 to 5.101). In this case, ensure bovine or other patch material is available.*

## Outcome of Surgical Repair

Longevity of the pulmonary autograft in the aortic position is superior to bioprostheses such as porcine valves, which tend to degenerate after only a few years in children and young adults. Valve replacement especially in young children is not ideal, however, studies compared outcomes between the Ross procedure and mechanical valve replacement in children with aortic valve

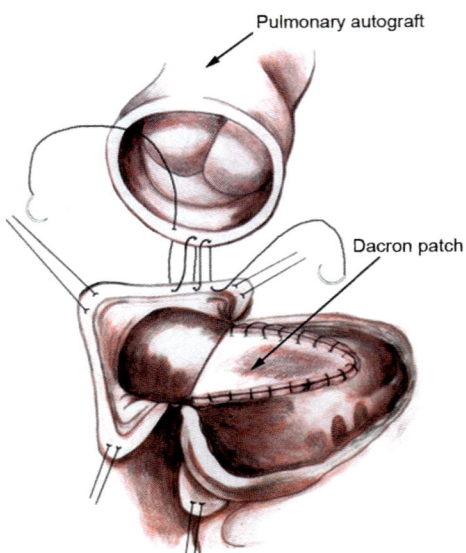

Pulmonary autograft

Dacron patch

**Fig. 5.99:** If the aortic root annulus is too small, then an aortoventri-culoplasty combined with the Ross procedure (commonly known as a *Ross-Konno procedure*) is performed

disease found that the Ross procedure is superior to mechanical valve replacement.[85] Furthermore, anticoagulation is not required as with mechanical valves. Thus, individuals can lead an active life without the risks associated with anticoagulation therapy. This is especially important for young children but also for women of childbearing age needing aortic valve replacement, as anticoagulation is contraindicated in pregnancy.

## The Konno Procedure—Overview

The Ross procedure is a technically difficult and long procedure, as it requires two-valve replacements. The surgeon's experience with this procedure will affect the decision-making. The Ross procedure is contra-indicated in children with Marfan syndrome[xiii] and pulmonary valve pathology. Some surgeons may opt for alternative procedures if there is significant dilatation of the aortic root (which is often the case in children with Marfan syndrome, Fig. 5.100), compared to the pulmonary annulus, whereas others may still decide on the Ross procedure along with aortic annular reduction. In case of severe left ventricular outflow tract obstruction (associated with aortic stenosis), enlargement of the aortic annulus with a patch is necessary together with valve replacement. This is referred to as the Konno procedure (Fig. 5.101).

## Bentall Procedure—Overview

The Bentall procedure is a surgical repair of an ascending aortic or aortic root aneurysm in combination with aortic valve disease.

---

[xiii]Marfan syndrome occurs in approximately 1 in every 10,000 people. It is a genetic condition that weakens the structural connective tissue of the body that provides a frame for the muscles. Children with Marfan syndrome tend to be unusually tall, with long limbs and long thin fingers. The syndrome affects the heart, blood vessels, eyes and skeleton. There is no specific cure for this syndrome. In 75% of cases, the gene for Marfan syndrome is inherited, passed down from parents who have the disease. In the remaining 25% of cases, neither parent may have the disease and the cause or reason for this genetic mutation is unknown.

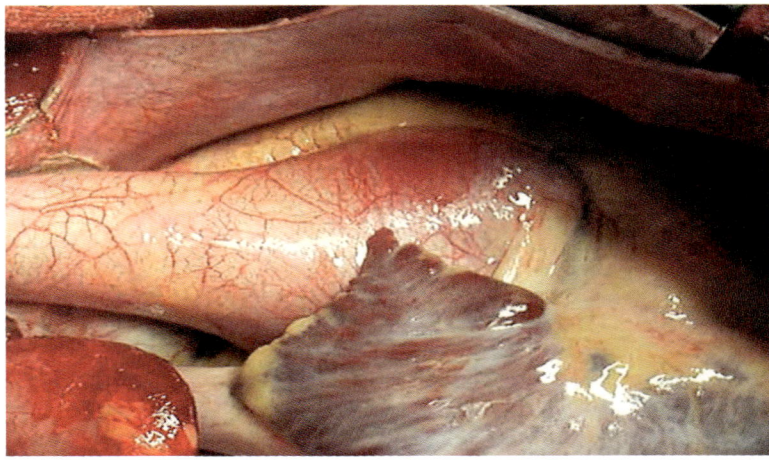

**Fig. 5.100:** Aortic root aneurysm in an adolescent with Marfan syndrome

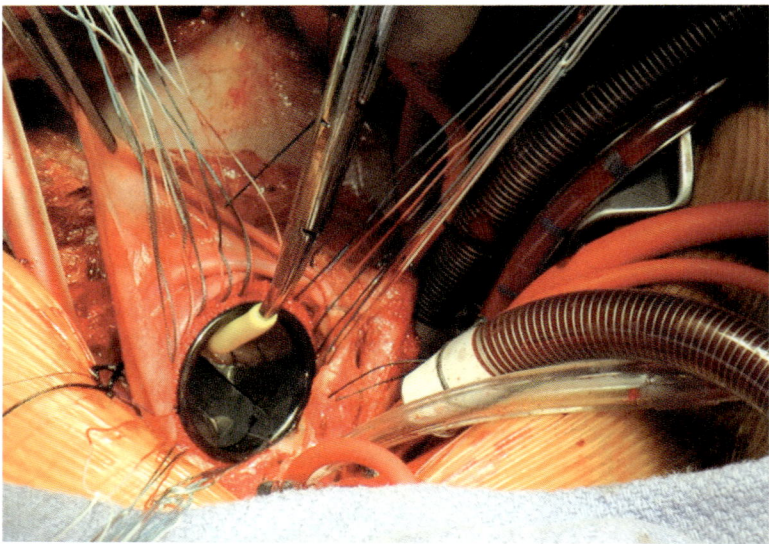

**Fig. 5.101:** The Konno procedure—a Dacron patch or autologous pericardium (the latter can be seen in the picture) is used to widen the left ventricular outflow tract. The diseased aortic valve is replaced with a mechanical valve. *(Photo by EDJ, courtesy of KAMC, National Guard Hospital, Riyadh, Saudi Arabia)*

First described by Bentall and DeBonno in 1968.[86] During the procedure, a composite aortic valve graft is used to replace the proximal ascending aorta and aortic valve (Figs 5.105 and 5.106).

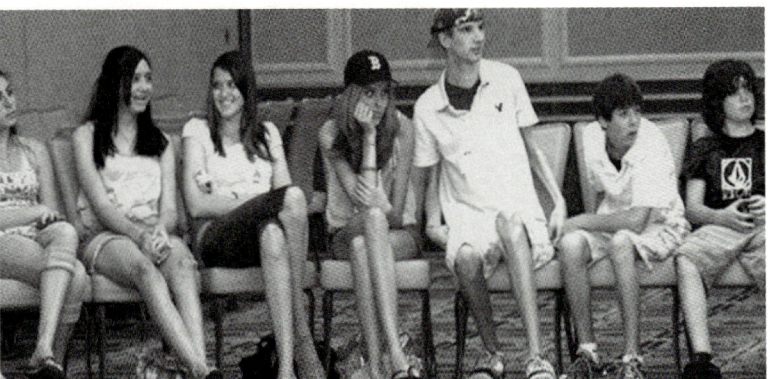

**Fig. 5.102:** Children with Marfan syndrome tend to be unusually tall, with long limbs and long thin fingers

Pectus excavatum

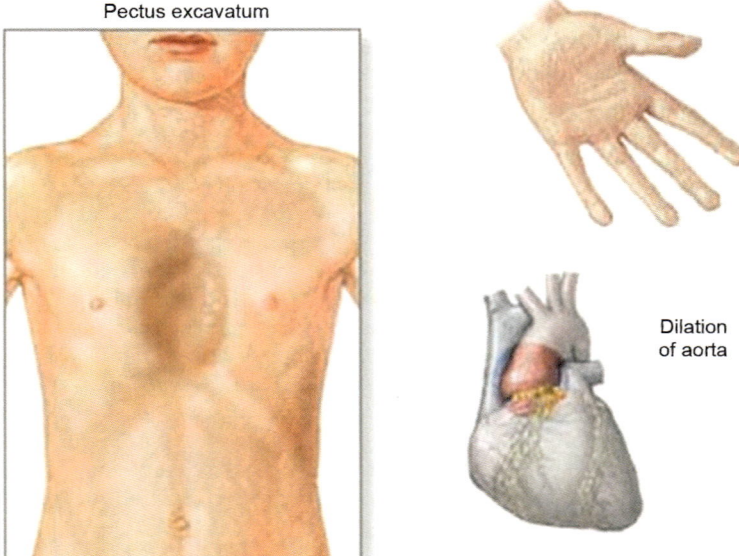

Dilation
of aorta

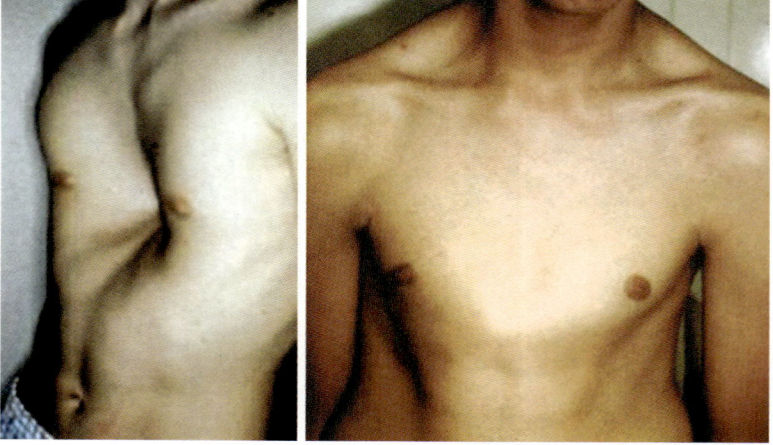

**Fig. 5.103:** The syndrome affects the heart, blood vessels, eyes and skeleton

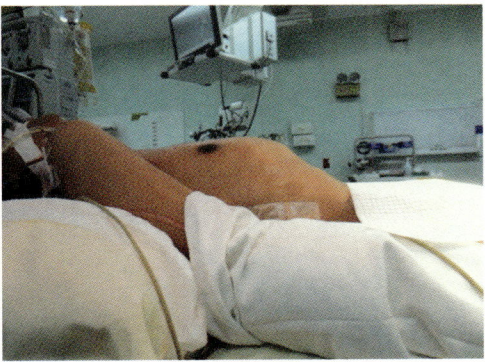

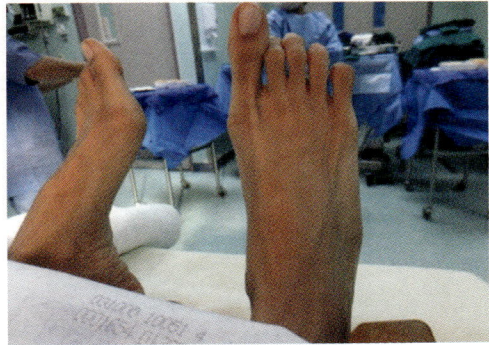

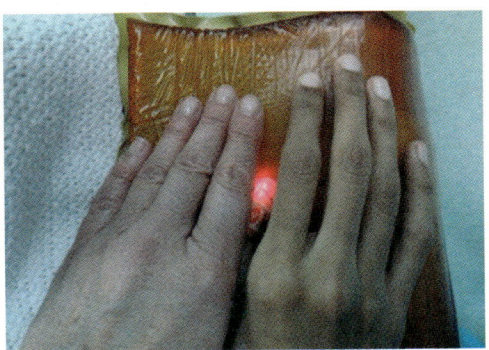

**Fig. 5.104:** The most common features of Marfan syndrome—pectus excavatum (sunken or funnel chest), pectus carinatum (an overgrowth of cartilage causing the sternum to protrude forward), arachnodactyly (long thin fingers), long toes and dilation of the aorta. *(Photos by EDJ, courtesy of KAMC, National Guard Hospital, Riyadh, Saudi Arabia)*

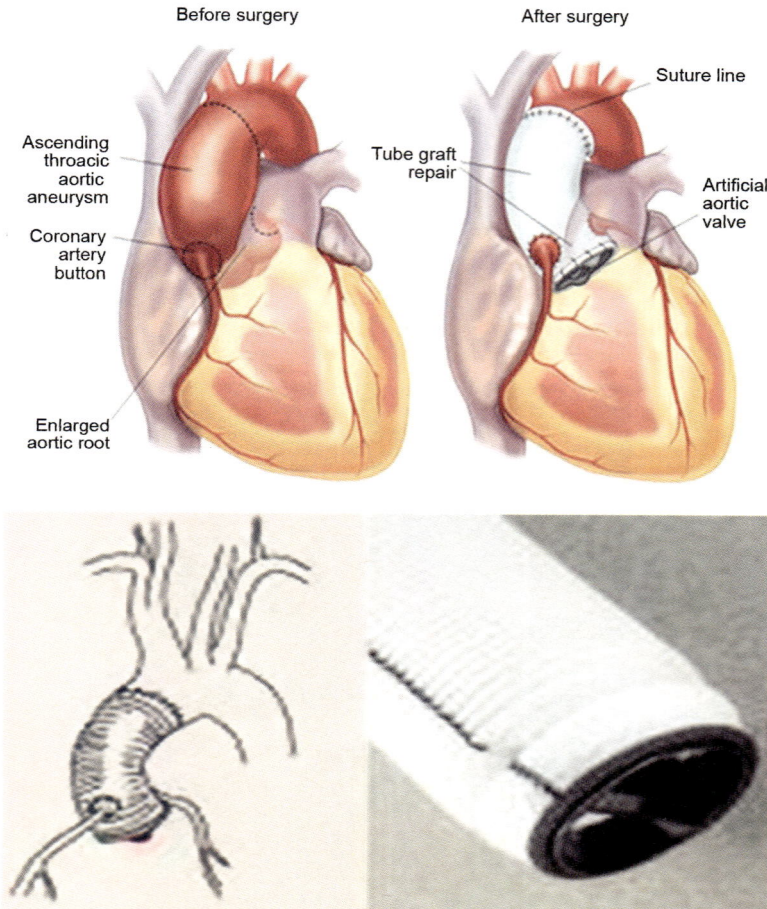

Before surgery

After surgery

Ascending throacic aortic aneurysm

Coronary artery button

Enlarged aortic root

Suture line

Tube graft repair

Artificial aortic valve

**Fig. 5.105:** During the Bentall procedure, a composite aortic valve graft is used to replace the proximal ascending aorta and aortic valve

### Bentall Procedure—Technique

1. Skin incision is made and the sternum is divided.
2. The procedure is carried out on cardiopulmonary bypass with usually a single venous cannula, cardioplegia (antegrade and retrograde), aortic cross clamping and a left atrial vent. Aortic cannulation depends on the anatomy and extent of the disease. Femoral arterial cannulation may be necessary.

3. Dissection is carried out around the aorta using forceps, diathermy and dissecting scissors to separate it from the pulmonary artery and then transected beyond the enlarged aortic root (Fig. 5.106a). The diseased aortic valve and proximal tissues are removed, leaving the right and left coronary arteries with a button of tissue to allow for suturing to the composite graft later (Fig. 5.106b).

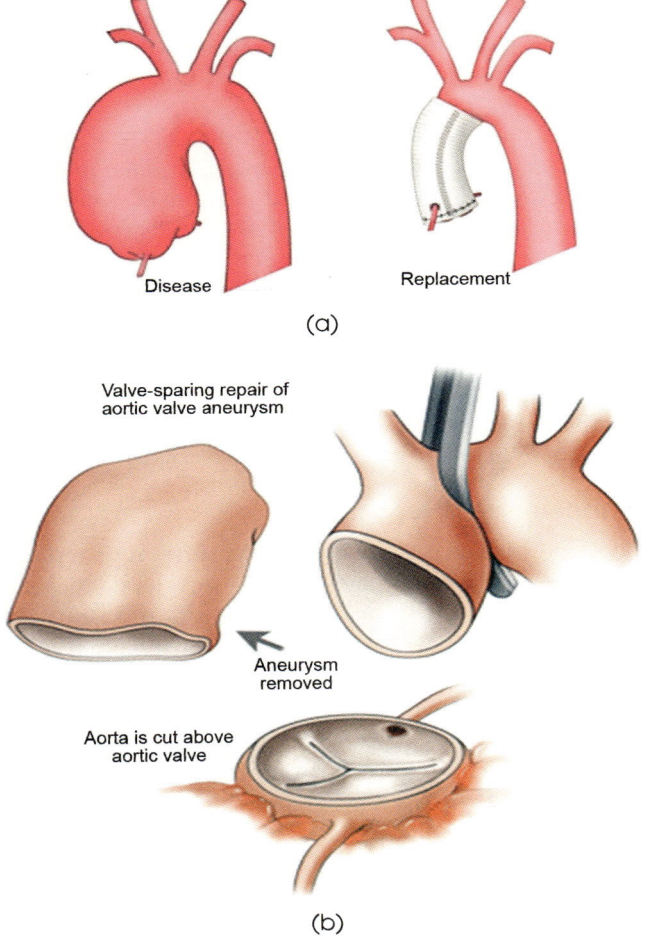

(a)

(b)

**Fig. 5.106:** The Bentall procedure—A composite aortic valve graft is used to replace the proximal ascending aorta and aortic valve (a). Both coronary arteries are reimplanted into the graft (b)

4. The aortic annulus is measured using aortic valve sizers and the appropriate size composite graft is sewn into the aortic annulus, using 2-0 ethibond or tycron 17 mm pledgeted sutures.
5. An eye cautery is used to make a neat circular opening into the graft and both left and right coronary arteries are sewn onto the graft using 6-0 polypropylene suture (Figs 5.105 and 5.106a).
6. The proximal length of the graft is then measured and cut to appropriate length. It is then sewn onto the aorta, using a continuous 4-0 polypropylene suture.

### NURSING OBSERVATION

*Aortic cannulation depends on the anatomy and extent of the disease. Check beforehand with the surgeon and perfusionist, whether femoral arterial cannulation is anticipated and prepare the necessary instruments such as small vascular clamps, or a put together special femoral cannulation instrument set, and purse string sutures for the femoral artery. Usually, when the femoral artery is cannulated, smaller snuggers and tourniquets are used for securing the cannula in place. If the aorta is cannulated, have a variety of different sizes aortic cross clamps available. For the re-implantation of the coronary arteries, have a so-called eye cautery available for making neat circular openings in the graft. Tissue glue and other haemostatic material may be required.*

## David Procedure—Overview

The David procedure is a valve-sparing aortic root replacement. Cardiac surgeon Dr. Tirone David (1944 –) developed the technique at the Toronto General Hospital. Children and young adults with aortic valve disease or an aortic aneurysm are often candidates for a David procedure. The David procedure can also be beneficial for those with Marfan syndrome. Since children with this disorder may also have problems with the adherence of a prosthetic valve, surgeons typically strive to repair, rather than replace their valves and often opt to perform a David procedure in aortic root disease with acceptable aortic valve pathology.

## David Procedure—Technique

1. The heart is cooled, stopped and a clamp is placed across the aortic valve. The aorta is transected (divided) just above where the coronary arteries originate. The coronary ostia (openings) are removed as small buttons of tissue. The remainder of the ascending aorta is removed except for the valve tissue (Figs 5.107 and 5.108a).

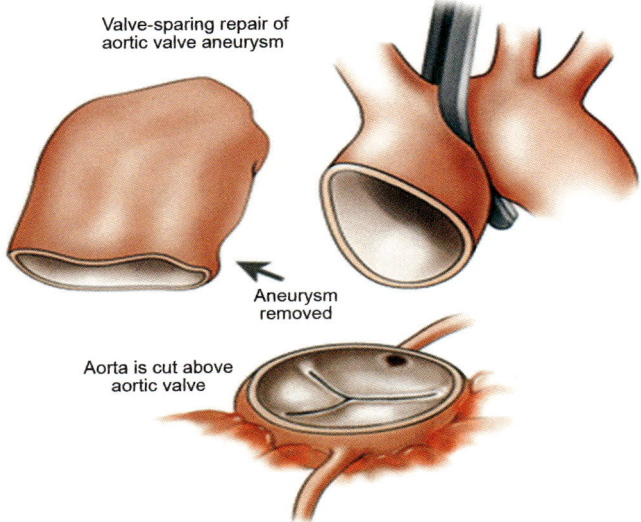

Valve-sparing repair of
aortic valve aneurysm

Aneurysm
removed

Aorta is cut above
aortic valve

**Fig. 5.107:** The heart is cooled, stopped and a clamp is placed across the aortic valve. The aorta is transected (divided) just above where the coronary arteries originate. The coronary ostia (openings) are removed as small buttons of tissue. The remainder of the ascending aorta is removed except for the valve tissue

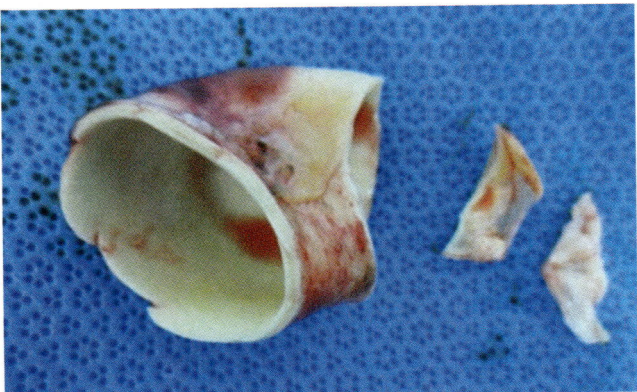

**Fig. 5.108a:** Aortic aneurysm tissue

2. Sutures are placed under the valve and passed outside of the aortic annulus (ring of tissue surrounding the valve). A proper size vascular graft is selected and attached to the heart with the prepared sutures (Fig. 5.108b).

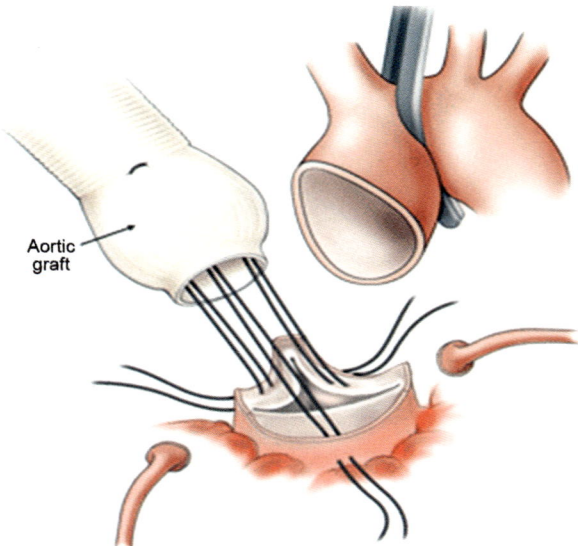

Aortic graft

**Fig. 5.108b:** Sutures are placed under the valve and passed outside of the aortic annulus. A proper size vascular graft is selected and attached to the heart with the prepared sutures

3. The valve is then carefully positioned within the graft to eliminate leaking. A fair bit of customized tailoring is then performed to ensure that the valve leaflets will open and close properly. The valve tissue is completely attached to the graft with a continuous suture technique. Two small holes are created in the graft for re-attachment of the coronary arteries. Finally, the end of the graft is attached to the aortic arch (Figs 5.109 and 5.110).

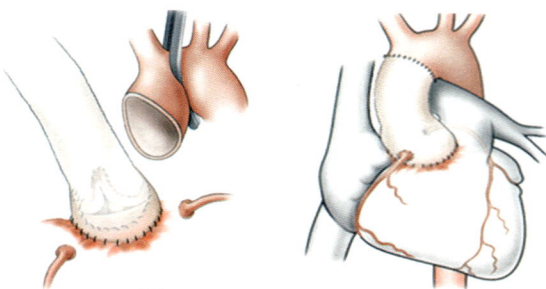

**Fig. 5.109:** The valve is then carefully positioned within the graft to eliminate leaking.

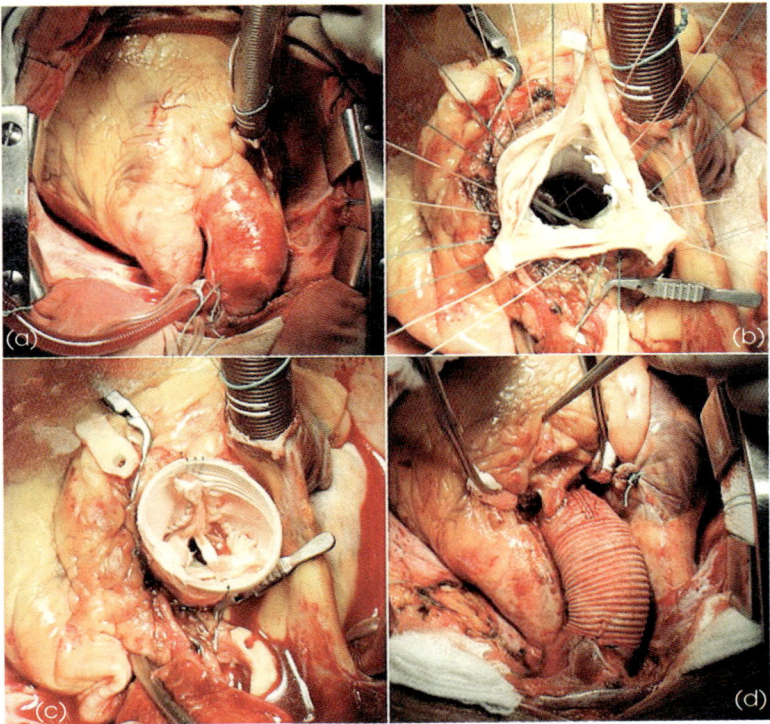

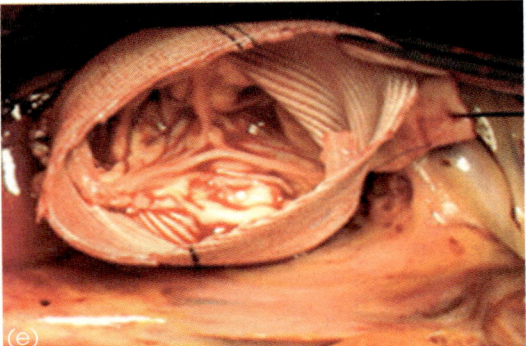

**Fig. 5.110:** Initial view before the procedure (a). The aortic root has been dissected and the stitches are put in for prosthesis implantation (b). Aortic valve has been resuspended in the polyester graft to replace aortic root. Coronary arteries ostia are also seen (c). Final view of the procedure (d).

Section 3

## WHEN CHAMBERS AND VALVES ARE NOT IN NORMAL SEQUENCE AND NORMAL POSITION—ATRIOVENTRICULAR DISCORDANCE AND VENTRICULOARTERIAL DISCORDANCE

In the following section, cardiac anomalies will be discussed in which the heart valves and chambers are not in their normal position, referred to as *atrioventricular discordance*. As well as anomalies in which the great arteries are connected to the *wrong* ventricle. This is referred to as *ventriculoarterial discordance*. Anomalies of the relationship between the atria and the ventricles frequently result in univentricular hearts (see also previous section). Such hearts may have both atrioventricular valves entering a single ventricle or there may be an absent left or right atrioventricular connection. Examples of these anomalies are double inlet left ventricle (DILV), double inlet right ventricle (DIRV) and congenitally corrected transposition of the great arteries (cc-TGA). Examples of anomalies of the relationship between the ventricles and the great arteries are: tetralogy of Fallot (TOF), double outlet right ventricle (DORV), double outlet left ventricle (DOLV), truncus arteriosus and transposition of the great vessels (TGA). Each anomaly will be discussed in the following section.

### DOUBLE INLET LEFT VENTRICLE AND DOUBLE INLET RIGHT VENTRICLE (ATRIOVENTRICULAR DISCORDANCE)

### Introduction

Double inlet ventricle is a rare congenital anomaly in which both atrioventricular valves (tricuspid and mitral valve), or a single atrioventricular valve, open into a single ventricle, which usually resembles the morphological left ventricle. Double inlet right ventricle (DIRV) in which both atrioventricular valves open completely into the right ventricle is very rare.

In most forms of DILV, the positions of the aorta and the pulmonary artery, and the left and the right ventricles are the reverse of the normal heart (Fig. 5.111), although it can also occur with normal positioned great arteries. The right ventricle is often small and both the mitral and tricuspid valves open into an enlarged left ventricle. Usually, there is an atrial septal and a

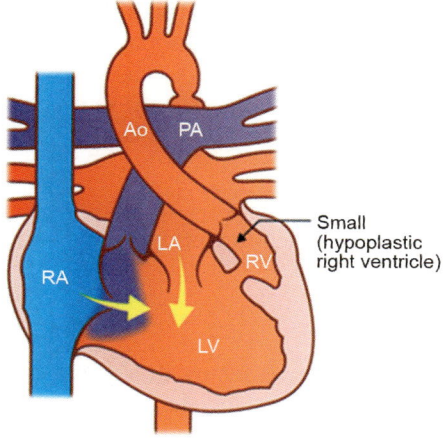

Double inlet (yellow arrows) left ventricle
from right and left atriums

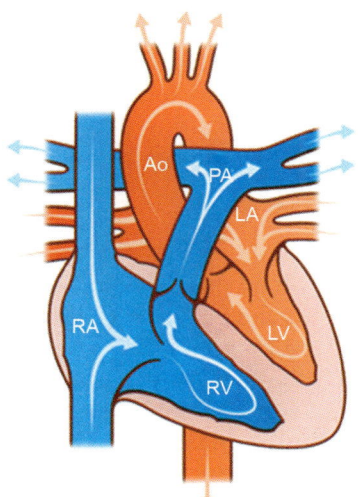

Normal heart and circulation

**Fig. 5.111:** Double inlet left ventricle (DILV)—in most forms of DILV, the
positions of the aorta and the pulmonary artery, and the left and the
right ventricles are the reverse of the normal heart

ventricular septal defect. Other associated anomalies are coarctation of the aorta and pulmonary stenosis or atresia. Both DILV and DIRV are also referred to as a univentricular heart, or single ventricle, since either the right ventricle (in DILV) or the left ventricle (in DIRV) is underdeveloped.[87]

## What Causes DILV and DIRV?

The exact cause of double inlet left ventricle and double inlet right ventricle are unknown.

## Prevalence

Double inlet left ventricle occurs in about 5 to 10 of 100,000 live births. Double inlet right ventricle is very rare.

## Symptoms

In this defect, pulmonary blood flow is excessive, leading to pulmonary hypertension and congestive heart failure. Affected infants usually cannot feed normally, and usually, have difficulty gaining weight. In some babies, there is mild obstruction to either systemic or pulmonary blood flow. Blood flow through the aorta to the body may become restricted if the size of the ventricular septal defect is too small, resulting in serious illness as the only route of blood flow to the aorta is across the ventricular septal defect.

## Treatment

Excessive pulmonary blood flow in double-inlet left ventricle may initially be corrected by the insertion of a pulmonary artery band before, further and definite surgery. The Damus-Kaye-Stansel procedure, in which the aorta and pulmonary artery are joined using a patch, is one surgical option (Fig. 5.112). To restore the pulmonary circulation, a Blalock-Taussig shunt is connected between the subclavian artery and the right pulmonary artery. Alternatively, a right ventricle-to-pulmonary artery (conduit) is placed.

The most common surgery for DILV and DIRV is the 3-staged surgical approach; Blalock-Taussig shunt, Glenn and the final Fontan procedure. Ventricular septation in which the single ventricle is divided into two ventricles by means of the placement

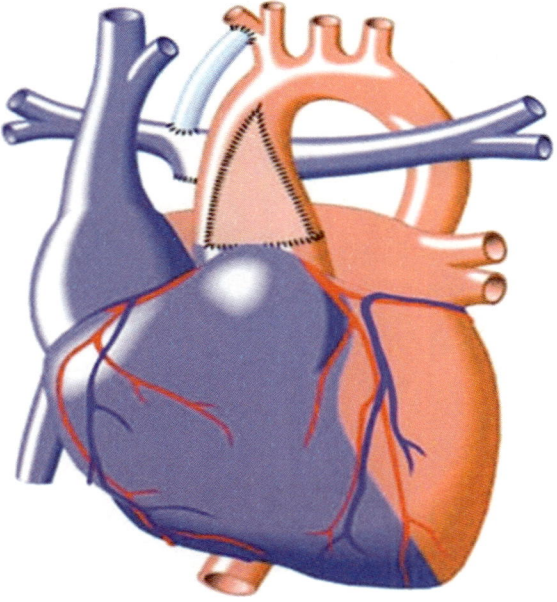

**Fig. 5.112:** The Damus-Kaye-Stansel procedure in which the aorta and pulmonary artery are joined together using a patch, is one surgical option for the treatment of DILV. To restore the pulmonary circulation, a Blalock–Taussig shunt is connected between the subclavian artery and the right pulmonary artery.

of a patch may be an alternative to the Fontan operation for selected patients with DILV (Fig. 113). This is referred to as a biventricular repair.

### Outcome of Surgical Treatment

The treatment and outcome of double inlet left ventricle depends on the severity of the disease. If a biventricular repair is feasable, this would be the most favourable option rather than the Fontan procedure. The Fontan operation does not create normal circulation in the body, but it creates the type of circulation a child can live and grow with. Advances in surgical technique allow many infants to reach adulthood. The impact of various management strategies for the treatment of DILV on the long-term outcomes of these children remains unknown.

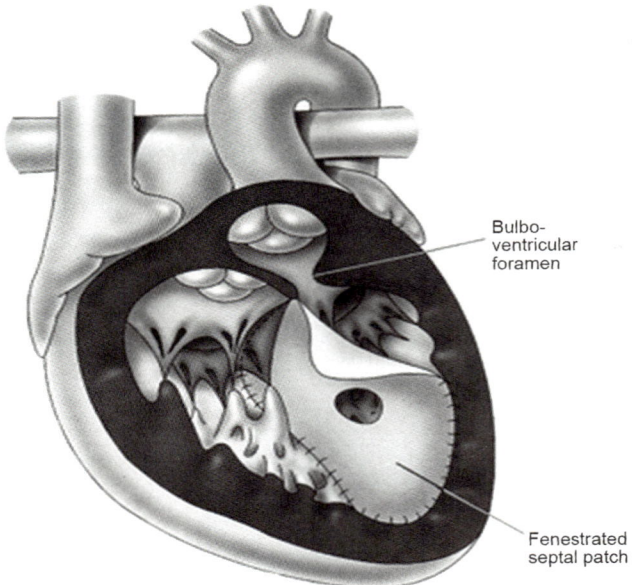

Bulbo-
ventricular
foramen

Fenestrated
septal patch

**Fig. 5.113:** Double inlet left ventricle—dividing the univentricular heart into 2 functional ventricles

---

**SURGEON'S COMMENT**

*Most children with double-inlet left ventricle and transposition of great arteries (DILV/TGA) go through univentricular pathways. Damus-Kaye-Stansel procedure is done when there is obstruction of blood flow from single ventricle to the aorta and thus the systemic blood flow becomes uninterrrupted. Lungs are supplied by construction of a systemic-pulmonary shunt. This procedure becomes the first stage of the univentricular pathway, which leads them to a Glenn and then a Fontan procedure at later stages.*

---

## CONGENITALLY CORRECTED TRANSPOSITION OF THE GREAT ARTERIES (ATRIOVENTRICULAR AND VENTRICULOARTERIAL DISCORDANCE)

### Introduction

Congenitally corrected transposition of the great arteries (cc-TGA or l-TGA) is a rare congenital heart defect, often associated with multiple cardiac abnormalities and conduction defects. Children with congenitally corrected transposition have both atrioventricular and ventriculoarterial discordance, and therefore, also have a morphological right ventricle (RV) and delicate tricuspid valve in the systemic circulation. Associated defects, such as abnormalities of the tricuspid valve, ventricular septal defect, and pulmonary stenosis, occur in the majority of these children. Heart block occurs with increasing age. Progressive tricuspid regurgitation occurs with age and is associated with deterioration of RV function. Surgical treatment should be considered at the earliest sign of RV dilatation or dysfunction.

### What Causes Congenitally Corrected Transposition of Great Arteries (TGA)

During the embryological development the heart tube looped to the left (levo or l-transposition) instead of to the right, resulting in atrioventricular discordance (ventricular inversion). This means that the right ventricle is connected to the left atrium and the left ventricle is connected to the right atrium. In addition, the aorta is connected to the right ventricle and the pulmonary artery is connected to the left ventricle, (transposition) (Figs 5.114 and 5.115).

Thus, venous blood returns from the body into the right atrium, passes through the mitral valve into a morphological left ventricle (mitral valve is related to the left ventricle). Blood then flows through the pulmonary valve into the pulmonary artery (pulmonary valve is related to the pulmonary artery) and to the lungs. Pulmonary venous blood returns to the left atrium and then passes through the tricuspid valve into a morphological right ventricle (tricuspid valve is related to the right ventricle). Blood then flows through the aortic valve into the aorta (aortic valve is related to the aorta). Therefore, blood flows in an effective sequence, hence the name corrected transposition (aorta and pulmonary artery connected to the wrong ventricles (transposition), but left and right ventricles are transposed (connected to the wrong atria) resulting in normal pulmonary and systemic circulation. Nevertheless, in this anomaly, the right ventricle supports the systemic circulation, except it is not build to support the systemic circulation.

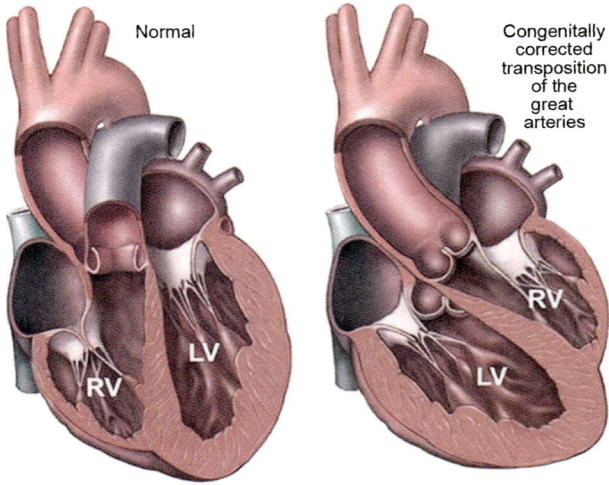

**Fig. 5.114:** Congenitally corrected transposition of the great arteries (cc-TGA or I-TGA) is a rare congenital heart defect in which the heart twists abnormally during fetal development and the ventricles reversed. *Note:* The aorta lies anterior and to the left of the pulmonary artery (the normal position of the aorta is posterior (behind) the pulmonary artery)

## Prevalence

Congenitally corrected transposition of the great arteries accounts for less than 1% of all congenital heart defects and is rare. The literature reports fewer than 1000 cases worldwide. The aetiology of congenitally corrected transposition is currently unknown, often with an increase in incidence reported among families with previous cases of congenitally corrected transposition.

## Treatment

In the past congenitally corrected transposition of the great arteries was left untreated. This approach, however, does not solve the problem of the right ventricle having to do the work that is normally done by a larger, stronger left ventricle; pushing oxygen-rich blood throughout the body. The right ventricle has a different structure than the left ventricle. The right ventricle normally pumps blood to the lungs and works at a low pressure. The left ventricle normally pumps blood to the body and pumps at a much

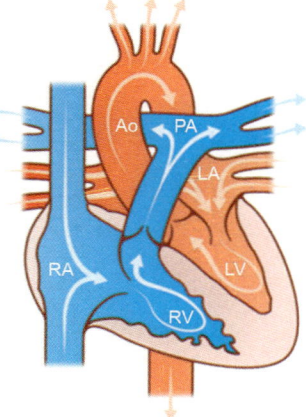

Normal heart and circulation

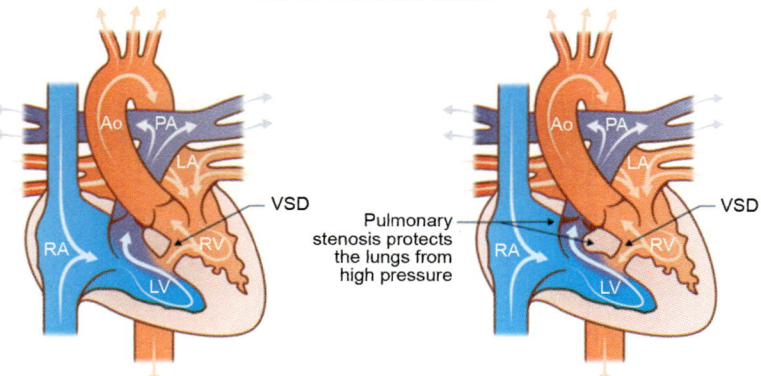

cc TGA with a ventricular septal defect

cc TGA with a ventricular septal defect and pulmonary stenosis

**Fig. 5.115:** In this complex malformation the ventricles are on the opposite side of the heart to the usual. The atria are connected to the incorrect ventricles and the great arteries also come from the wrong ventricles (transposition). Despite these problems, blood from the lungs passes to the aorta, so the child is not blue. In individuals who have no other heart defects the heart may function well enough for the affected person to survive to adult life without symptoms. In many cases an associated VSD is present (as shown in the illustration). This allows excessive blood flow and pressure in the lung circulation. Other heart defects are commonly present, (e.g. valve abnormalities, coarctation, pulmonary stenosis). Many children develop heart block, which may necessitate a pacemaker

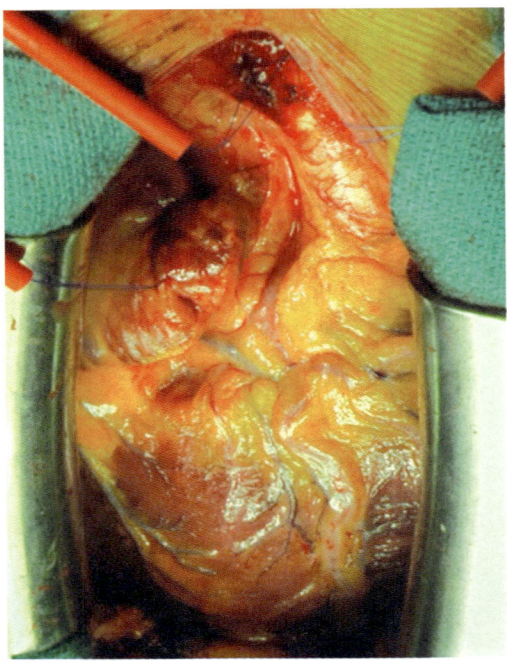

**Fig. 5.116:** In individuals who have no other heart defects, the heart may function well enough for the affected person to survive into adult life without symptoms. Photo is of a 33-year-old male who was diagnosed at the age of 21 with I-TGA and underwent tricuspid valve replacement at the age of 33. *Note:* The right atrium attached to the left ventricle (LV) with the pulmonary artery arising from the LV (Frontal view of the heart). *(Photo by EDJ, courtesy of KAMC, National Guard Hospital, Riyadh, Saudi Arabia)*

higher pressure. Over time, this extra burden on the right ventricle results in gradual deterioration of function of the right ventricle and can lead to congestive heart failure.

Another problem that may occur if left untreated is tricuspid valve disease. The valve that enters the right ventricle is the tricuspid valve (tricuspid valve is committed to the right ventricle, the mitral valve is committed to the left ventricle) and is a thin and delicate structure. In a normal heart, it functions in the low-pressure pulmonary circulation. In this anomaly, however, since the ventricles are switched or transposed, the valve is exposed to high pressure in the right ventricle. This pressure may cause the valve to leak blood backwards (regurgitation). If the ventricular pump working is reduced, contraction may not return to normal even after a perfect valve replacement. The valve needs to be replaced before severe symptoms develop since symptoms occur late in the course of decreasing heart function. If the function of the right ventricle has become severely compromised, valve replacement surgery may no longer be possible or recommended.

Last but not least, because the ventricles are reversed, the conducting pathways in the heart are thin and fragile and may not conduct the electrical impulses around the heart normally. Thus, there is an increased chance of interruption of the electrical impulses before they reach the ventricles. This is called complete heart block and these children may need a pacemaker at a young age.

In conclusion, children with corrected transposition and no other associated abnormalities may not require treatment because their life expectancy has been reported to be near normal. At the other end of the spectrum, a double-switch procedure, as described below, would be contraindicated in children with severe hypoplasia of either ventricle, or severe pulmonary stenosis. These children should be considered for a Fontan repair, or a Senning and Rastelli.

When pulmonary stenosis is associated, an arterial switch is not suitable because the pulmonary stenosis would then become aortic stenosis. Instead, the left ventricle can be routed to the aorta by a baffle, closing the VSD in such a way that blood is directed from the left ventricle to the aorta and the right ventricle is connected to the pulmonary artery with a homograft.

The best surgical option for congenitally corrected transposition of the great arteries remains controversial. Since surgeons gain greater experience with the double switch operation and surgical risk decreases, there is increasing enthusiasm for this approach (Fig. 5.117). The double switch procedure was first performed in 1989. It consists of an atrial switch in combination with an arterial switch operation. An operation such as this essentially ensures that the left ventricle becomes the systemic ventricle and the right ventricle becomes the pulmonary ventricle.

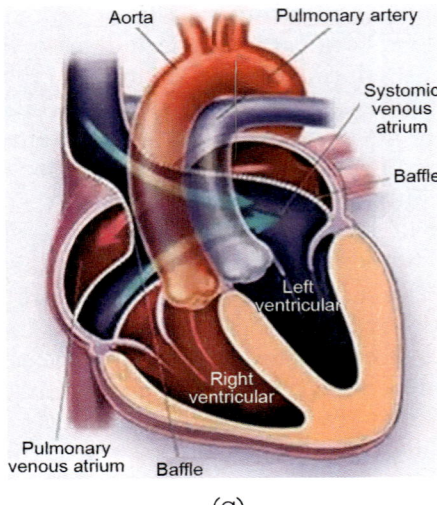

(a)

(b)

**Fig. 5.117:** The senning or mustard operation diverts double-switch operation for I-TGA using the mustard atrial baffle technique (a) and arterial switch procedure. The VSD has been closed with a patch. Venous blood from the superior and inferior vena cava (SVC, IVC) is directed to the RV and then to the pulmonary trunk, and pulmonary venous blood is directed to the LV and then to the aorta (b)

**SURGEON'S COMMENT**

*Children with corrected transposition have normal circulation unless there is an associated ventricular septal defect. But they have a higher risk of arrhythmias and heart block. At later stages, the right ventricle starts showing signs of failure, as it is not used to systemic workload. Double switch (Atrial and arterial) is the corrective surgery but it is a complex operation and a high-risk undertaking.*

## TETRALOGY OF FALLOT (VENTRICULOARTERIAL DISCORDANCE)

### Introduction

Tetralogy of Fallot (TOF) is the most common form of cyanotic congenital heart defects **(blue baby syndrome)**.

In this condition, there are typically four abnormalities, hence the name tetralogy, **tetra** means *four*, and are as follows (Fig. 5.118):

1. Right ventricular outflow tract (RVOT) obstruction,
2. Ventricular septal defect, usually large and just below the aortic valve;
3. Overriding aorta, (abnormal location of the aorta, positioned across the ventricular septal defect);
4. Right ventricular hypertrophy, (thickening of the right ventricular wall).

Children with tetralogy of Fallot are more likely to have chromosome disorders, such as Down's syndrome and Digeorge syndrome.[xiv]

### What Causes Tetralogy of Fallot?

Tetralogy of Fallot is caused by the anterior malalignment of the aortopulmonary septum, resulting in the clinical combination of a ventricular septal defect, pulmonary stenosis, and an overriding

---

[xiv]DiGeorge syndrome is an inherited condition (also known as CATCH22 or 22q 11.2 deletion syndrome) that occurs when a part of the DNA on chromosome 22 is missing. Several different genes are lost, resulting in a collection of different features, including problems with the immune system, congenital heart defects (commonly affecting the pulmonary and aortic artery) and abnormalities of the parathyroid glands.

There may be a typical facial appearance with features such as a small jaw, small, low-set ears with abnormal folds, unusual eyes, small mouth, a rather bulbous nose and square nasal tip, and hypernasal speech with a cleft palate.

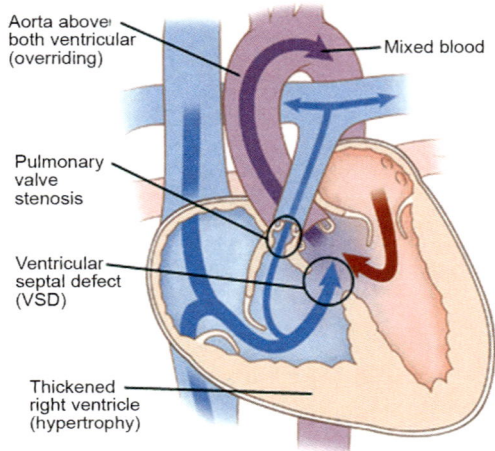

**Fig. 5.118:** Tetralogy of Fallot—there are typically four anomalies namely: overriding aorta, pulmonic stenosis, ventricular septal defect, and right ventricular hypertrophy

aorta. Right ventricular hypertrophy develops progressively from resistance to blood flow through the right ventricular outflow tract. In some cases there is also an atrial septal defect and the anomaly is then referred to as pentalogy of Fallot (POF). TOF was first described by the French physician Louis Arthur Fallot (1850–1911) who published his findings in 1888.

### Prevalence

TOF is estimated to account for 4 to 9% of all congenital heart defects, (3–6 in 10,000 live births). It is slightly more common in males than females.

### Symptoms

Cyanosis is the most common symptom and is caused by inadequate blood flow to the lungs. The right ventricular outflow tract obstruction combined with a large ventricular septal defect causes blood to enter the aorta from both the right (right-to-left shunt) and left ventricles and is significantly deoxygenated. Severe cyanosis may present at birth in babies with severe ventricular outflow tract obstruction and associated pulmonary stenosis or atresia. In children who have less severe pulmonary stenosis, cyanosis may not be visible (pink Tetralogy). The symptoms of tetralogy of Fallot are generally typical. A classic symptom of suspected tetralogy of Fallot is the so-called *tet spells.* Infants with tetralogy of Fallot may suddenly develop deep blue skin, nails and lips after crying, feeding, crawling, or upon awakening. In addition, those children may develop rapid and difficult breathing due to shortness of oxygen, as the result of severe pulmonary stenosis. These episodes are called *hypoxic spells* or *tet spells.* Tet spells are potentially lethal and sometimes unpredictable. It is thought to be caused by a sudden spasm of the ventricular septum, which worsens the right ventricular outflow tract obstruction, thus less blood flow to the lungs. Older children, will often squat during a tet spell (Fig. 5.119). Squatting increases peripheral vascular resistance[xv] and reduces stystemic venous return thus decreases the amount of blood flowing across the ventricular septal defect (right-to-left-shunt). This increases blood flow to the lungs and hence relieves shortness of breath (cyanosis).

## Tetralogy of Fallot Repair—Overview

### History

Palliative treatment for tetralogy of Fallot became available in the 1940's when cardiologist Helen Taussig recognised that cyanosis worsened and led to death in these children. She spectulated that cyanosis was due to inadequate blood flow to the lungs. Working together with Blalock this led to the first type of palliation for these infants. In 1944, Blalock operated on an infant with tetralogy of Fallot and created the first Blalock-Taussig shunt between the subclavian artery and the pulmonary artery (*see* also Blalock-Taussig shunt). Definite or curative repair of TOF was not possible till the 1950's with the invention of the cardiopulmonary bypass machine.

TOF can be associated with severe pulmonary valve stenosis or absent pulmonary valve (pulmonary atresia). Survival of children with pulmonary atresia depends on the presence of a number of naturally occurring connecting blood vessels (collaterals) between the aorta and pulmonary arteries in the lungs. This is referred to as major aortopulmonary collateral arteries or MAPCAs.

---

[xv]Peripheral vascular resistance, a resistance to the flow of blood determined by the tone of the vascular musculature and the diameter of the blood vessels. It is responsible for blood pressure when coupled with stroke volume.

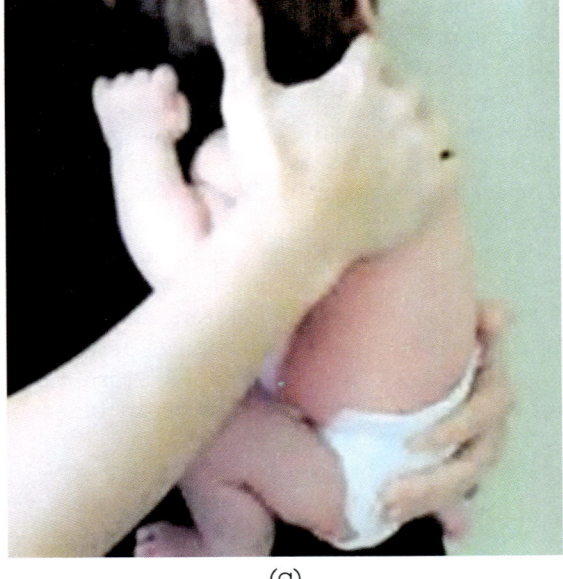

(a)

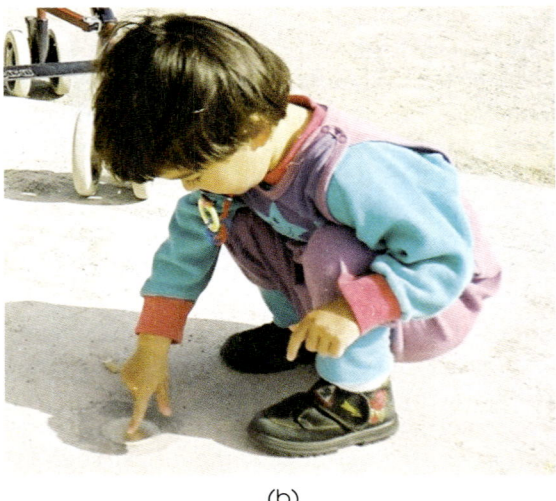

(b)

**Fig. 5.119:** Placing the child in the knee-chest position either lying supine or over the parent's shoulder (a). This calms the infant, reduces systemic venous return and increases systemic vascular resistance. Older children will often squat during a tet spell (b)

Corrective surgery for simple or classic TOF is usually performed at the age of 3 to 6 months involves closure of the ventricular septal defect and enlargement of the narrow area of the right ventricular outflow tract (RVOT) (Figs 5.120 and 5.21). In severe RVOT obstruction, the child may need a pulmonary-valved conduit. Infants with tetralogy of Fallot who are severely cyanosed (caused by severe pulmonary stenosis) their blood flow to the lungs will initially depend on a patent ductus arteriosus. Once the ductus arteriosus closes, these infants may initially need a systemic-to-pulmonary shunt (Blalock-Taussig shunt) to maintain blood flow to the lungs to improve cyanosis (Fig. 5.122).

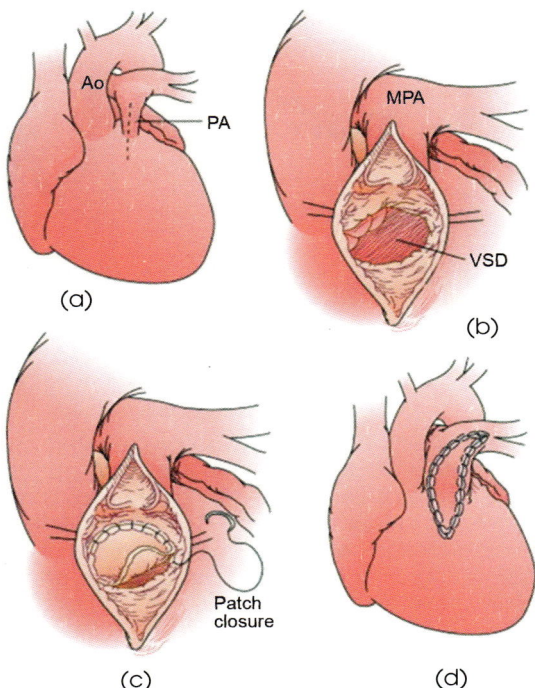

**Fig. 5.120:** Complete repair of tetralogy of Fallot. Enlargement of the right ventricle to main pulmonary artery (PA) connection with a transannular incision if necessary (a). Resection of muscle from the outflow tract and identification of edges of the ventricular septal defect (VSD) (b). MPA, main pulmonary artery. Patch closure of the VSD (c). Placement of a transannular patch if required (d)

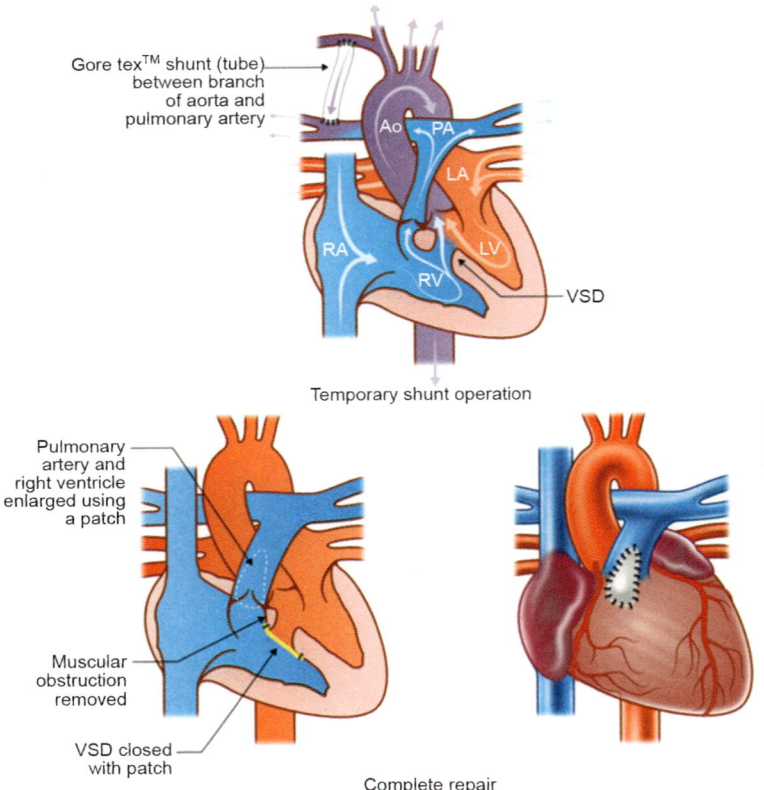

**Fig. 5.121:** Some affected children, who are severely blue, need a temporary operation (BT shunt), which is carried out in infancy to increase lung blood flow and improve cyanosis. Corrective surgery is usually performed at about six months. Correction involves closure of the VSD with a patch and enlargement of the narrow area of the right ventricle and pulmonary artery (pulmonary stenosis), often requiring a further patch (complete repair)

## Tetralogy of Fallot Repair—Technique

1. After sternotomy, which may be a re-sternotomy if a palliative shunt is in place, the pericardium is opened and suspended with silk sutures (thymus may have been removed if previous palliative surgery was performed).
2. In the case of the presence of a palliative shunt, or a patent ductus arteriosus, these are divided.

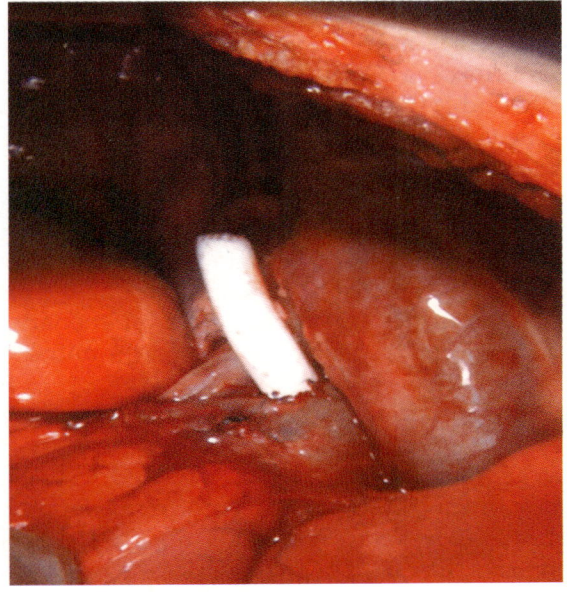

(a)

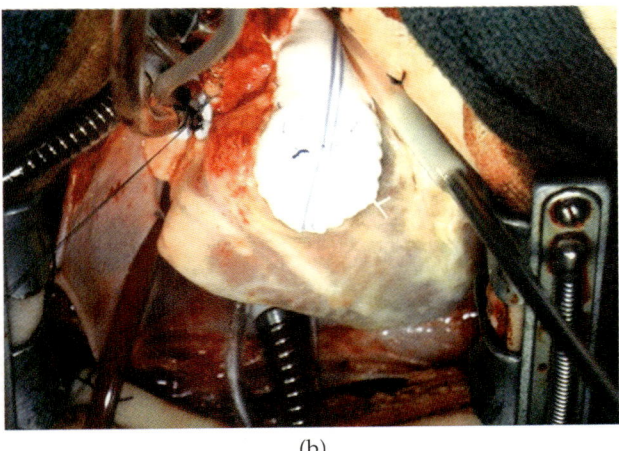

(b)

**Fig. 5.122:** Some affected children, who are severely blue, need a Blalock-Taussig shunt during infancy (a), complete repair with enlargement of the narrow area of the right ventricle and pulmonary artery (pulmonary stenosis), often requiring a further patch (b) is carried out at a later stage

3. The patient is cannulated with an aortic cannula in the ascending aorta and bicaval venous cannulation in both superior vena cava (SVC) and inferior vena cava (IVC).
4. Both SVC and IVC are encircled with caval tapes and snared.
5. The aortic is then cross-clamped and cardioplegia is administered.
6. A left ventricular vent is inserted. Some surgeons may insert it through the right atrium, across the atrial septum, and advance the vent across the mitral valve into the left ventricle. Other surgeons may insert the vent through a purse string suture at the junction of the right upper pulmonary vein and the left atrium and then advance it across the mitral valve into the left ventricle.
7. Next, the right atrium is opened and suspended with silk sutures.
8. The tricuspid valve is carefully retracted with small vein retractors which will allow the surgeon excellent visualization of the ventricular septal defect (VSD) and the right ventricular outflow tract (RVOT). The diameter of the pulmonary valve annulus is assessed with calibrated dilators. Obstructing muscle bundles are resected. The VSD is inspected and closed, in most cases, with a patch using the infant's own pericardium, commercially available bovine or porcine pericardium, or synthetic material (Gore-Tex™, Dacron).
9. If the RVOT obstruction is severe, the pulmonary artery is also opened from the outside, further muscle is resected and an additional transannular patch may be used to accomplish adequate annulus size.

**NURSING OBSERVATION**

*The nurse should have knowledge whether a previous Blalock-Taussig shunt has been placed in which case a redosternotomy will be performed. In addition, calibrated dilators or Hegar dilators should be available to assess the diameter of the pulmonary valve annulus. Furthermor, have patch material available for possible repair of the right ventricular outflow tract (RVOT). In severe tetralogy of Fallot the pulmonary stenosis may be severe and the surgeon may decide to place a right-to-pulmonary artery conduit. The type of conduit should be discussed with the surgeon in advance as well as patch material used in the case of RVOT obstruction repair.*

### SURGEON'S COMMENT

*The consistent feature of tetralogy of Fallot is a large-sized ventricular septal defect. However, the degree of right ventricular outflow tract obstruction varies from patient to patient. Some patients only have infundibular obstruction with muscle bundles and mild degree of pulmonary stenosis. They can be repaired by just opening the right atrium (transatrial repair). Others require further opening of the main pulmonary artery as well (transatrial, transpulmonary repair). However, if the pulmonary valve annulus is also narrow, the incision has to be carried out across the pulmonary annulus and a large patch is then used to widen the area of the annulus (transannular repair). In some patients, the branch pulmonary arteries are also narrowed and they require patch repair of these branches in addition. The cannulation routine for this operation is similar to the standard technique for VSD closure but you should be aware of the need for preparation of autologous pericardium, and ensure availability of other patch material (Gore-Tex™ bovine pericardium, etc.). In some cases, where there are abnormal coronary arteries or absent pulmonary valve syndrome, a right ventricle to pulmonary artery conduit (Contegra or homograft) may also be required.*

## Outcome of Surgical Repair of Tetralogy of Fallot

Prognosis depends on the severity of the right ventricular outflow tract obstruction. Without surgery, the natural progression of the anomaly suggests a poor outcome. Mortality rates range from 30% at age 2 years to 50% by age 6 years, if not surgically treated. The mortality rate seems highest in the first year. Most children with tetralogy of Fallot can be corrected with surgery. After surgical correction, many children are without symptoms and are able to lead a normal life. Individual surgeons opinions vary whether or not tetralogy of Fallot should be primarily repaired at an early age (at the age of 3–6 months or even within the first few days of life), or treated with a two-stage approach (palliative shunt, Blalock-Taussig shunt) and definite repair at the age of 1–2 years. Palliative surgery with a systemic-to-pulmonary shunt may be considered, e.g. when the infant has severe hypoplastic pulmonary arteries to promote their growth.

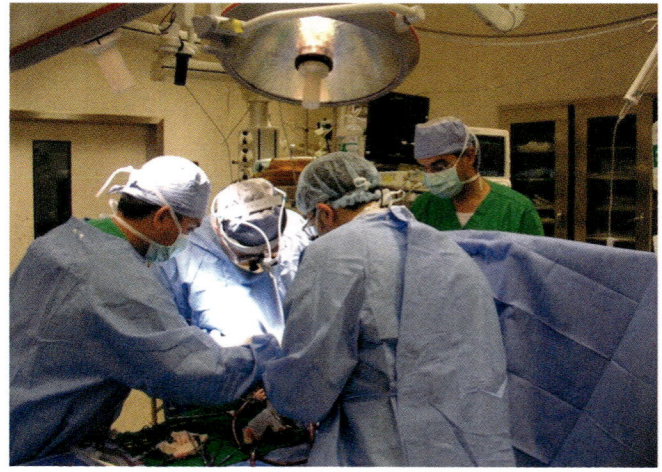

Dr. Jamjoom MD, Chairman, paediatric and adult cardiac surgeon and Dr. Burhani MD at the King Faisal Specialist Hospital and Research Centre-Gen. Org, Jeddah, Saudi Arabia

## DOUBLE OUTLET RIGHT VENTRICLE (VENTRICULOARTERIAL DISCORDANCE)

### Introduction

In double outlet right ventricle (DORV), the aorta and the pulmonary artery both originate entirely or predominantly from the right ventricle (Figs 5.123 and 5.124). This is a problem because the right ventricle carries desaturated blood, which then flows through the aorta and the rest of the body. There is usually a large ventricular septal defect, pulmonary valve stenosis or atresia.[92]

The literature suggest that based on the location of a ventricular septal defect (VSD) in relation to the great arteries, double outlet right ventricle can be classified into four main categories (Fig. 5.124).

1. **Double outlet right ventricle with subaortic VSD:** In double outlet right ventricle with subaortic VSD the VSD is located just below the aortic valve.

2. **Double outlet right ventricle with subpulmonary VSD:** In double oulet right ventricle with subpulmoonary VSD the VSD is located just below the pulmonary artery. This is also called Taussig-Bing anomaly.

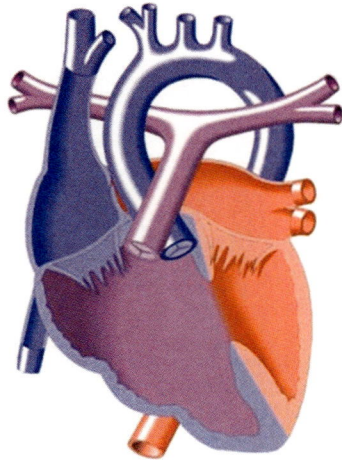

**Fig. 5.123:** Double outlet right ventricle (DORV)—the aorta and the pulmonary artery both originate entirely or predominantly from the right ventricle

3. **Double outlet right ventricle with a doubly committed VSD:** In this anomaly the VSD is located below both aortic and pulmonary valves, hence the name doubly committed VSD.
4. **Double outlet right ventricle with noncommitted VSD:** As the name suggests the VSD in this anomaly is located neither near the aortic nor the pulmonary artery.

## Symptoms

Thus, the pathophysiology of DORV varies. Clinical manifestations may range from that of a large ventricular septal defect (VSD) to that of transposition of the great arteries and mostly depend on the position of the VSD in relation to the great vessels (whether it is subpulmonary or subaortic) and the presence or absence of pulmonary valve stenosis (PS). Both of these factors contribute substantially to the haemodynamics of this congenital heart defect. If the ventricular septal defect is subaortic, which occurs in 60–70% of patients, the VSD is closer to the aortic valve, thus oxygenated blood from the left ventricle is directed to the aorta and desaturated blood from the right atrium is directed mainly to the pulmonary artery.

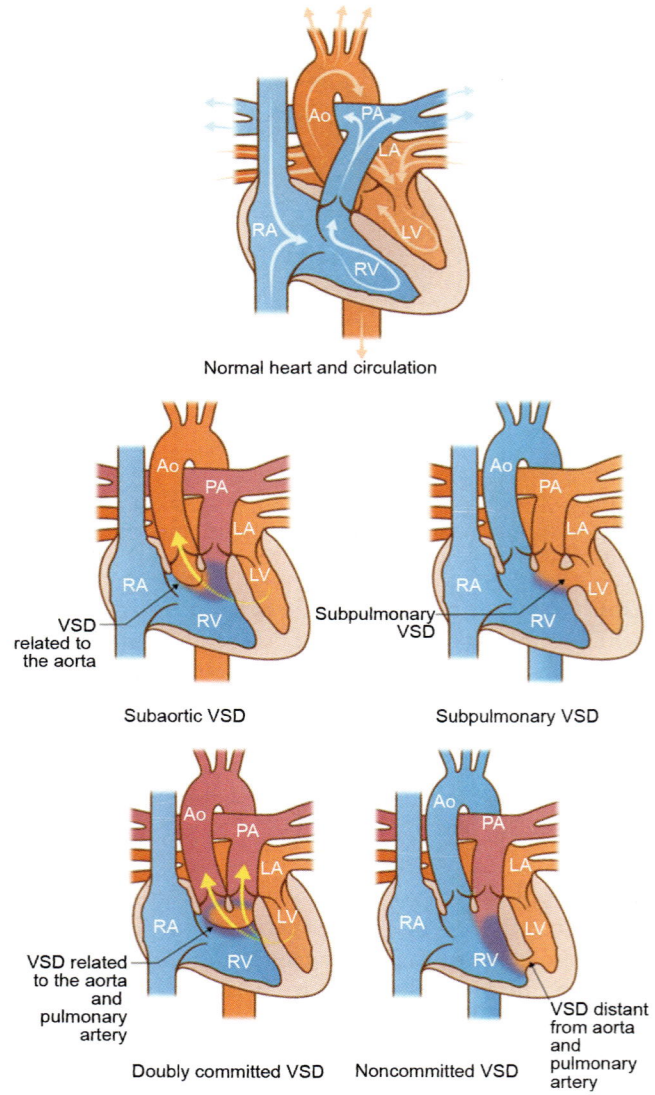

Normal heart and circulation

Subaortic VSD

Subpulmonary VSD

VSD related to the aorta

Subpulmonary VSD

Doubly committed VSD

Noncommitted VSD

VSD related to the aorta and pulmonary artery

VSD distant from aorta and pulmonary artery

**Fig. 5.124:** In double outlet right ventricle (DORV) the two great arteries (aorta and pulmonary artery) both originate from the right ventricle and blood from the left ventricle passes across a VSD into the RV to reach the great arteries. The lung circulation is often exposed to very high pressure and increased blood flow (as with a large VSD). There are many different varieties of this abnormality

With a subpulmonary VSD (Taussig-Bing anomaly, called after cardiologist Helen Taussig (1898–1986), and cardiologist Richard Bing (1909–2010), which occurs in 10% of patients, oxygenated blood from the left ventricle is directed to the pulmonary artery and desaturated blood from the right atrium is directed to the aorta. This physiology resembles transposition of the great arteries with a VSD; thus, the child presents with cyanosis and congenital heart failure.

### Prevalence

In the United States, the incidence of double outlet right ventricle is 0.09 cases per 1000 live births. Double outlet right ventricle comprises about 1–1.5% of all congenital heart disease.

### Treatment

Surgical options are based on correcting the specific combination of anatomic defects of this anomaly and may vary from a simple ventricular septal defect closure to more complex surgery, where the surgeon has the choice between a biventricular or univentricular repair.

In other words, repair of double outlet right ventricle may be amendable for a corrective operation that leads to a biventricular repair. If this cannot be achieved, univentricular repair will be the only other option. In such cases, palliative operations such as, banding of the pulmonary artery in the case of excessive pulmonary blood flow, can be used to palliate excessive pulmonary flow and protect the pulmonary vascular bed until definitive management can be undertaken. In the case of inadequate pulmonary blood flow, an aortopulmonary shunt, typically a Blalock-Taussig shunt can be used to palliate inadequate pulmonary flow and promote growth for the pulmonary vascular bed and acceptable oxygenation until definitive management can be undertaken. This definite repair will consist of a Glenn procedure followed by the Fontan.

The site of the VSD may vary and can affect the clinical manifestations and the options for surgery.

When referring to (Fig. 5.124) the upper left diagram, DORV with a subaortic VSD shows an abnormality similar to tetralogy of Fallot, but without obstruction to flow to the lungs. Repair involves placement of a patch within the right ventricle to direct left ventricular (LV) flow to the aorta (biventricular repair).

In the type called the Taussig-Bing anomaly (top right diagram, and (Fig. 5.125) blood from the LV passes through the VSD to the pulmonary artery, whilst blood from the right ventricle tends to be directed mainly to the aorta. This is similar in many ways to transposition with a VSD and it may be treated with an arterial switch operation along with a patch within the right ventricle to direct flow to the arterial valve adjacent to the VSD (biventricular repair).

The illustration labelled doubly committed VSD shows a rare variant, which may be suitable for repair in a similar way to the first type. The fourth diagram shows a non-committed VSD in which the VSD is distant from both arteries and blood *mixes* in the right ventricle. This is sometimes suitable for repair but in some cases a Glenn and Fontan procedure may be considered.

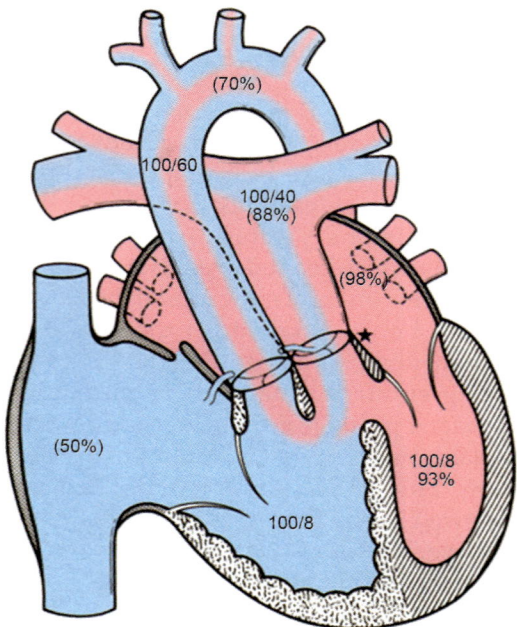

**Fig. 5.125:** Double outlet right ventricle with subpulmonary VSD; Taussig–Bing anomaly. *Note:* The Ao and PA are positioned side-by-side

---

**NURSING OBSERVATION**

*Surgical options are based on correcting the specific combination of anatomic defects of this anomaly and may vary from a simple ventricular septal defect closure to more complex surgery, where the surgeon has the choice between a biventricular or univentricular repair.*

*In Taussig-Bing anomaly, the scrub nurse should prepare as for an arterial switch operation. Have patch material available for the ventricular septal defect (VSD) closure. The scrub nurse should be familiar with the surgeon's technique for closing the VSD (interrupted pledgeted sutures or continuous suture technique), as well as which material is used for the VSD closure. As multiple anastomoses need to be tested during the haemostasis phase, a good supply of irrigation fluid, irrigation syringes and fine sutures should be available.*

---

**SURGEON'S COMMENT**

*In cases of subaortic VSD, a large patch of pericardium or Gore-Tex™ will be used to form an intraventricular tunnel, directing the left ventricular blood through the VSD to the aorta. The VSD is also enlarged if it is small in size. In cases of subpulmonary VSD, when the VSD is closed with a patch, the anatomy of the heart becomes like that of a transposition of great arteries (TGA) with aorta now arising from right ventricle. That is why an arterial switch is necessary to completely correct the congenital defect.*

*In cases of doubly committed or non-committed VSD, if the heart cannot be divided into two chambers, it is treated like a univentricular heart. In these cases, a pulmonary artery band is applied to prepare these patients for future Glenn and Fontan procedures.*

## DOUBLE OUTLET LEFT VENTRICLE (VENTRICULOARTERIAL DISCORDANCE)

### Introduction

Double outlet left ventricle (DOLV) is a very rare cardiac anomaly in which more then 50% of both the aorta and the pulmonary artery originate from the left ventricle. In this anomaly, there is almost always a ventricular septal defect to allow mixing of blood. Furthermore, the great arteries may be malposed (l-TGA, congenitally corrected transposition of the great arteries). Most children with DOLV will have pulmonary outflow tract obstruction and present soon after birth with cyanosis. DOLV with two well-developed ventricles is surgically treated with closure of the VSD, and placement of a conduit between the right ventricle and

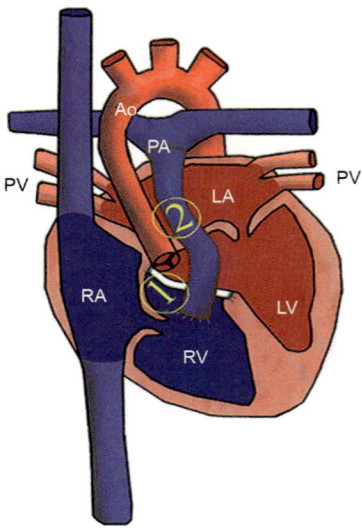

**Fig. 5.126:** Rastelli repair for DOLV with VSD closure (1) and placement of a conduit between the right ventricle and the pulmonary artery (2), AO, aorta; LA, left atrium; LV, left ventricle; PA, pulmonary artery; PV, plumonary veins; RA, right atrium; RV, right ventricle

the pulmonary artery (Rastelli) (Fig. 5.126). Children with DOLV and a single functional ventricle will require a Fontan operation.

## TRUNCUS ARTERIOSUS (VENTRICULOARTERIAL DISCORDANCE)

### Introduction

Persistent truncus arteriosus or truncus arteriosus is a rare congenital heart disease in which the embryological structure fails to properly divide into the pulmonary artery and the aorta. In this defect a single vessel, the truncus arteriosus arises from normally formed right and left ventricles (Figs 5.127 and 5.128). This single vessel or common trunk usually has one large valve, which may have between two to five leaflets, and is frequently abnormal and/or incompetent. There is almost always a ventricular septal defect (VSD). Truncus arteriosus is often associated with Di-George syndrome. Pulmonary arteries may arise from the common trunk in one of several patterns, which are used to classify subtypes (Figs 5.129–5.133).

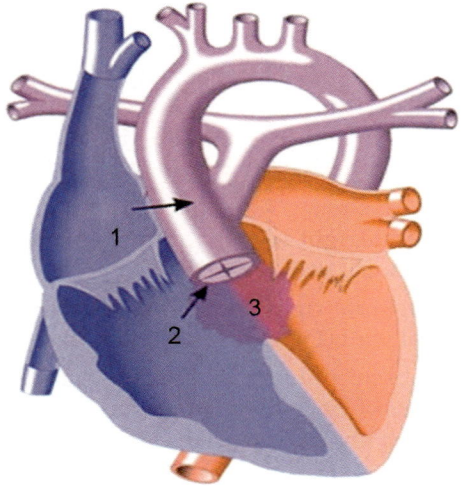

**Fig. 5.127:** Truncus arteriosus: (1) Main trunk (truncus arteriosus), (2) large valve with 4–5 leaflets, (3) large VSD

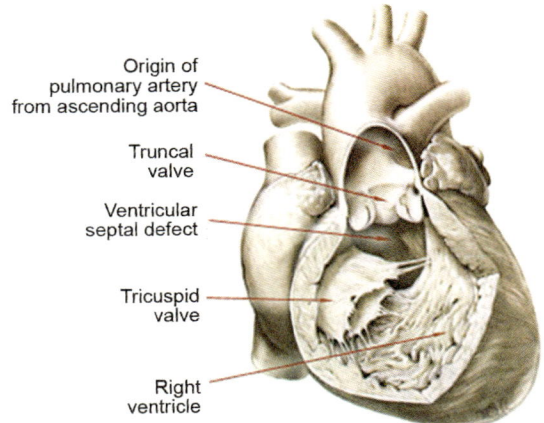

Origin of pulmonary artery from ascending aorta

Truncal valve

Ventricular septal defect

Tricuspid valve

Right ventricle

**Fig. 5.128:** In the normal heart there are two main vessels leaving the pumping chambers: the aorta, which carries blood to the body from the left side; and the pulmonary artery, which carries blood to the lungs from the right heart. In the defect known as truncus, the two main vessels are fused into one large channel into which both pumping chambers empty. There is a ventricular septal defect (VSD), which allows both to pump into the common channel

Truncus arteriosus is almost always associated with a large ventricular septal defect. There are 4 types.

1. **Type I:** A single main pulmonary artery originates from the lateral wall of the truncus just above the truncal valve. This single trunk then divides into the right pulmonary artery and the left pulmonary artery. This is the most common type (Fig. 5.219a).

2. **Type II:** A separate right and left pulmonary artery arising from the posterior truncal wall (Fig. 5.129b).

3. **Type III:** A separate right and left pulmonary artery arising from the lateral wall (Fig. 5.129c).

4. **Type IV**: An absent pulmonary artery is rare. It is probably a severe tetralogy of Fallot with pulmonary atresia and aortic collaterals supplying the lung. This type is also called pseudo-truncus arteriosus (Fig. 5.129d).

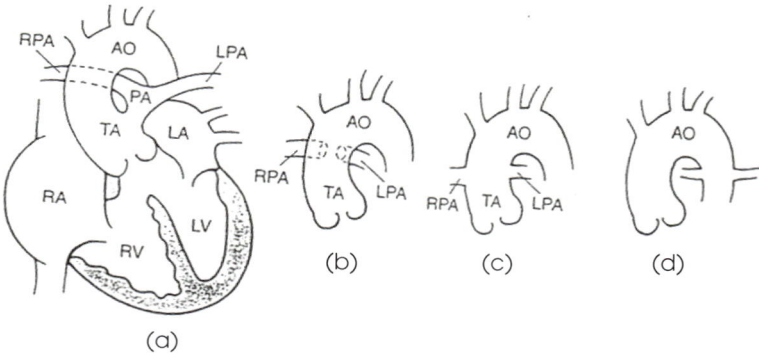

**Fig. 5.129:** Classification of truncus arteriosus.

Type I has a single main PA that originates from the lateral wall of the truncus just above the truncal valve. This single trunk then divides into the RPA and LPA. This is the most common type (a).

Type II has a separate right and left PA arising from the posterior truncal wall (b).

Type III has a separate right and left PA arising from the lateral wall (c).

Type IV has absent PA and is rare. It is probably a severe TOF with pulmonary atresia and aortic collaterals supplying the lung. This type is also called pseudo-truncus arteriosus (d).

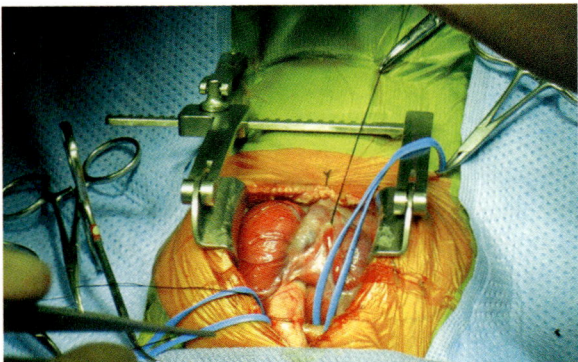

**Fig. 5.130:** Truncus arteriosus type II—the left and right pulmonary arteries are encircled with vessel loops. Right pulmonary artery can be seen. Picture taken standing at the head of the child. *(Photo by EDJ, courtesy of KAMC, National Guard Hospital, Riyadh, Saudi Arabia)*

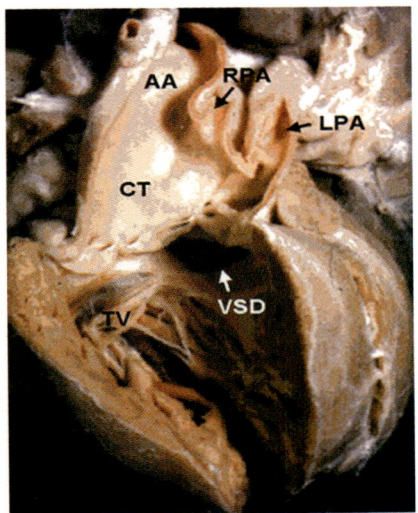

**Fig. 5.131:** Pathologic specimen with truncus arteriosus (TA), viewed through the opened right ventricle and truncal valve. The common trunk (CT) can be seen giving off the ascending aorta (AA) as well as the left (LPA) and right pulmonary arteries (RPA). The truncal valve straddles the ventricular septal defect (VSD). The tricuspid valve (TV) is also labelled

## What Causes Truncus Arteriosus

The anomaly is thought to result from incomplete or failed separation of the embryonic truncus arteriosus into the aorta and the pulmonary artery, hence the name, truncus arteriosus.

## Prevalence

Truncus arteriosus represents 1–2% of congenital heart defects in live born babies. Interestingly among aborted foetuses and stillborn infants with cardiovascular anomalies, truncus arteriosus represents almost 5%.

## Symptoms

As the common channel leaves the heart, there is branching with vessels going to the lungs, while the main channel continues to the body. The major problem in truncus arteriosus is that the lungs are flooded with blood and the heart muscle is overloaded (Fig. 5.132). These infants usually are in distress in the first few days of life because of the severe overcirculation of the lungs, and early surgical attention is required.

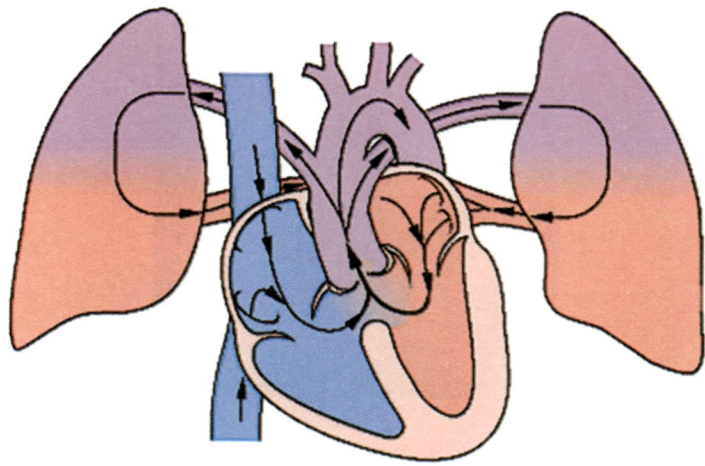

**Fig. 5.132:** The major problem in truncus is that the lungs are flooded with blood and the heart muscle is overloaded. Outflow from both ventricles is directed into the truncus arteriosus. Pulmonary blood flow typically is at least three times higher than systemic blood flow, resulting in pulmonary overcirculation and congestive heart failure

## Treatment

The operation for truncus involves separating the pulmonary blood vessels from the truncal vessel. Then a synthetic tube (conduit) is connected to the right ventricle at one end, and to the pulmonary artery at the other end (Rastelli). The VSD also must be closed with a patch of synthetic material. Nowadays, in most centres, truncus arteriosus is primary repaired in the neonatal period.

### Truncus Arteriosus Repair—Overview

#### History

The earliest classification was developed by Collett and Edwards in 1949. In 1965, Van Praagh proposed a slightly different classification (Fig. 5.133).

### Truncus Arteriosus Repair—Technique

Main surgical steps in the truncus arteriosus repair (Rastelli):
1. The pulmonary artery is separated from the truncus and the defect is closed either with a patch (commercially available bovine or porcine pericardium), synthetic material (Gore-tex™, Dacron) or a part of a homograft leaving the common trunk-committed to the left ventricle; aorta.

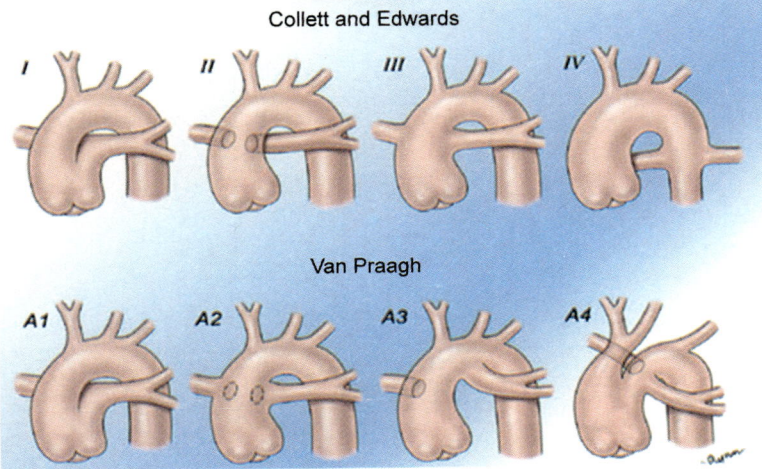

**Fig. 5.133:** The earliest classification was developed by Collett and Edwards in 1949. In 1965, Van Praagh proposed a slightly different classification

2. Repair of the VSD is through an incision in the right ventricle.
3. Placement of a conduit between the right ventricle (same incision through which the VSD is repaired) and the pulmonary artery is carried out to re-establish the pulmonary circulation. In most centres, a cryopreserved valved aortic or pulmonary allograft (homograft) is used for the conduit. Alternatively, a Gore-Tex™ or Dacron graft may be used.

The operation can be performed either with the child on continuous cardiopulmonary bypass or by utilizing deep hypothermic circulatory arrest:

1. The heart is exposed through a standard median sternotomy. Thymus tissue may be absence if the child has Di-George syndrome. Harvesting of pericardium may be performed for the VSD closure.
2. The left and right pulmonary arteries are mobilized and isolated with vessel loops.
3. The aorta is cannulated high, well above the bifurcation of the truncus, or common trunk.
4. Both SVC and IVC are cannulated. If the technique of deep hypothermic circulatory arrest is used, a single right atrial

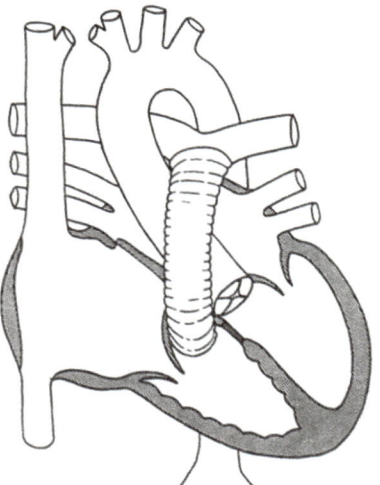

**Fig. 5.134:** Rastelli repair for truncus arteriosus—creating a connection between the right ventricle and the main pulmonary artery

cannula may be inserted in the right atrial appendage instead.

5. Cardiopulmonary bypass is started, and the patient is cooled to 18–20°C for circulatory arrest or 34°C for continuous bypass.

6. During the cooling period, the left and right pulmonary arteries are further mobilized.

7. The coronary arteries are identified, and the bifurcation of the truncal root is carefully examined by the surgeon.

8. Cardioplegia purse string is placed next, followed by cardioplegia needle. Aortic cross clamp is placed and cardioplegia is given. Both pulmonary arteries are clamped or snared to prevent cardioplegia flowing into the pulmonary circulation.

9. Next, the pulmonary arteries are excised from the truncal root. Adequate tissue should surround the orifices of the branch pulmonary arteries in order to facilitate the subsequent conduit anastomosis. Great attention is given to the location and origin of the coronary arteries so as to not injure them during excision of the pulmonary arteries. If there is a main pulmonary artery segment before the bifurcation of the pulmonary artery branches, the pulmonary artery is easily excised from the truncal root. This is the case in Type I truncus arteriosus, which is the most common Fig. 5.133). The defect in the truncal root is closed with a nonabsorbable 5-0 or 6-0 polypropylene suture. Careful attention to the truncal valve and the coronary ostia is critical to this phase of the operation. The defect is closed primarily in the majority of cases. Alternatively, autologous pericardium, a bovine patch, or a piece of homograft may be used for repair.

10. If there is little or no main pulmonary artery tissue, then some of the truncal tissue surrounding the branch pulmonary arteries must also be removed. This is the case in Type II and Type III; if the branch pulmonary arteries originate quite separately from each other, then the truncal root is transected proximally and distally to the take-off of the branch pulmonary arteries (Fig. 5.135). This not only facilitates the excision of the pulmonary arteries, but also provides adequate tissue for the distal conduit anastomosis.

11. The ventricular septal defect is closed next by means of a longitudinal incision into the right ventricle, beginning just below the truncal valve annulus. This exposes the ventricular septal defect (Fig. 5.136). The incision is extended into the right ventricle just far enough to expose the defect and create a right ventricular opening of appropriate size for the conduit.

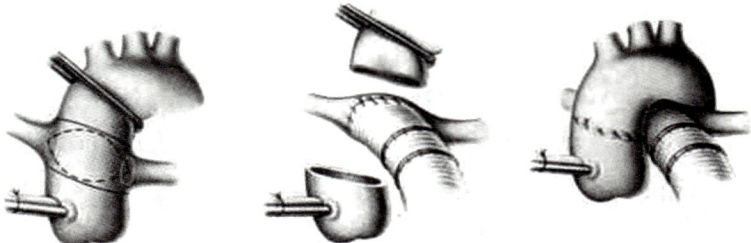

**Fig. 5.135:** Repair of truncus arteriosus type II and type III; truncal transection, and primary end-to-end anastomosis of the truncal root to the ascending aorta is performed

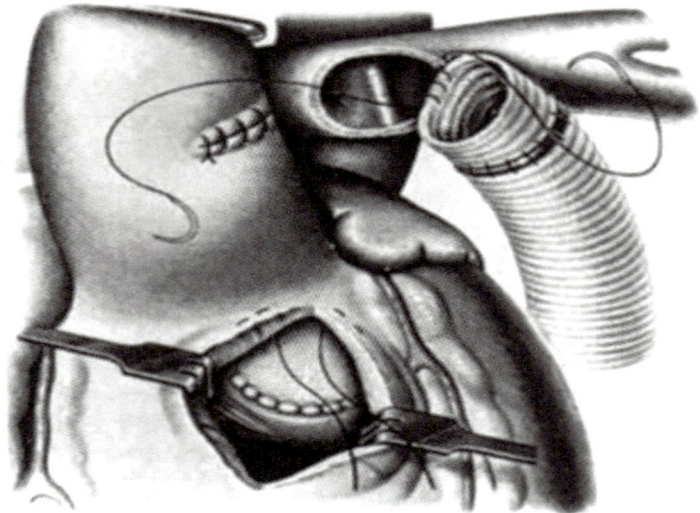

**Fig. 5.136:** Incision made in the right ventricle through which the VSD is repaired. Distal part of graft is sewn on to the main pulmonary artery

12. If there is an atrial septal defect this defect is closed next. The atrial septum is closed either retrograde through the tricuspid valve or through a small right atriotomy.

13. If a patent foramen ovale (PFO) is present, it is left alone to serve as a *vent*. If there is no PFO, the surgeon may decide to create one and a tiny incision may be made into the atrial septum, to create a *pop-off vent*. The atriotomy is then closed.

14. Aortic cross clamp is removed and core rewarming is then started.

15. Placement of a conduit between the right ventricle (same incision through which the VSD is repaired) and the pulmonary artery is carried out to re-establish the pulmonary circulation (Figs 5.136 and 5.137).

16. After completion of the repair, the child is weaned from cardiopulmonary bypass.

17. Pacing wires and chest drains are inserted in a standard fashion. The sternum is closed if the child is stable.

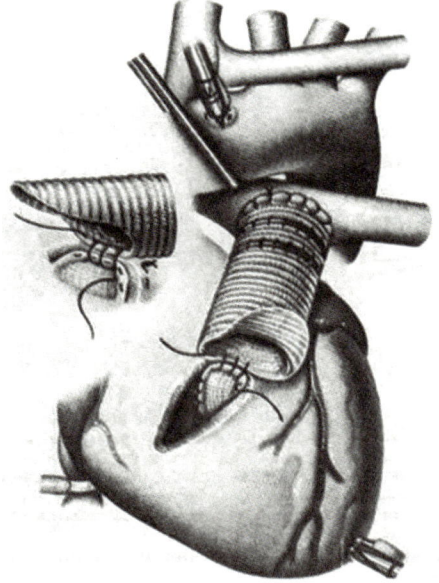

**Fig. 5.137:** Placement of a conduit between the right ventricle (same incision through which the VSD is repaired) and the pulmonary artery is carried out to re-establish the pulmonary circulation

**NURSING OBSERVATION**

*Surgical option for truncus arteriosus repair is most commonly a Rastelli procedure.*

*Have patch material available for the ventricular septal defect (VSD) closure. The scrub nurse should be familiar with the surgeon's technique for closing the VSD (interrupted pledgeted sutures or continuous suture technique), as well as which material is used for the VSD closure and the way it is prepared. For the conduit between the right ventricle and the pulmonary artery it is the surgeon's preference which material is used. This may be a Gore-Tex™ graft, homograft, or a valved conduit (Contegra). As multiple anastomoses need to be tested during the haemostasis phase, a good supply of irrigation fluid, irrigation syringes and fine sutures should be available.*

**SURGEON'S COMMENT**

*Standard cannulation procedures are followed. In addition, snares with vessel loops are placed around the pulmonary artery branches to avoid flooding of lungs when on bypass and also to avoid cardioplegia loss into the pulmonary circulation.*

*Availability of the conduit of the choice of the surgeon for right ventricle to pulmonary artery should be ensured beforehand as well as the patch material for closure of ventricular septal defect (in large size).*

*Closure of ventricular septal defect is carried out through right ventriculotomy with continuous polypropylene sutures. Coronary probes should be available in case the surgeon wants to assess the coronary arteries.*

*In most cases, left atrial pressure monitoring line will be placed.*

*In some cases, the chest may be left open especially if the child's pericardial cavity is small to accommodate the conduit.*

## Outcome of Surgical Repair

Primary surgical repair has improved the survival of children with truncus arteriosus despite an overall perioperative mortality of 10%. In a report from the Society of Thoracic Surgeons Congenital Heart Surgery Database of 572 children who underwent primary repair at 49 centres, the overall in-hospital mortality was 11%.[98] This may vary at single cardiac institutions. The long-term survival following primary repair as demonstrated by one study was 90, 85, and 83% at 5, 10, and 15 years, respectively.[99] Predictably, conduit replacement or revision is almost invariably necessary. Children with truncal insufficiency who do not undergo truncal valve repair or replacement at initial truncus repair are at significantly higher risk for late truncal valve replacement.

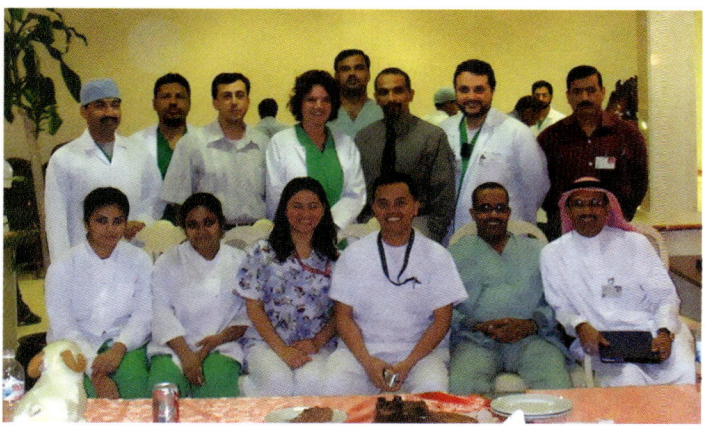

Cardiac team at the King Faisal Specialist Hospital and Research Centre-Gen. Org, Jeddah, Saudi Arabia

## TRANSPOSITION OF THE GREAT ARTERIES (VENTRICULOARTERIAL DISCORDANCE)

### Introduction

Transposition of the great arteries (TGA) is a congenital heart defect in which there is a reversal, or transposition of the aorta and the pulmonary artery, that is, the aorta arises from the right ventricle instead of the left ventricle and the pulmonary artery arises from the left ventricle instead of the right ventricle (Fig. 5.138). As a result, oxygen-rich blood from the lungs is sent back to the lungs, and oxygen-poor blood from the body is sent back to the body. It is a cyanotic congenital heart disease. Symptoms of TGA usually become obvious in the first 24 hours of life, as the ductus arteriosus closes. When this happens, the flow of oxygen-rich blood will be severely restricted and serious symptoms may rapidly manifest themselves. In many cases, TGA is accompanied by other heart defects, which are actually beneficial in this case. The most common type being intracardiac shunts such as atrial

---

**NURSING OBSERVATION**

*Tetralogy of Fallot, truncus arteriosus and transposition of the great arteries are among the most common cyanotic heart disease. The perioperative nurse should have knowledge of the clinical symptoms of cyanotic heart disease in order to give expert nursing care to these children.*

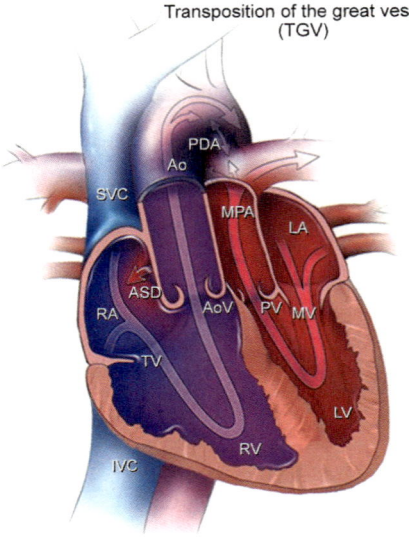

Transposition of the great vessels (TGV)

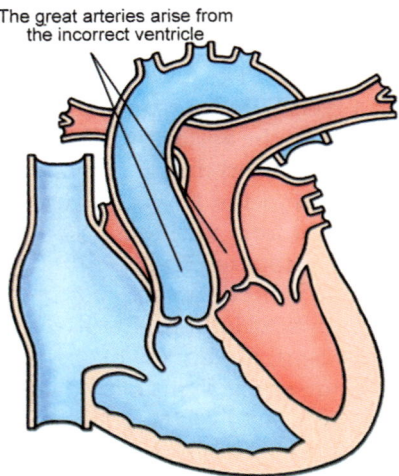

The great arteries arise from the incorrect ventricle

**Fig. 5.138:** Transposition of the great arteries—the aorta arises from the right ventricle instead of the left ventricle and the pulmonary artery arises from the left ventricle instead of the right ventricle. RA, right atrium; RV, right ventricle; LA, left atrium; LV, left ventricle; SVC, supprior vena cava; IVC, inferior vena cava; MPA, main pulmonary atery; AO, aorta; TV, tricusped valve; MV, mitral valve; AoV, aortic valve; ASD, atrial septal defect; PDA, patent ductus arteriosis

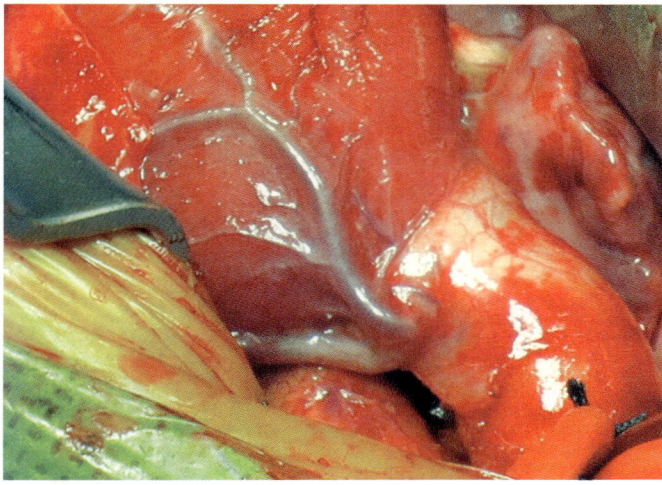

**Fig. 5.139:** Frontal view of the aorta attached to the right ventricle. The pulmonary artery can be seen to the left of the aorta. The right atrium can be seen to the right. Note the coronary artery. Picture taken standing at the head of the child. *(Photo by EDJ, courtesy of KAMC, National Guard Hospital, Riyadh, Saudi Arabia)*

septal defect (ASD), patent foramen ovale (PFO), ventricular septal defect (VSD), and patent ductus arteriosus (PDA). Stenosis, or other defects, of valves and/or vessels may also be present.

### History

In 1950, Blalock and Hanlon described the first palliative procedure for transposition of the great arteries (TGA), in which an atrial septectomy was performed to allow mixing of blood within the heart and hence improve arterial oxygen levels. With the invention of cardiopulmonary bypass, Senning, a Swedish cardiac surgeon (1915–2000), performed the first complete repair for TGA in 1957.[100] He used the native atrial tissue to create a baffle or tunnel within the atria that directed desaturated blood from the right atrium, through the mitral valve into the left ventricle, the pulmonary artery and the lungs. Saturated blood from the left atrium is redirected, through the tricuspid valve, into the right ventricle and aorta (Fig. 5.140). Although, blood flow through the heart is redirected into the correct great arteries, the right ventricle continues to act as the systemic pump, and the left ventricle as the pulmonary pump.

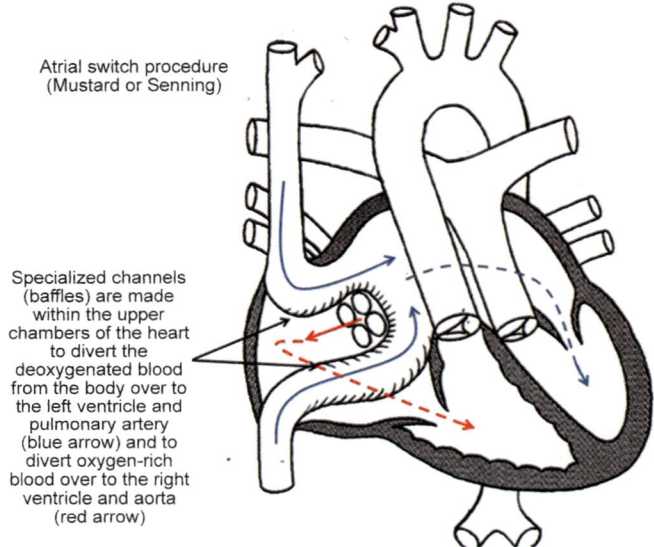

Atrial switch procedure
(Mustard or Senning)

Specialized channels
(baffles) are made
within the upper
chambers of the heart
to divert the
deoxygenated blood
from the body over to
the left ventricle and
pulmonary artery
(blue arrow) and to
divert oxygen-rich
blood over to the right
ventricle and aorta
(red arrow)

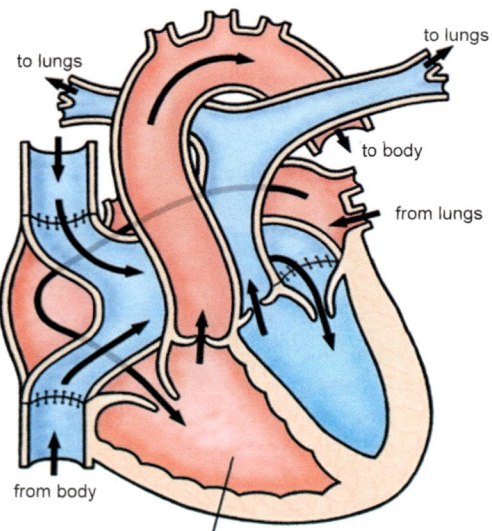

to lungs

to lungs

to body

from lungs

to lungs

from body

The morphologic right ventricle
acts as the systemic ventricle

**Fig. 5.140:** Atrial switch and Senning repair, in which the blood flow is redirected at the atrial leve

In 1964, Mustard, a Canadian cardiac surgeon (1914–1987), described a simpler technique; he excised the atrial septum and used a patch to create the *baffle* within the atria.[101] Both techniques are referred to as atrial switch *since the switch* occurs at the *atrial* level. In 1966, Rashkind and Miller pioneered the first interventional catheterization technique to create a large atrial septal defect, by means of a balloon catheter. This procedure is referred to as the Rashkind procedure and still in use today for TGA with absence of atrial septal and or ventricular septal defect to allow mixing of blood. The Senning and Mustard techniques still have a small role in the treatment of d-TGA in children with fixed subpulmonary obstruction and as part of the double switch type of repair used in the treatment of congenitally corrected transposition.

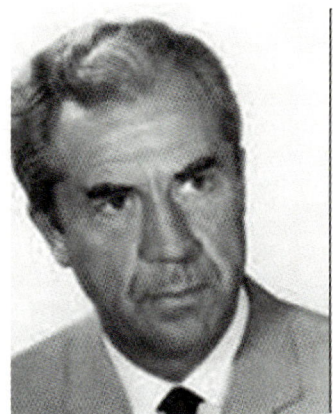

Dr Senning 1915–2000

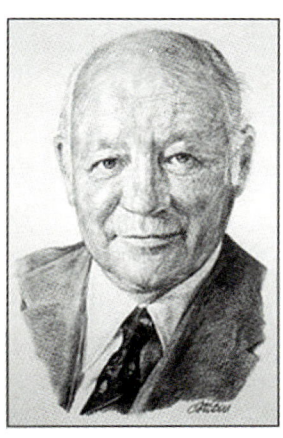

Dr Mustard 1914–1987

The Brazilian cardiac surgeon, Jatene, reported the first successful arterial switch operation in 1975 (Fig. 5.141).[102, 103] The arterial switch operation (ASO) corrects the anatomy of the discordant ventriculoarterial connections. Following repair, the right ventricle is connected to the pulmonary artery and the left ventricle is connected to the aorta, the way a normal heart is designed. Both Senning and Mustard tried this technique in the 1950s without success. This was due to the inability to transfer the coronary arteries successfully, but moreover, mortality rates in small infants in the early era of cardiopulmonary bypass were very high.

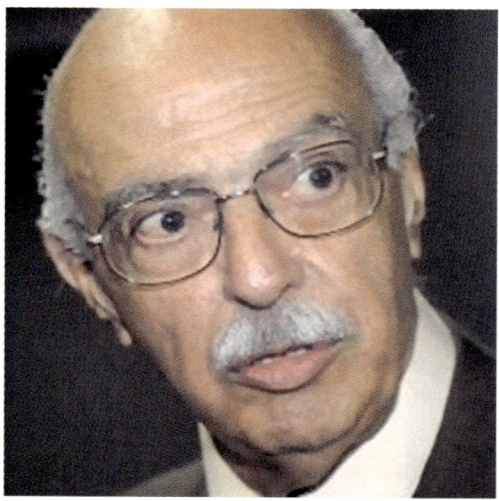

**Fig. 5.141:** Adib Domingos Jatene (1929–2014) was a Brazilian physician of Lebanese background, university professor, scientist and thoracic surgeon, one of the founders of the University of São Paulo Heart Institute and internationally respected as the inventor of the Jatene operation, a technique to correct transposition of the great vessels in the newborn

## Transposition of the Great Arteries Repair—Overview

In approximately 60% of patients with transposition of the great arteries (TGA), the aorta is anterior (in front) and to the right of the pulmonary artery. This is referred to as dextro-TGA or d-TGA, which means that the ventricles are in their normal position. For these patients, an arterial switch operation (ASO) is performed.

The surgical steps for the arterial switch or Jatene procedure for d-TGA will be described here, as this is the most frequently performed operation for d-TGA (Fig. 5.142). The surgery is usually performed in the first month of life, to avoid adjustment of the left ventricle to the lower pulmonary pressure, which would be unable to support the systemic circulation after the switch, if surgery is performed at a later stage. In neonates, who are too sick to have the surgery and in children who present late, (which may be common in underdeveloped countries, where healthcare may not be readily available), pulmonary artery banding may be the initial procedure to train the left ventricle for future arterial switch operation.

### Transposition of the Great Arteries Repair—Technique

Surgical steps in the arterial switch operation:

1. Transection of both the aorta and the pulmonary artery,
2. Detachment of the coronary arteries along with a button from the aortic wall;
3. The great arteries are then switched into their new position (LeCompte manoeuver (Fig. 5.143); the pulmonary artery is moved in front of the aorta),
4. Transfer of the coronary arteries buttons to the neo (new) aorta;
5. Neo-aorta anastomosis;
6. Reconstruction of the neo-pulmonary artery (with autologous pericardium).

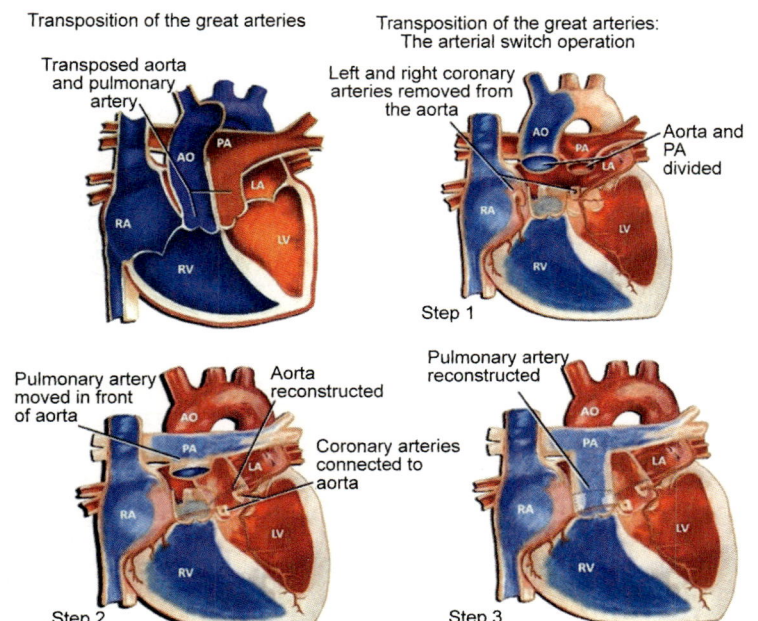

**Fig. 5.142:** Surgical steps for arterial switch operation

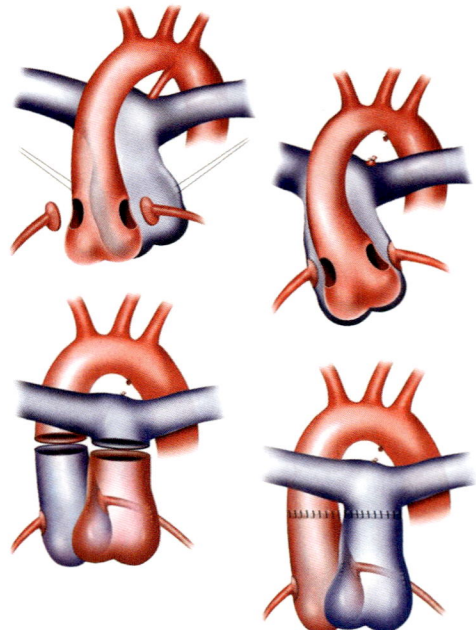

**Fig. 5.143:** Surgical steps for the arterial switch operation. Transection of both the aorta and the pulmonary artery. Detachment of the coronary arteries along with a button from the aortic wall. The great arteries are then switched into their new position (LeCompte manoeuver; the aorta is moved behind the pulmonary artery). Transfer of the coronary arteries buttons to the neo (new) aorta anastomosis. Reconstruction of the neo-pulmonary artery (with autologous pericardium)

The procedure is performed with a median sternotomy incision, or, if the infant had a previous palliative procedure, the child is prepared for redo sternotomy. Individual surgeons may perform the surgery with circulatory arrest, depending on the child's age and anatomy.

1. After the sternotomy incision is made, a generous portion of the pericardium is excised for use as an autologous patch for the reconstruction of the neo-pulmonary artery.

2. The ductus arteriosus and both the pulmonary arteries (PA) and the aorta are mobilised. Some surgeons may place vessel loops around the right and left PA to isolate these structures.

3. The aorta and both superior and inferior vena cava are cannulated in a standard fashion and the child is placed on cardiopulmonary bypass. Ductus arteriosus is then ligated and divided to facilitate further mobilization of the left pulmonary artery. Cardioplegia needle is inserted into the aortic root, aorta is cross clamped and cardioplegia is administered.

4. The child is cooled to target temperature, during which time, the surgeon may further mobilise the PA and aorta.

5. If an atrial or ventricular septal defect is present, this will be repaired next. Usually, when the right atrium is opened a left ventricular vent will be placed in the left ventricle.

6. The aorta and pulmonary arteries are transected and some surgeons may place a traction or marking suture in the neo-aorta to mark the position of the coronary arteries transfer.

7. The coronary arteries are examined closely and the ostia (openings) and course of the coronary arteries are identified with a calibrated 1 mm coronary probe.

8. The coronary ostia and a large button of the aortic wall are excised (Fig. 5.144). The proximal sections of the coronary

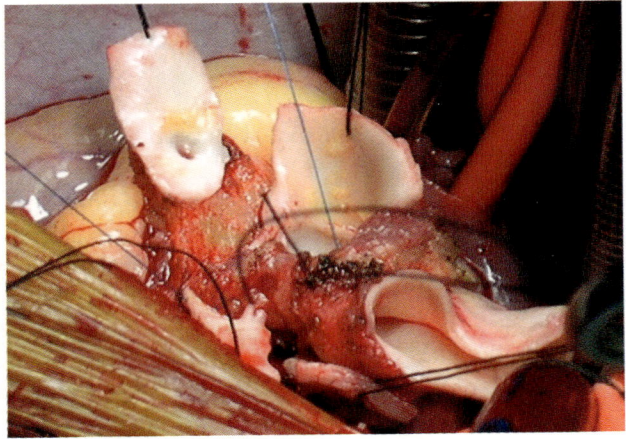

**Fig. 5.144:** The coronary ostia and a large button of surrounding aortic wall is excised. *(Photo by EDJ, courtesy of King Faisal Specialist Hospital, Jeddah, Saudi Arabia)*

arteries are separated from the surface of the heart, to prevent tension and distortion, after reimplantation into the neo-aorta.

9. Triangular buttons of similar size are made at the site of the PA root, to which the coronary arteries will be transferred.

10. The great arteries are then switched into their new position (LeCompte manoeuvre) (Fig. 5.146).

11. If at this stage, more cardioplegia needs to be given, a small coronary ostial cannula is placed in the left and right coronary ostia and cardioplegia is administered directly.

12. Next, the coronary arteries buttons are transferred to the neo (new) aorta.

13. Then, the distal aorta is sutured to the PA root to form the neo-aorta.

14. Some surgeons would like to reconstruct the neo-aorta first and then transfer the coronary arteries to the openings made to the sides of the neo-aorta.

15. Once the neo-aorta is reconstructed and the coronary arteries are transferred to it, the coronary arteries are occluded with fine clamps (e.g. neuroclips or coronary clamp) and haemostasis of all these anastomoses is checked. Extra sutures are applied if needed. The coronary clamps are then removed and this marks the end of cross clamp time. Systemic rewarming is commenced.

16. Recovery of normal ECG, good perfusion of all segments of the heart and good myocardial contractility are the signs of satisfactory coronary anastomoses.

17. If the surgeon is not satisfied with the perfusion of the heart at this stage, he may decide to apply the cross-clamp again, give cardioplegia and revise one or both coronary anastomoses.

18. Finally, the neo-pulmonary artery is reconstructed with autologous pericardium or other patch material depending on the surgeon's preference (Fig. 5.145).

19. After completion of the repair, the infant is weaned off the cardiopulmonary bypass machine. Left atrial pressure monitoring line, pacing wires and chest drains are inserted in a standard fashion. The sternum is closed.

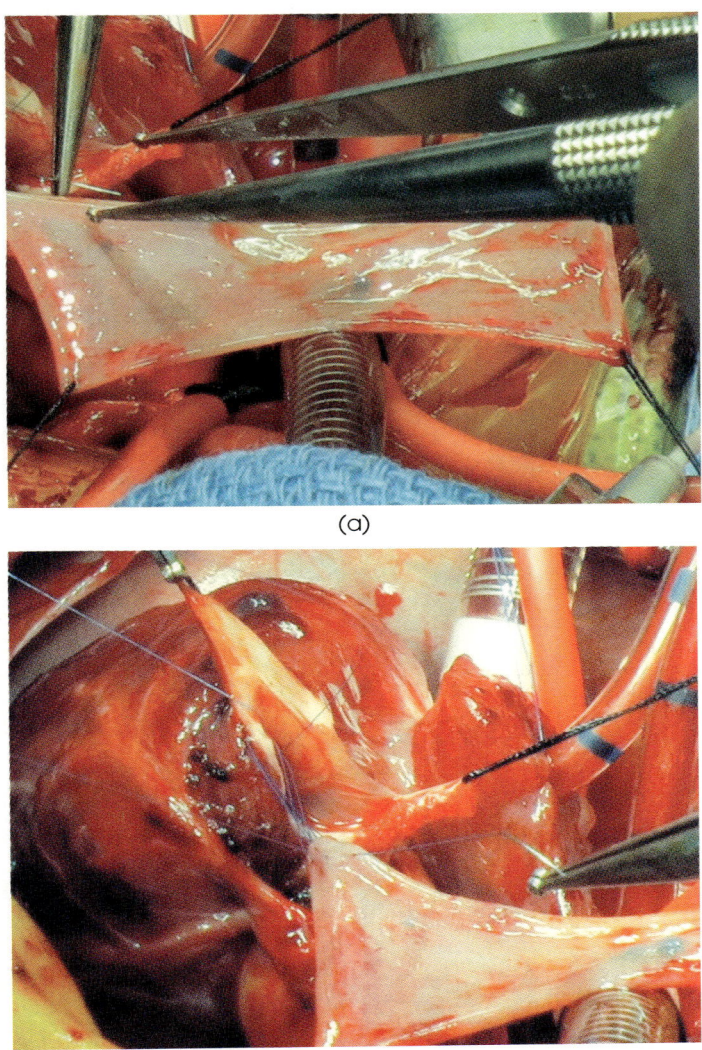

(a)

(b)

**Fig. 5.145:** The neopulmonary artery is reconstructed with autologous pericardium (a) or other patch material depending on the surgeon's preference and sewn onto the aortic root (neo-PA) with a 6–0 or 7–0 polypropylene suture  (b). *(Photo (a), (b) by EDJ, courtesy of KAMC, National Guard Hospital, Riyadh, Saudi Arabia)*

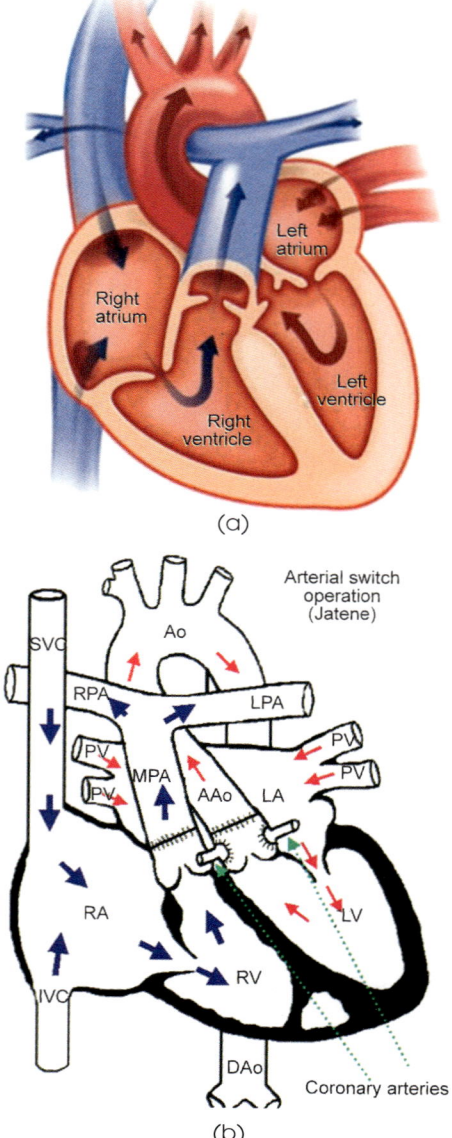

(a)

(b)

**Fig. 5.146:** The Jatene arterial switch procedure. *Note:* The aorta lies behind the pulmonary artery (LeCompte Manoeuver, (b)); compare normal position of the aorta and pulmonary artery as shown in picture (a).

*The perioperative scrub nurse should be familiar with the surgeon's preference regarding the use of autologous pericardium and in which way the surgeon prefers the autologous patch to be preserved. Some surgeons may prefer to use a pulmonary homograft patch or other material for reconstruction of the neo-pulmonary artery. Have fine coronary probes available for checking the patency and course of the coronary arteries.*

*Furthermore, have knowledge whether the child has a ventricular septal defect, and some children with TGA may have an atrial septal defect, either will be repaired during initial correction of TGA. Tissue glue and other haemostatic material may be required.*

*The arterial switch operation is a fascinating procedure and can be well observed by the perioperative nurse, since the repair is outside the heart, making it an excellent opportunity for the perioperative scrub nurse to advance in assisting the surgeon in more complex surgical procedures.*

*Standard cannulation procedure for a neonate is observed with bicaval cannulation and snares around the vena cavae. First cardioplegia delivery is done with usual an aortic root cannula but subsequent doses have to be gives by a non-traumatic fine coronary cannula (e.g. olive-tip cannula).*

*Fine instruments are required for coronary anastomoses. Thus, full coronary set usually, used by the surgeon for coronary artery surgery should be available including fine coronary probes and coronary suckers.*

*As multiple anastomoses need to be tested during the haemostasis phase, a good supply of irrigation fluid, irrigation syringes and fine sutures should be available. Interruption of flow at this stage is usually very frustrating for the surgeon and also increases the cross clamp and myocardial ischaemia time unnecessarily.*

*As mentioned above, the scrub nurse should be mentally prepared that the surgeon might re-apply the cross clamp, repeat cardioplegia dose and re-do one or the other coronary anastomosis if he is not happy with the recovery of the heart.*

*Left atrial monitoring line is a must as it shows the performance of the left ventricle at the time of weaning from bypass and later in the intensive care unit.*

## *Outcome of Surgical Repair*

The Jatene procedure is an anatomic correction of transposition of the great arteries. After the operation the left ventricle becomes the systemic ventricle, which is better suited for the systemic circulation than the right ventricle. Children do very well after the Jatene procedure especially, if performed early in infancy. Long-term problems, may be coronary stenosis, distortion of the pulmonary arteries, dilatation of the neo-aortic root, and aortic valve regurgitation.

## Rastelli Procedure—Overview

### History

The Rastelli procedure was initially used for the repair of *d*-transposition of the great arteries (*d*-TGA) with a ventricular septal defect and pulmonary stenosis. In such infants, an arterial switch repair is not amendable since the pulmonary stenosis, would convert to aortic stenosis. In the Rastelli procedure, the ventricular septal defect is closed with a patch, in such a way, that it redirects the blood flow from the left ventricle (which is connected to the pulmonary artery in *d*-TGA) to the aorta. The pulmonary valve is oversewn and an extracardiac conduit is placed between the right ventricle and the pulmonary artery (usually the pulmonary confluence). However, if this procedure is performed early in infancy, the child will outgrow the conduit and will need a second operation to replace it.

Giancarlo Rastelli (1934–1970) whom the procedure is named after, was a pioneer cardiac surgeon (Fig. 5.147). He was born in Italy. The Rastelli procedure was first performed at the Mayo Clinic, USA in 1968. It was first described as a possible repair of truncus arteriosus and then evolved into an operation applicable to children born with *d*-TGA with a VSD and pulmonary stenosis, VSD with pulmonary stenosis, double outlet right ventricle, and also for *l*-TGA with pulmonary stenosis. Long-term outcomes of the Rastelli may not always be good due to conduit related problems.

## Rastelli Repair—Technique

1. The patient is cannulated with an aortic cannula in the ascending aorta and bicaval venous cannulation in both superior vena cava (SVC) and inferior vena cava (IVC).
2. Both SVC and IVC are encircled with caval tapes and snared.
3. The aorta is then cross clamped and cardioplegia is administered.

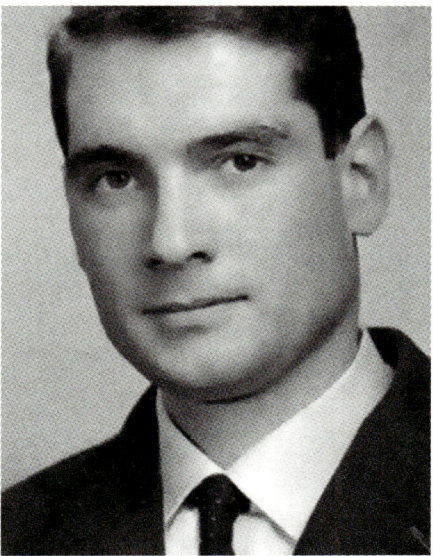

**Fig. 5.147:** Giancarlo Rastelli (1934–1970) was an Italian cardiac surgeon. He was the creator of the Rastelli procedure. He died of cancer at just 36 years of age. At the time of his death he was the head of cardiovascular surgical research at the Mayo Clinic, USA

4. A left ventricular vent is inserted through a purse string suture at the junction of the right upper pulmonary vein and the left atrium and then advanced across the mitral valve into the left ventricle.
5. Next, the ventricular septal defect (VSD) is visualized through a right ventriculotomy.
6. Obstructive left ventricular muscle is excised, and a large intra-ventricular baffle is sutured into place closing the VSD and redirecting left ventricular outflow to the more anteriorly placed aortic valve.
7. The pulmonary valve is oversewn and an extracardiac conduit is placed between the right ventricle and the pulmonary artery (usually the pulmonary confluence) (Fig. 5.148).
8. After completion of the repair, the child is weaned from cardiopulmonary bypass.
9. Pacing wires and chest drains are inserted in a standard fashion. The sternum is closed if the child is stable.

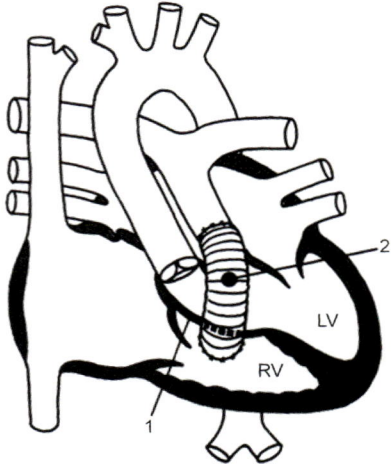

**Fig. 5.148:** The Rastelli operation—the VSD is patched to tunnel blood from the LV into the aorta (1). The pulmonary valve is oversewn, and a valved conduit is inserted from the RV to the pulmonary artery (2)

---

**NURSING OBSERVATION**

*The perioperative scrub nurse should be familiar with surgeon's preference regarding material used for the baffle, the infant's own pericardium, commercially available bovine or porcine pericardium, or synthetic material (Gore-Tex™, Dacron).*

*The pulmonary valve is oversewn and an extracardiac conduit is placed between the right ventricle and the pulmonary artery. Be familiar with which material is used for the conduit and suture material used for the anastomosis. As multiple anastomoses need to be tested during the haemostasis phase, a good supply of irrigation fluid, irrigation syringes and fine sutures should be available. Tissue glue and other haemostatic material may be required.*

## Outcome of Surgical Repair

Statisfactory postoperative haemodynamics are dependent on free unobstructed blood flow from both the left and right ventricles. Obstruction to either outflow tract will contribute to ventricular failure. Arrhythmia is a potential postoperative complication and temporary atrioventricular pacing capability must be readily available. Uncomplicated recovery from the Rastelli operation should result in a hospital stay of one to two weeks. Late postoperative complications include recurrent left ventricular outflow tract obstruction, early conduit obstruction and arrhythmias. If the

Rastelli procedure is performed early in infancy, the child will outgrow the conduit and will need a second operation to replace it.

## Nikaidoh Procedure—Overview

### History

An alternative to the Rastelli procedure for $d$-TGA with VSD and pulmonary stenosis is the Nikaidoh procedure. This procedure was first reported by Nikaidoh (Fig. 5.149) in 1984.[106] In this procedure the aorta, including the native aortic valve and the coronary arteries is translocated from the right ventricle to the left ventricle, without transferring the coronary arteries separately, as in the arterial switch operation. The left ventricular outflow tract obstruction is excised before the aorta is sutured onto the pulmonary annulus (left ventricle). The ventricular septal defect is closed. The pulmonary artery, including the native pulmonary valve is sutured onto the right ventricle, often requiring an additional patch.

Modifications to the original technique may be individual coronary artery transfer, the use of the Lecompte manoeuvre, the placement of a conduit between the right ventricle and the pulmonary artery (Rastelli).

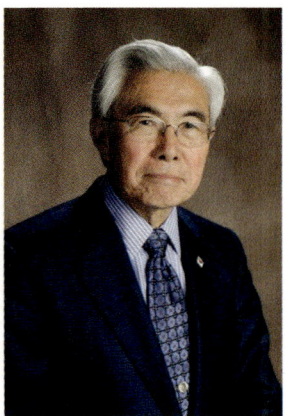

**Fig. 5.149:** Dr Hisashi Nikaidoh a world-renowned paediatric cardiac surgeon. Born in Tokyo, Nikaidoh is a legend among his fellow surgeons for pioneering what has come to be known as the Nikaidoh procedure. First performed in 1983, this surgery has gained worldwide acceptance for the treatment of children with TGA, VSD and PS

## Nikaidoh Operation—Technique

1. Via a standard median sternotomy incision cardiopulmonary bypass is established with a single right atrial cannula or with bicaval cannulation and a left ventricular vent.
2. The child is cooled to 28–30°C.
3. A piece of pericardium is harvested to use for reconstruction of the right ventricular outflow tract.
4. Extensive mobilization of both left and right coronary arteries is carried out (Fig. 5.150) before the aorta including the aortic valve is harvested from the right ventricle. The proximal pulmonary artery and pulmonary valve is also divided (Fig. 5.151).
5. The left ventricle is then opened, the outflow tract obstruction is excised and the aortic root including the coronary arteries (Fig. 5.152) and the aortic valve is sutured (translocated) to the pulmonary annulus (Fig. 5.153). The posterior aspect of the aortic root is sutured to the pulmonary annulus first.

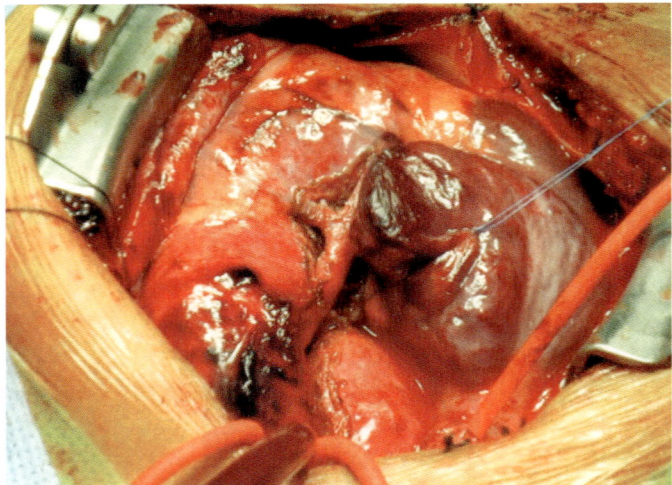

**Fig. 5.150:** Extensive mobilization of both left and right coronary arteries is carried out. This can be done on a beating heart to shorten the bypass and cross clamp time. The aorta attached to the right ventricle and mobilization of right coronary artery can be seen in the picture. The right atrium is retracted with a suture. Picture is taken standing at the head of the child. *(Photo by EDJ, courtesy of KAMC, National Guard Hospital, Riyadh, Saudi Arabia)*

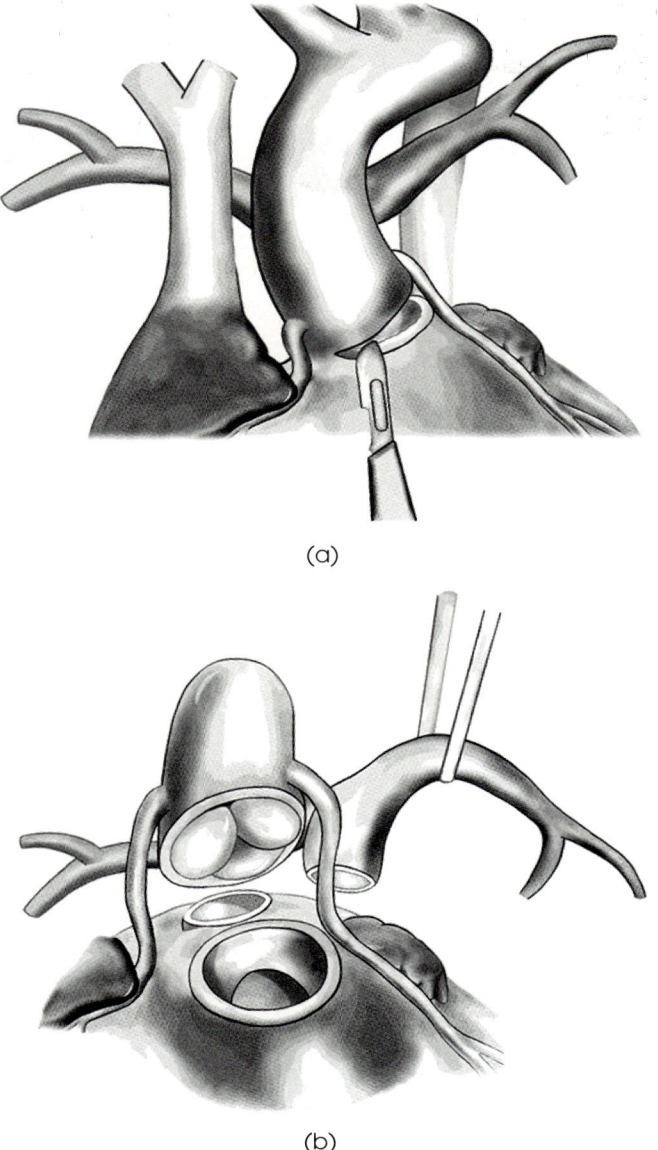

(a)

(b)

**Fig. 5.151:** The aortic root including the native valve and the coronary arteries is transected from the right ventricle (a). The pulmonary artery including the pulmonary valve is transected from the left ventricle (b)

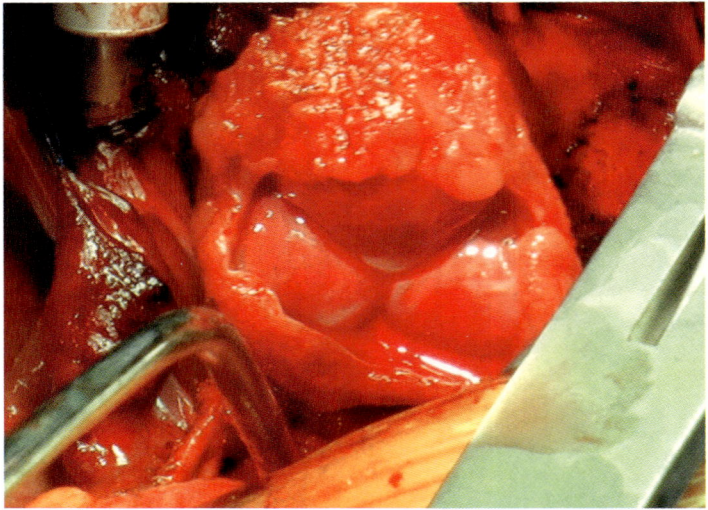

**Fig. 5.152:** The aorta including the coronary arteries, the aortic valve (as shown in picture) is harvested from the right ventricle. *(Photo by EDJ, courtesy of KAMC, National Guard Hospital, Riyadh, Saudi Arabia)*

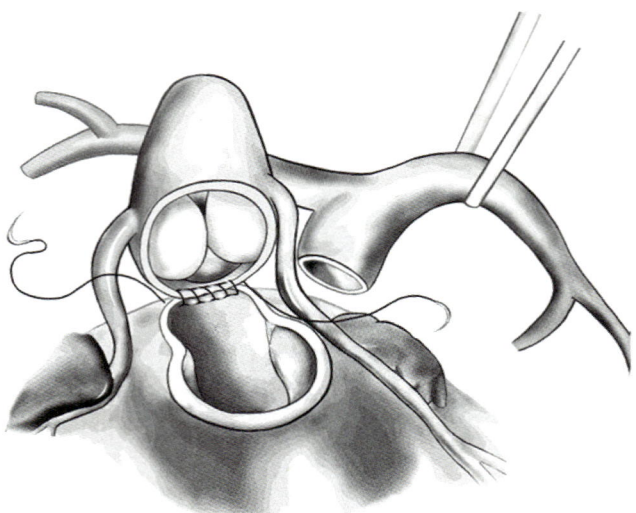

**Fig. 5.153:** The left ventricular outflow tract obstruction is excised, the aortic root including the coronary arteries is sutured on to the left ventricle

6. Then the ventricular septal defect is closed with a patch (Fig. 5.154). The aorta is transected more proximally to perform the LeCompte manoeuvre and reanastomosed with a poly-propylene suture. Then the anterior aspect of the aortic root is sutured onto the left ventricular outflow tract, completing the aorta translocation.

7. Finally, the proximal main pulmonary artery is connected directly to the right ventricle and augmented with an additional piece of pericardial patch (Fig. 5.156).

8. After repair the child is weaned off the cardiopulmonary bypass, pacing wires and chest drains are inserted and the chest is closed in a standard fashion.

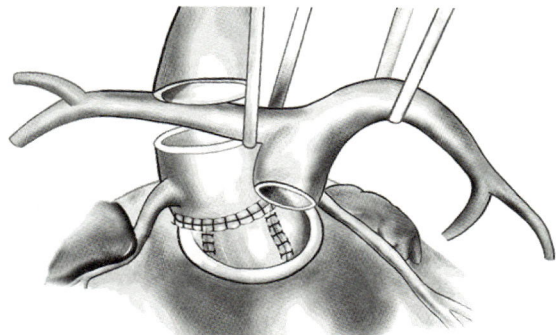

**Fig. 5.154:** The VSD is closed with a patch. The aorta is transected more proximally to perform the LeCompte manoeuver

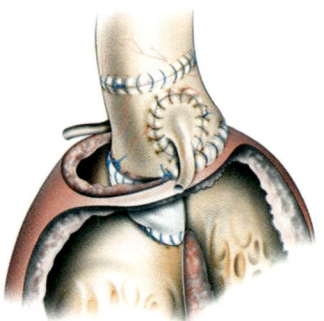

**Fig. 5.155:** In some cases, one of the coronary arteries may have to be harvested and reinserted depending on the anatomy of the child

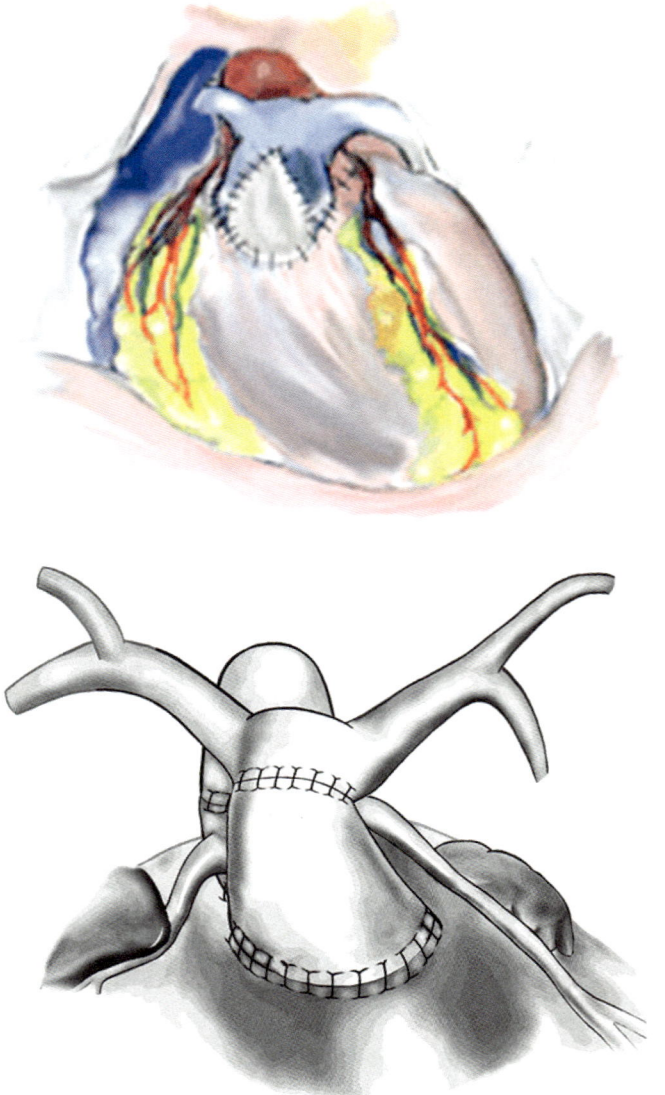

**Fig. 5.156:** The pulmonary artery including pulmonary valve is sutured to the right ventricle outflow tract opening. A further pericardial patch is used to complete the anastomosis of the pulmonary artery to the right ventricle

## NURSING OBSERVATION

The Nikaidah operation is a technically complex procedure and has only been performed in a few centres worldwide at present. Most Nikaidoh procedures have been performed by Nikaidoh himself. For the scrub nurse to prepare and assist the surgeon in a Nikaidoh procedure will demand from the nurse to be focussed at all times and have the knowledge and experience in assisting the surgeon with what can be a daunting procedure not only for the surgeon but for the whole team. The number of techniques that surgeons have developed for successfully transferring coronary arteries in the arterial switch procedure can be directly applied in the aortic translocation technique, if the coronary arteries appear kinked at the time of the translocation and the scrub nurse should have knowledge of the arterial switch operation, in which the coronary arteries are routinely transferred and use this knowledge in the Nikaidoh procedure. The experience of harvesting the pulmonary autograft for the Ross procedure in a similar fashion has trained the surgeon to perform aortic translocation for the Nikaidoh procedure. As multiple anastomoses need to be tested during the haemostasis phase, a good supply of irrigation fluid, irrigation syringes and fine sutures should be available. Tissue glue and other haemostatic material may be required.

## SURGEON'S COMMENT

The Rastelli is more commonly performed than the Nikaidoh procedure for transposition with VSD and pulmonary stenosis. Standard bicaval cannulation is done and cardiopulmonary bypass is instituted with moderate hypothermia. Aorta is cross clamped and cardioplegia is given in the aortic root. A left atrial vent is placed.

An opening is made in the anterior wall of the right ventricle (Ventriculotomy) and through this ventriculotomy, a generous patch of treated autologous pericardium, bovine pericardium or Gore-Tex™ is placed around the VSD and the aortic root, forming an intraventricular tunnel that directs the left ventricular blood towards the aorta. If there is an ASD, it is closed. Air is then removed from the left heart and aortic cross clamp is removed.

The main pulmonary artery is then disconnected from the left ventricle and a conduit (Contegra or a pulmonary homograft) is then anastomosed on one side to the right ventriculotomy and on the other side to the pulmonary bifurcation (RV to PA conduit).

Usual material used are the large size VSD patch and RV to PA conduit of the surgeon's choice. Continuous polypropylene sutures are used for making the intraventricular tunnel).

## Outcome of Surgical Repair

The overall experience with the Nikaidoh operation is somewhat limited and there are just a few reports in the medical literature.[107] The Nikaidoh procedure results in a more normal anatomic repair. The left and right ventricular outflow tracts are better aligned then with the Rastelli repair.[108]

### Damus-Kaye-Stansel Procedure (DKS)—Overview

#### History

The Damus-Kaye-Stansel (DKS) was originally developed along with the Rastelli procedure. The DKS is reserved for patients with transposition of the great arteries with subaortic stenosis. The operation involves division of the main pulmonary artery and connection to the side of the ascending aorta, so that the left ventricle is reconnected to the aorta (Fig. 5.157). To re-establish pulmonary blood flow a Blalock-Taussig shunt, Glenn shunt or

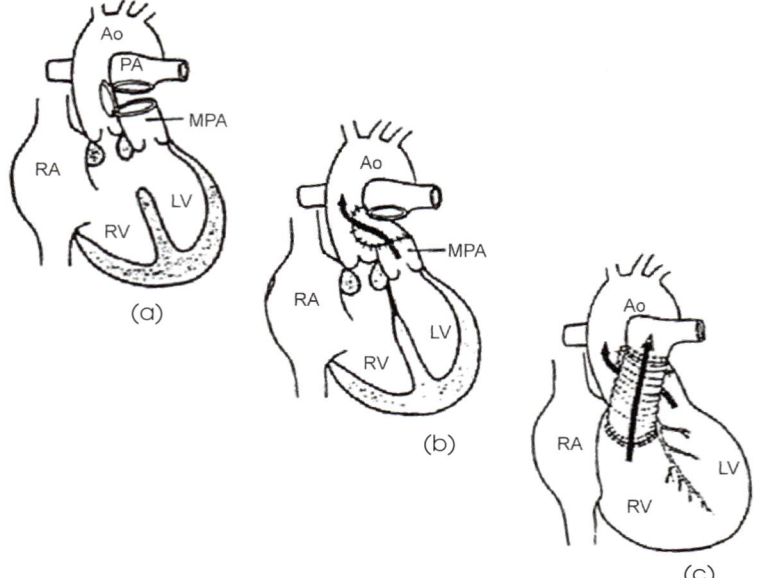

**Fig. 5.157:** Main pulmonary artery to ascending aorta (Damus-Kaye-Stansel) and a right ventricle-to-pulmonary artery anastomosis using a Gore-Tex™ graft to re-establish pulmonary blood flow (Rastelli), in a child with TGA and subaortic stenosis

right ventricle-to-pulmonary artery anastomosis with a conduit (Rastelli) procedure is performed. At a later stage, the Fontan procedure is performed, if previous Glenn procedure.

The DKS operation was first described in 1975 independently by 3 surgeons, Damus, Kaye and Stansel, and proved soon to be an effective method for patients with TGA and subaortic stenosis.[109–111]

The DKS may also be performed in children with other forms of complex congenital heart disease in which systemic outflow is obstructed (left ventricular outflow tract obstruction).

## DKS Procedure—Technique

1. Via a standard median sternotomy incision cardiopulmonary bypass is established with an arterial cannula in the aorta, bicaval venous cannulation and a left ventricular vent.
2. Both SVC and IVC are encircled with caval tapes and snared.
3. The aorta is then cross clamped and cardioplegia is administered.
4. A left ventricular vent is inserted through a purse string suture at the junction of the right upper pulmonary vein and the left atrium and then advanced across the mitral valve into the left ventricle.
5. Next, the ventricular septal defect (VSD) is visualized through a right ventriculotomy and closed with a patch (there is no need to excise right ventricular outflow tract obstructive muscle, since the subaortic stenosis will be bypassed by the anastomosis of the pulmonary artery-to-side of aorta proximal to the stenosis).
6. The pulmonary artery is then transected and the proximal end is anastomed to the side of the aorta. A conduit is placed between the right ventricle and the pulmonary confluence to re-establish the pulmonary circulation in the case of biventricular repair. Alternative, a BTS, Glenn and at a later stage the final Fontan procedure is performed in cases in which only a univentricular repair can be offered.
7. After completion of the repair, the child is weaned from cardiopulmonary bypass.
8. Pacing wires and chest drains are inserted in a standard fashion. The sternum is closed if the child is stable.

## *Outcome of Surgical Repair*

Late complications of the DKS procedure include recurrence of systemic ventricular outflow tract obstruction and regurgitaion of the pulmonary valve. If a conduit is used in the case of biventricular repair, late conduit obstruction may occur, and replacement of the conduit when procedure is carried out at a young age, is unavoidable.

**Section 4**

## ANOMALIES OF THE GREAT ARTERIES (ANOMALIES OF THE PULMONARY ARTERY AND AORTA)

In this section, the most common anomalies of the pulmonary artery and aorta will be discussed. Anomalous origin of the left coronary artery from the pulmonary artery (ALCAPA) is an example of an anomalous pulmonary artery. Coarctation, interrupted aortic arch, aortopulmonary window and hypoplastic left heart syndrome are examples of anomalies of the aorta.

## ANOMALOUS ORIGIN OF THE LEFT CORONARY ARTERY FROM THE PULMONARY ARTERY

### Introduction

Anomalous origin of the left coronary artery from the pulmonary artery (ALCAPA) is a heart defect in which the left coronary artery is connected to the pulmonary artery instead of the aorta (Fig. 5.158). This defect often results in myocardial ischaemia and infarction in infants and children. To compensate for the lack of the normal two coronary arteries, which supply the heart muscle with blood, collateral arteries may develop between the left and right coronary arteries and depending on their development,

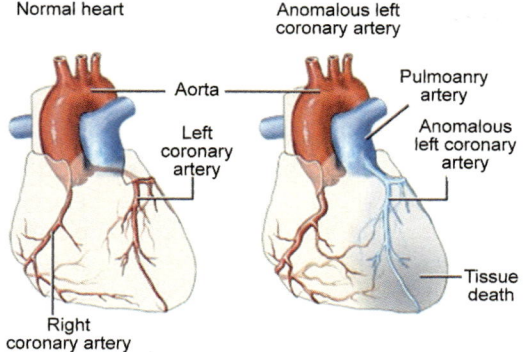

Normal heart

Anomalous left coronary artery

Aorta

Left coronary artery

Right coronary artery

Pulmoanry artery

Anomalous left coronary artery

Tissue death

**Fig. 5.158:** Anomalous origin of the left coronary artery from the pulmonary artery (ALCAPA)

myocardial ischaemia and/or infarction may not occur till adulthood. ALCAPA was first described in 1866. The first clinical description in conjunction with autopsy findings was described by Bland, White and Garland in 1933, hence the anomaly may also be referred to as the **Bland-White-Garland syndrome**.[112]

## What Causes ALCAPA?

The ALCAPA anomaly may result from abnormal septation of the conotruncus into the aorta and pulmonary artery.

## Prevalence

It is a rare but serious condition, affecting 1 in every 300,000 live births.[113] It usually manifests as an isolated heart defect but in 5% of cases it may be associated with an atrial septal defect, ventricular septal defect, and aortic coarctation. Occurrence is generally similar between males and females. No risk factors for the occurrence of ALCAPA in any individual family are known, and ALCAPA is not associated with any syndromes or noncardiac conditions.[114]

## Symptoms

ALCAPA is one of the most common causes of myocardial ischaemia and infarction in children. This is due to the fact that the left coronary artery is connected to the pulmonary artery instead of the aorta. Left coronary artery flow reverses and enters the pulmonary artery due to the low pulmonary vascular resistance (coronary steal phenomena). As a result, left ventricular myocardium remains underperfused. Consequently, the combination of left ventricular dysfunction with significant mitral valve insufficiency as a result, leads to congestive heart failure (CHF) symptoms (e.g., tachypnoea, poor feeding, irritability) in the young infant. Approximately 85% of children present with clinical symptoms of CHF within the first 1–2 months of life. About 90% of children diagnosed with this anomaly die within the first year without surgical intervention. The differences between the infant and adult types of ALCAPA syndrome, the importance of developing intercoronary collateral vessels, and the different clinical manifestations are summarized in a diagram (Fig. 5.159).

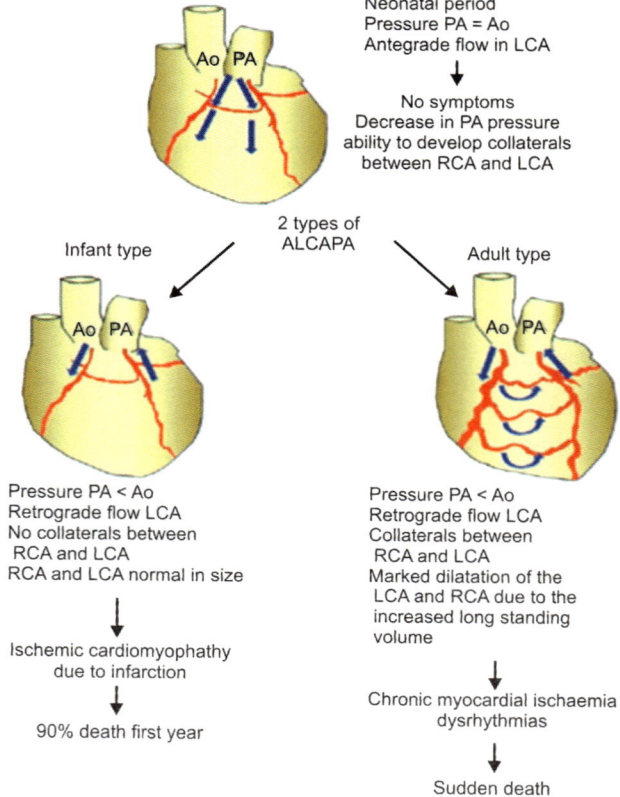

**Fig. 5.159:** Diagram shows the spectrum of pathophysiologic changes that take place after birth in patients with ALCAPA syndrome. The differences between the infant and adult types of ALCAPA syndrome, the importance of developing intercoronary collateral vessels, and the different clinical manifestations are summarized

## Treatment

Different surgical approaches have been reported, including ligation of the ALCAPA, direct reimplantation of the left coronary artery in the aorta, Takeuchi procedure, and the use of arterial grafts or saphenous vein grafts, to create a double coronary artery system. The direct implantation of the ALCAPA into the ascending aorta seems to be ideal but might be difficult in some children, for example, if the intramural course of the coronary artery or origin of the coronary artery is at great distance from the ascending aorta, making direct implantation impossible. In these children, an intrapulmonary aortocoronary tunnel may be considered. This approach was described by Takeuchi in 1979.[115] Fortunately in most children, the anomalous left coronary artery is situated in a position that allows for direct transfer of the anomalous coronary artery. Direct anastomosis of the anomalous left coronary artery from the pulmonary artery directly to the aorta was described in the 1970s and currently remains the procedure of choice. The experience gained in coronary artery transfer during the arterial switch operation has facilitated techniques for coronary transfer to repair the anomalous left coronary artery from the pulmonary artery.

### ALCAPA Repair—Technique

Implantation of the left anomalous coronary artery into the aorta is the operation of choice in most institutions. The aim is to provide a two-coronary artery system to achieve a complete recovery of myocardial ischaemia. The operation may be performed using either continuous low flow bypass with moderate hypothermia (25 to 28°C) or deep hypothermic circulatory arrest (18°C) in very small infants.

1. A median sternotomy is performed and the thymus is resected.
2. The pericardium is opened and suspended with silk sutures.
3. An aortic purse string is placed distally near the innominate artery (Fig. 5.160).
4. A purse string is placed in the right atrial appendage for a single venous cannula.
5. Heparin is administered, the aortic and right atrial cannulae are inserted, and cardiopulmonary bypass is commenced.
6. Anatomy of the pulmonary artery and epicardial course of the anomalous coronary artery are identified to determine whether direct reimplantation is possible.

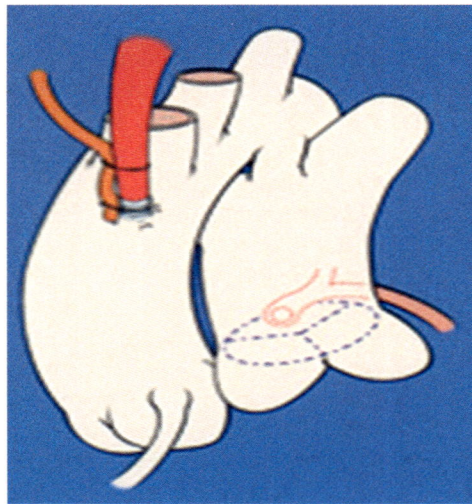

**Fig. 5.160:** The ascending aorta is cannulated very close to the innominate artery to provide a long length of ascending aorta for the cardioplegia site and for the orifice that is to be created on the side of the aorta for the aortic implantation

7. The aorta is fully mobilized as well as the right and left pulmonary arteries.
8. The ductus arteriosus is ligated and divided.
9. Tourniquets are placed around both the right and left pulmonary arteries (Fig. 5.161).
10. Cardioplegia purse string followed by cardioplegia needle is placed in the ascending aorta, aorta is cross clamped and cold cardioplegia solution is administered via the aortic root.
11. The aortic cross clamp will be carefully placed and a cardioplegia needle is being used to infuse cardioplegia into the proximal ascending aorta. The snares on the right and left pulmonary arteries create a closed chamber in the main pulmonary artery, and prevent run-off of cardioplegia solution into the lungs (most patients have collaterals from the right coronary artery (RCA) to the left main coronary artery (LMCA). This means that cardioplegia will flow through the RCA-collaterals-LMCA into the pulmonary artery and lungs unless the right and left pulmonary arteries are snared). The infant is cooled to 28°C.

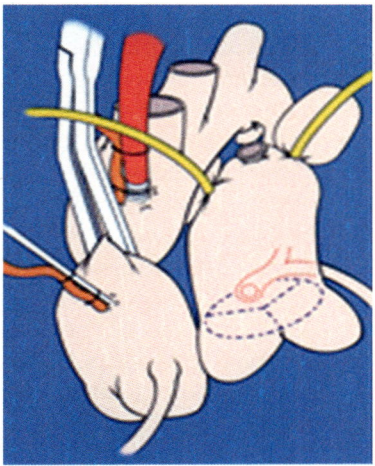

**Fig. 5.161:** The aortic cross clamp will be carefully placed and a cardioplegia needle is being used to infuse cardioplegia into the proximal ascending aorta. The snares on the right and left pulmonary arteries create a closed chamber in the main pulmonary artery, and prevent run-off of cardioplegia solution into the lungs

12. If circulatory arrest is used, the head vessels are occluded, circulation is arrested, venous blood is drained into the reservoir (of CPB machine) and both arterial and venous cannulae are removed.

13. The pulmonary artery is transected next (Fig. 5.162).

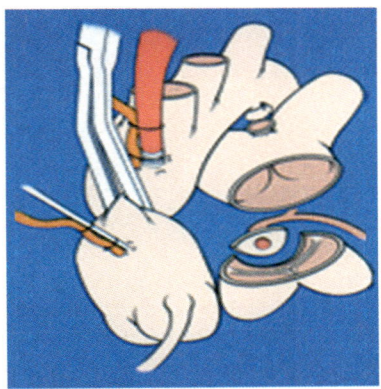

**Fig. 5.162:** The pulmonary artery is transected

14. After the first dose of cardioplegia, the main pulmonary artery is transected (the right and left pulmonary arteries are snared and the patent ductus arteriosus is ligated and divided). The coronary artery button is developed in a fashion similar to developing a button for a coronary transfer in the arterial switch operation. It may be necessary to leave a large amount of pulmonary artery tissue attached to the button to create adequate length for the transfer.

15. The aorta is opened as in the arterial switch operation. The coronary button is carefully aligned with the incision in the aorta to avoid twisting or kinking. The anastomosis is with a continuous 7-0 or 8-0 nonabsorbable polypropylene suture. The aorta is closed with a continuous 7-0 nonabsorbable polypropylene suture.

16. After completion of the aortic closure, cardioplegia may be administered and the anastomosis inspected to ensure adequate filling of the coronary and to asses haemostasis.

17. The pulmonary artery may be repaired with a patch of autologous pericardium as in the arterial switch operation. Cross clamp may be taken off and rewarming is begun before pulmonary artery repair (Fig. 5.163).

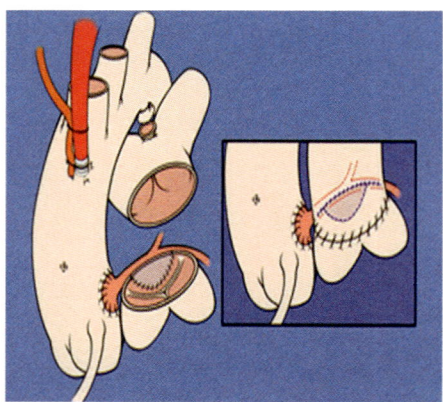

**Fig. 5.163:** The aortic cross clamp is now off. The posterior site of the pulmonary artery where the button was harvested is reconstructed with a patch of fresh autologous pericardium. The pulmonary artery is reanastomosed at the site of the transection as illustrated in the small inset. Reconstruction of the pulmonary artery with the cross clamp off, helps to minimize the aortic cross clamp time

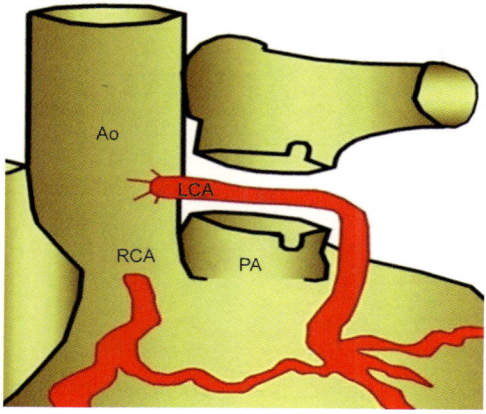

**Fig. 5.164:** Diagram shows coronary button transfer. In this procedure, the LCA is reimplanted into the aorta (Ao) with a button from the pulmonary artery (PA) wall. Coronary button transfer is the most commonly used procedure in newborns and is the most anatomic correction

18. Pulmonary artery is closed. The site of the pulmonary artery where the button was harvested is reconstructed with a patch, usually, autologous pericardium (Fig. 5.164).
19. As the child is slowly rewarmed, inotropic support is started.
20. Atrial and ventricular pacing wires are inserted.
21. Chest drains are inserted and chest closed if child is stable.

In some cases, when the ALCAPA is farthest away from the aorta or in which the anomalous coronary artery takes an intramural course between the great arteries, direct implantation is technically not possible. In these situations, other surgical approaches have been reported to combat this problem. Takeuchi and colleagues reported the creation of an intrapulmonary baffle to direct the left coronary artery into the ascending aorta (Fig. 5.165). In the original procedure, an aortopulmonary window was created and a portion of the anterior pulmonary artery wall used to create a baffle that directed blood from the aorta to the ostium of the anomalous coronary artery. In the modified Takeuchi procedure the baffle is constructed with a piece of bovine pericardium. However, this technique has drawbacks, such as baffle obstruction and pulmonary artery obstruction.

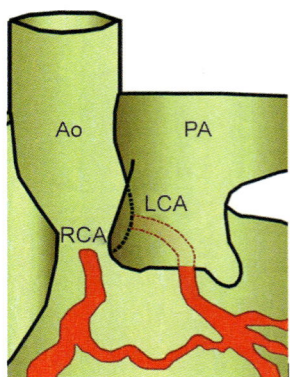

**Fig. 5.165:** Takeuchi approach—an intrapulmonary aortocoronary tunnel is created in infants in which direct implantation of the ALCAPA is technically not possible

### Nursing Observation

*The ALCAPA procedure is somewhat similar to the arterial switch operation with translocation of the coronary arteries. Because of the preoperative left ventricular dysfunction, inotropic support may not be adequate and support with extracorporeal membrane oxygenation (ECMO) may be necessary. The Takeuchi repair involves creation of an aortopulmonary window and an intrapulmonary tunnel that baffles the aorta to the ostium (opening) of the anomalous left coronary artery. Again this type of surgery has similarities with the arterial switch operation. For the baffle a piece of autogolous pericardium or bovine patch can be used. During the haemostasis phase, a good supply of irrigation fluid, irrigation syringes and fine sutures should be available. Tissue glue and other haemostatic material may be required.*

### Surgeon's Comment

*These patients usually have very poor left ventricular function due to abnormal coronary flow. Thus, they are high-risk for anaesthesia induction, for development of arrhythmias and for need of inotropes and ECMO.*

*Cannulation is standard with aortic and right atrial cannula. Critical part of surgery is transfer to coronary artery without any kinks or twists. Fine coronary instruments and coronary probes will be required.*

### *Outcome of Surgical Repair*

Nowadays, the prognosis for children with ALCAPA has dramatically improved due to a result of both early diagnosis and improvements in surgical techniques, including myocardial preservation. Most babies do well with timely treatment and can expect a normal life.

## Section 4.1: Anomalies of the Aorta

Development of the aorta takes place during the third week of gestation. It is a complex process that can lead to a variety of congenital variants and pathological anomalies. This section presents the most common anomalies of the aorta and aortic arch. The aorta comprises of the ascending aorta, tranverse or aortic arch and the descending aorta. Three major arteries originate from the aortic arch: the brachiocephalic or innominate artery, the left common carotid artery and the left subclavian artery which all supply blood to the brain and head (Figs 5.166 and 5.167).

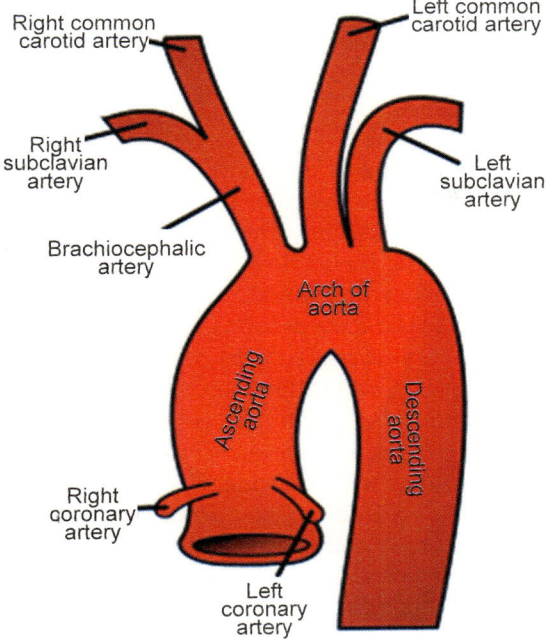

**Fig. 5.166:** Three major arteries originate from the aortic arch: the brachiocephalic or innominate artery, the left common carotid artery and the left subclavian artery, which supply blood to the brain and head

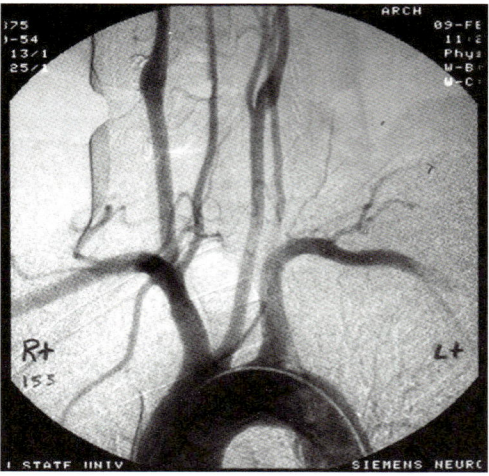

**Fig. 5.167:** Angiogram of the aortic arch with the three major vessels

## COARCTATION OF THE AORTA (CoA)

### Introduction

Coarctation of the aorta is a constricted segment of the aorta typically just distal to the origin of the left subclavian artery and close to the level of the ductus arteriosus (Fig. 5.168). It increases resistance to the aortic blood flow resulting in the left ventricle having to work harder to maintain flow through the narrowed segment. Pressure in the aorta proximal to, or before the narrowing is high, whereas pressure distal to or beyond the narrowing segment is often low. Coarctation may be detected by evaluating blood pressure and pulses in all four extremities. Blood pressure in the extremities perfused by the aorta proximal to the coarctation will be high, and pulses will be strong, whereas the blood pressure in the extremities perfused by the aorta distal to or beyond the coarctation will be low, and pulses will be weaker. It may occur as an isolated defect or with other lesions, most commonly bicuspid aortic valve or a ventricular septal defect. Sometimes, coarctation is a complicating feature of a more complex congenital heart defect, such as transposition of the great arteries, and hypoplastic left heart syndrome.

Aortic arch hypolasia coexist in varying degrees depending on the severity of the coarctation.

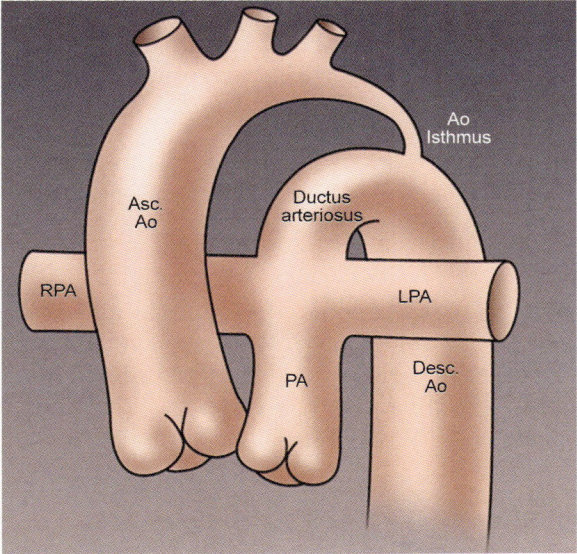

**Fig. 5.168:** Coarctation of the aorta is a constricted segment of the aorta typically just distal to the origin of the left subclavian artery and close to the level of the ductus arteriosus

## What Causes Coarctation?

### Two-Coarctation Theories

Firstly, the ductal tissue theory suggests that ductal tissue migrates into the aorta and causes constriction and consequent narrowing of the aortic lumen similar to that which occurs when the ductus constricts and closes soon after birth. This theory would explain, that the neonate will demonstrate cyanosis, and signs of poor systemic perfusion and shock, soon after birth, when the ductus begins to close and if the coarctation is located proximal to (before) the ductus arteriosus (preductal coarctation) and descending aortic blood flow is dependent on the ductus arteriosus.

Secondly, the haemodynamic theory suggests that reduced blood flow due to for instance, malformation of the aortic valve, causes underdevelopment of the aortic isthmus. The aortic isthmus is a slight constriction of the aorta immediately distal to or beyond the left subclavian artery at the point of attachment of the ductus arteriosus.

The diagnosis of coarctation may be missed until the patient develops signs of congestive heart failure, usually within the first weeks of life, in severe coarctation, or hypertension, which usually does not develop until adulthood. Coarctation is the most common heart defect associated with Turner syndrome.[xvi]

## Prevalence

Coarctation of the aorta is a relatively common defect that accounts for 5–8% of all congenital heart defects. Coarctation is more common in males than in females (3:1).

## Symptoms

In the neonate, the patent ductus arteriosus may allow for adequate blood flow to the lower body. However, when the patent ductus arteriosus closes, as typically occurs after 10 to 24 hours after a full term birth, the child may present as an emergency, as blood flow to the lower body will be severely compromised.

## Treatment

Most surgical repairs for coarctation of the aorta are closed heart procedures, without the use of cardiopulmonary bypass. The operation is generally performed via a left thoracotomy. The original coarctation repair is accomplished by resection of the coarctation section and end-to-end anastomosis of the proximal and distal segments. In infants, where the narrowing of the aorta extends into the aortic arch, the anastomosis can be fashioned in a manner that it uses the under side of the aortic arch to enlarge the

---

[xvi]Turner syndrome is a chromosomal abnormality in which all or part of one of the sex chromosomes is absent (unaffected humans have 46 chromosomes, of which two are sex chromosomes). Normal females have two X chromosomes, but in Turner syndrome, one of those sex chromosomes is missing or has other abnormalities. In some cases, the chromosome is missing in some cells but not others. It occurs only in females with a prevalence of in 1 in 2000 to 1 in 5000. The syndrome manifests itself in a number of ways. There are characteristic physical abnormalities, such as short stature, swelling, broad chest, low hairline, low-set ears, and webbed necks. Girls with Turner syndrome typically experience gonadal dysfunction (non-working ovaries), which results in amenorrhoea (absence of menstrual cycle) and sterility. Concurrent health concerns are also frequently present, including congenital heart disease, hypothyroidism (reduced hormone secretion by the thyroid), diabetes, vision problems, hearing loss, and many autoimmune diseases. Finally, a specific pattern of cognitive deficits is often observed, with particular difficulties in visuospatial, mathematical, and memory areas.

anastomosis area. This technique is referred to as extended end-to-end anastomosis (Fig. 5.169). Other nowadays less frequently used approaches to surgical repair of coarctation are shown in Fig. 5.170.

## Coarctation of Aorta Repair—Technique

1. The patient is positioned in a right lateral position.
2. Left thoracotomy is performed: the left pleural cavity is entered and the area of aortic isthmus is exposed by retracting the lung anteriorly and downwards. Surgeons may ask for a moist raytec swab and a malleable retractor to retract the lung.
3. Next, the isthmus of the aorta is exposed by dividing the overlying pleura and the edges of the pleura are retracted with silk stay sutures.
4. The coarctation of the aorta is identified and the aorta proximal and distal to the coarctation is fully mobilized. The ductus arteriosus is also dissected.
5. Some surgeons may place vessel loops around the patent ductus arteriosus and the descending aorta to isolate these structures.
6. Vascular clamps are placed on the proximal and distal aorta and the ductus arteriosus is excised and the stump is closed with a polypropylene suture.
7. The aorta is divided above and below the site of ductus arteriosus site and the excess ductal tissue is removed.
8. An end-to-end anastomosis is performed with a polypropylene suture.
9. After completion of repair the vascular clamps are carefully removed and haemostasis ensured (Figs 5.171–5.177).
10. Generally one chest drain is inserted and the thoracotomy incision is closed in a standard fashion.

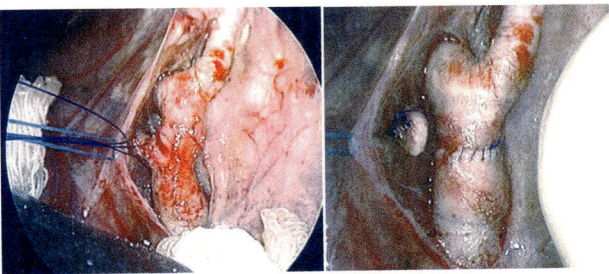

**Fig. 5.169:** Ductal tissue is seen on photo on the left. Photo on the right shows an end-to-end repair. *(Photo by EDJ, courtesy of King Faisal Specialist Hospital, Jeddah, Saudi Arabia)*

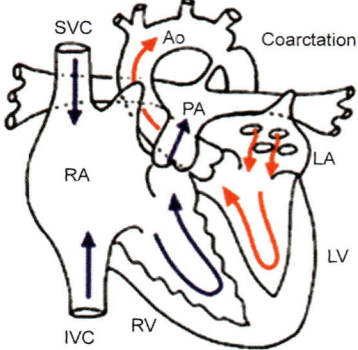

1. Left subclavian flap angioplasty

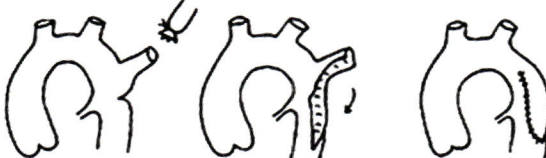

2. End-to-end repair with resection of coarctation segment

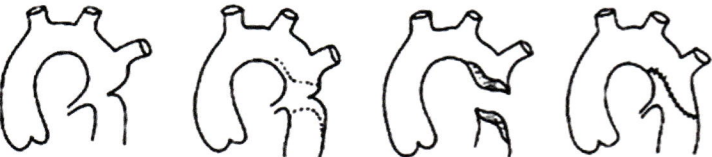

3. Left subclavian translocation angioplasty

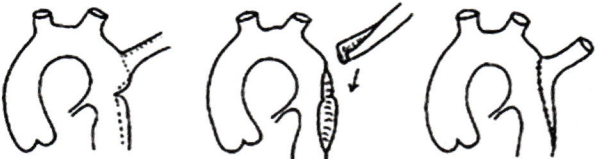

**Fig. 5.170:** Surgical approaches to repair of coarctation of aorta

## Outcome of Surgical Repair of Coarctation

Surgical results are excellent. However, reports show long-term prognosis is recurrent coarctation, recurrent hypertension which is common, and is the major factor of cerebrovascular disease, aortic aneurysm and rupture, heart failure, as well as coronary artery disease in adults, who underwent coarctation repair in childhood.

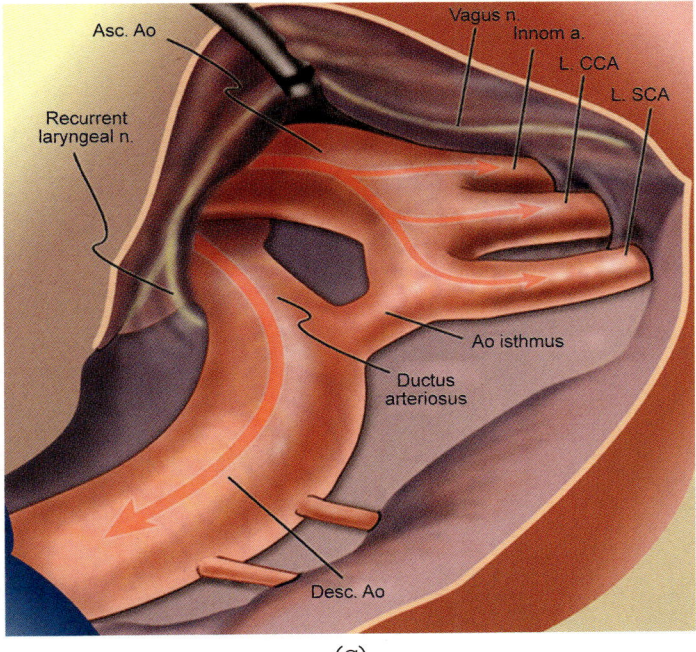

(a)

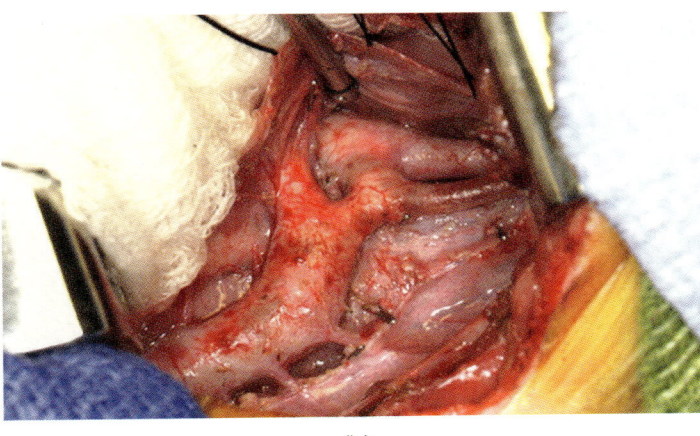

(b)

**Fig. 5.171:** The ascending aorta, transverse aortic arch and its branches, ductus arteriosus and descending aorta must be aggressively mobilized to effect a primary coarctation repair. Care should be taken to avoid injury to the recurrent laryngeal nerve

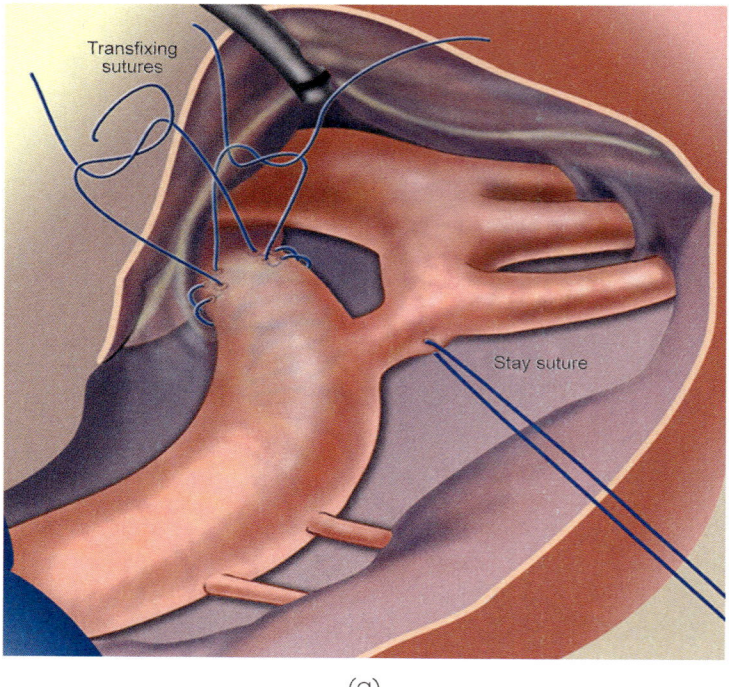

(a)

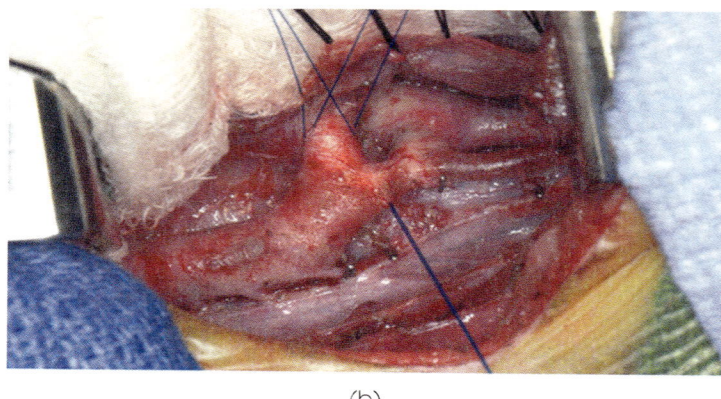

(b)

**Fig. 5.172:** In this picture the ductus arteriosus is controlled with two 5-0 polypropylene transfixing sutures. A stay suture is placed in the adventitial layer of the aortic isthmus. The ductus is then ligated with the two transfixing sutures

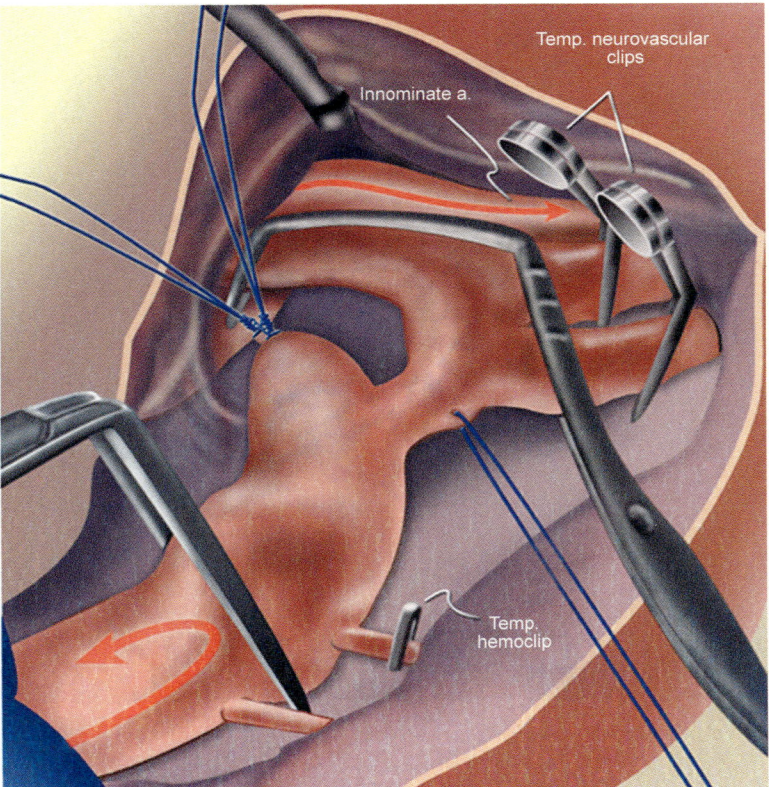

**Fig. 5.173:** Schematic picture of a partial occluding clamp is applied across the entire transverse aortic arch

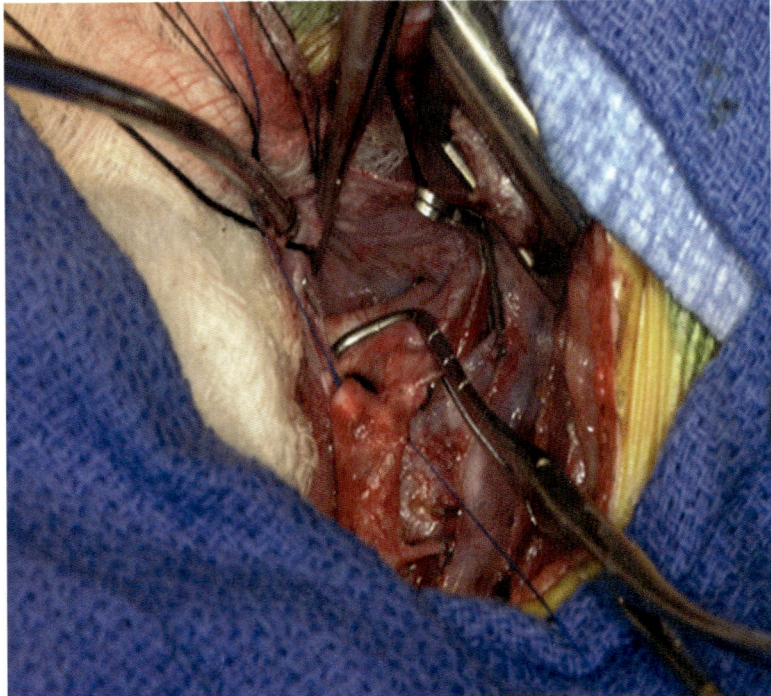

**Fig. 5.174:** A Castañeda or similar partial occluding clamp is applied across the entire transverse aortic arch. The clamp is positioned onto the ascending aorta, allowing blood flow through a partially occluded innominate artery. Adequacy of blood pressure is assessed with either a radial or an axillary arterial cannula. Care must be taken to avoid distortion of the innominate artery throughout the repair and close attention is paid to the right radial artery pressure when the clamp is on. The two clamps are held by the same assistant to allow for tension free anastomosis and good exposure. Any small change in position of the proximal clamp can result in inadequate blood flow through the innominate artery. Neurovascular clips are used to occlude backflow from the left carotid and left subclavian artery. Temporary medium titanium hemoclips are used to control intercostal arteries that will not be adequately controlled with an angled aortic cross clamp on the descending aorta. The hemoclips are later removed by squeezing the rounded end with a heavy needle holder. The clamps are stabilized by the first assistant throughout the case. The second assistant (or the perioperative nurse) will follow the suture used for the anastomosis and keep the field dry with the suction device

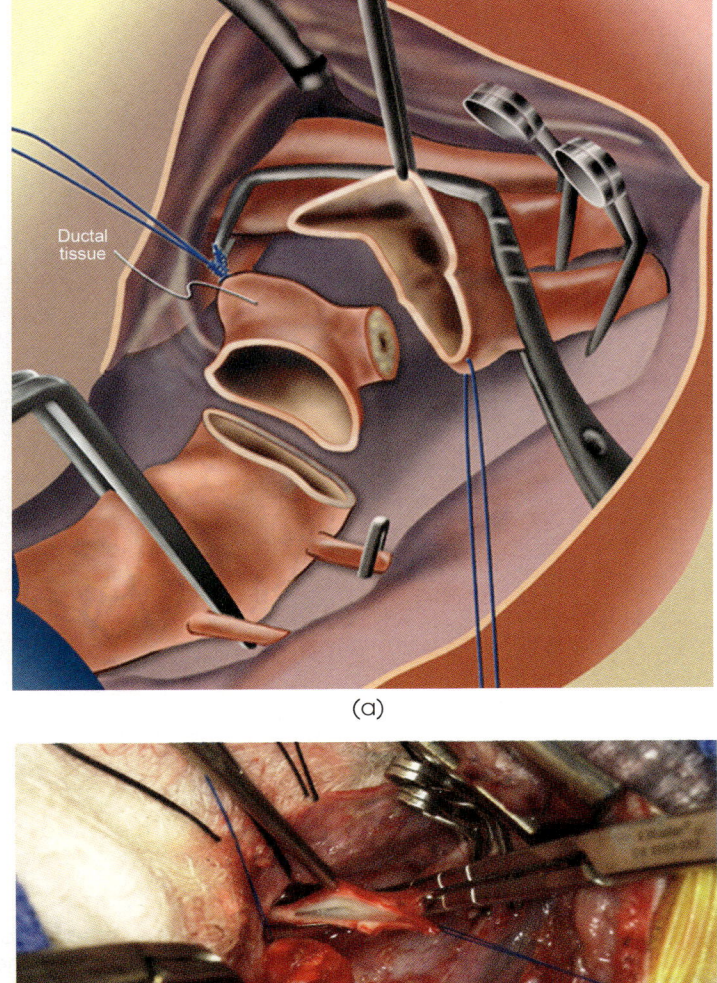

(a)

(b)

**Fig. 5.175:** Once the clamps have been applied, the ductal tissue is excised

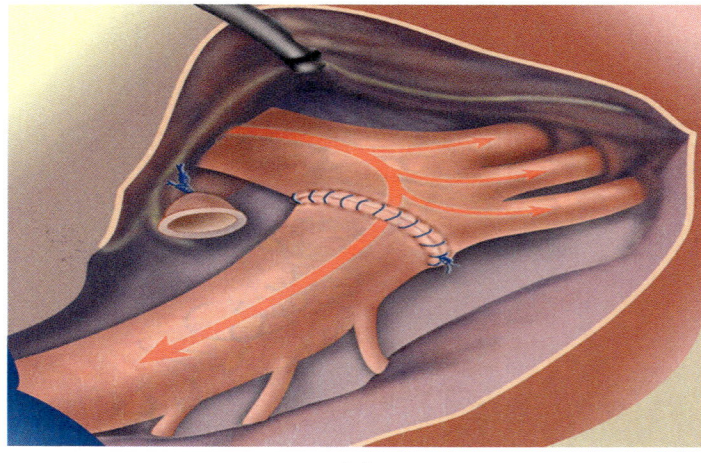

(a)

(b)

**Fig. 5.176:** The parietal pleura is closed over the aorta with a running suture. This is done to create an extra layer should bleeding occur

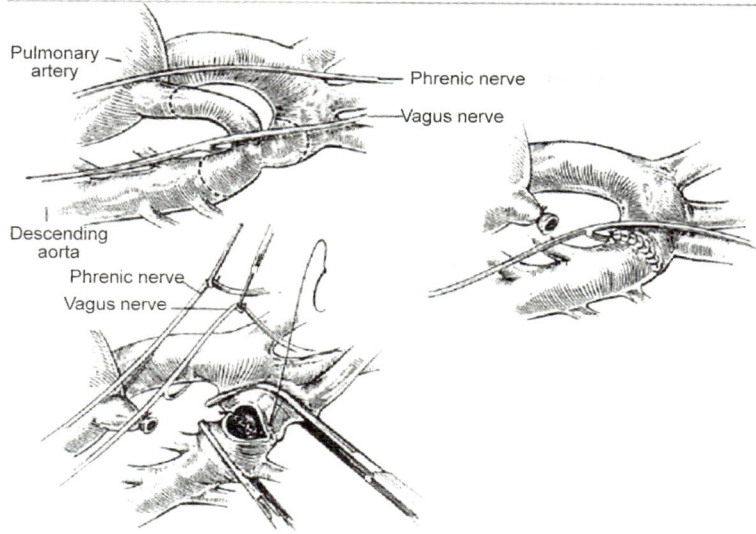

**Fig. 5.177:** Surgical repair of coarctation with resection and end-to-end anastomosis

## INTERRUPTED AORTIC ARCH (IAA)

### Introduction

Interruption of the aortic arch (IAA) is a congenital anomaly characterized by complete discontinuity of blood flow between two portions of the aorta. Thus, the aorta is divided into two parts that are not connected to each other. Blood supply proximal to the interruption is provided by the ascending aorta. Blood

---

**NURSING OBSERVATION**

This procedure can be tense,once the vascular clamps are placed on the aorta, as blood flow to the lower body is discontinued. Most surgeons attempt to limit the aortic cross clamp time and generally try to perform the repair with clamp time of less than 20 to 30 minutes. The vascular clamps are stabilized by the first assistant throughout the case. The second assistant (or a second scrub nurse) will follow the suture used for the anastomosis and keep the field dry with the suction device. During the haemostasis phase, a good supply of irrigation fluid, irrigation syringes and fine sutures should be available. Tissue glue and other haemostatic material may be required.

supply distal to the interruption is provided by a patent ductus arteriosus (Figs 5.178 and 5.179). So, oxygen saturation proximal to the interruption is normal, while the oxygen saturation distal

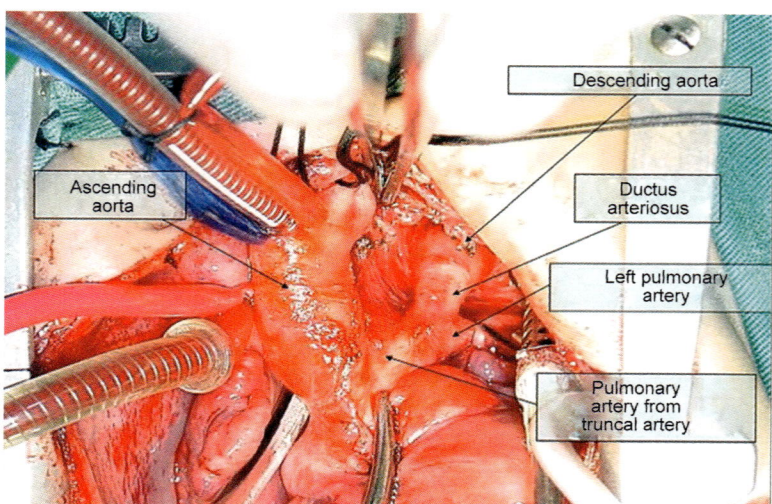

**Fig. 5.178:** Common associated anomalies with IAA are ventricular septal defect (VSD), truncus arteriosus (shown here), transposition of the great arteries with a VSD, and various forms of single ventricle

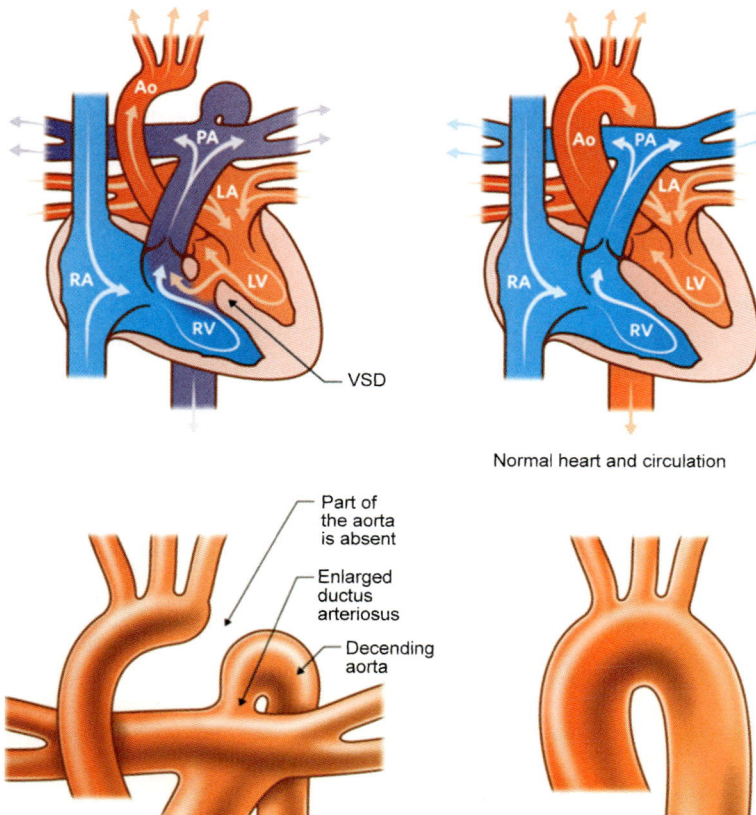

Normal heart and circulation

Part of the aorta is absent

Enlarged ductus arteriosus

Decending aorta

Interrupted aortic arch

Normal aorta

**Fig. 5.179:** Interrupted aortic arch: Interruption of aortic arch, descending aorta connected to pulmonary artery by large patent ductus arteriosus, ventricular septal defect (VSD)

to the interruption is lower than normal. IAA is typically associated with other intracardiac anomalies.[116] When two ventricles are present, there is almost always a ventricular septal defect.[117]

Part of the aorta is absent and this leads to severe obstruction to blood flow to the lower part of the body. The ductus allows flow to the lower circulation before birth but as it closes in the newborn period, blood pressure in the lower circulation becomes inadequate and major symptoms develop. Most affected infants develop severe symptoms (difficulty breathing and impaired kidney function) in the first week of life and need urgent surgery. Most affected infants also have a large VSD. Sometimes other defects may be present. Flow patterns are normal to the upper body. However, there is no flow of oxygenated blood to the lower body unless there exist, as in this drawing, shunts such as a ventricular septal defect that allows oxygenated blood into the pulmonary artery, and a patent ductus arteriosus that allows the partially oxygenated blood to travel from the pulmonary artery to the descending aorta.

Interrupted aortic arch has been classified into three types, based on the site where the interruption of the aorta is present (Fig. 5.180).

1. **Type A:** The aorta is interrupted distal to the origin of the left subclavian artery.

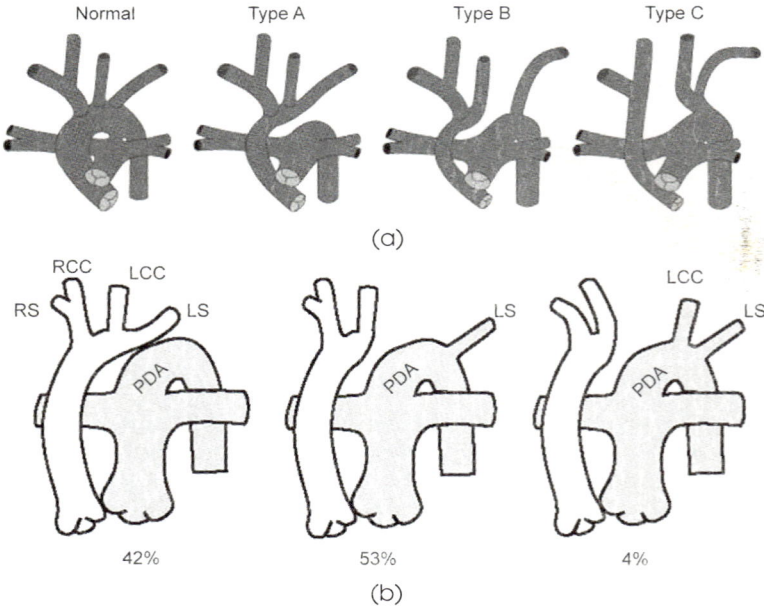

**Fig. 5.180:** Classification of interrupted aortic arches. Type A: Interruption distal to the left subclavian artery; Type B: Interruption distal to the left common carotid artery; Type C: Interruption distal to the brachiocephalic artery (a). Prevalence of each type of IAA (b). RS, Right subclavian; RCC, right common carotid; LCC, left common carotid; LS, left subclavian

2. **Type B:** The aorta is interrupted distal to the origin of the left common carotid artery.

3. **Type C:** The interruption occurs proximal to the origin the left common carotid artery.

Type B is the most common type of interrupted aortic arch, accounting for 84% of children with IAA.

Interrupted aortic arch (IAA) is usually diagnosed when the ductus arteriosus begins to close. Prostaglandin is given to keep the ductus arteriosus open until surgery is performed, usually as soon after birth as possible.

## Prevalence

IAA is a relatively rare cardiac anomaly, with an incidence of two cases per 100,000 live births. It is often associated with children with DiGeorge syndrome. Approximately 29% of children with IAA have DiGeorge syndrome.[119]

## Symptoms

In newborns with IAA, the only way for blood to bypass the blockage is via the patent ductus arteriosus. Closure of the patent ductus arteriosus in children with interrupted aortic arch results in lower body hypoperfusion and can be life-threatening.

## Treatment

Techniques for surgical correction are similar to those of coarctation repair and include end-to-end anastomosis of the remaining segments with or without patch augmentation, end-to-side anastomosis of the arch vessel with either the proximal or distal segment, or use of an interposition graft to take the place of the missing segment (Fig. 5.181). Most IAA repairs require cardiopulmonary bypass support.

### Outcome of Surgical Repair

Long-term probability for reintervention remains high regardless of operative technique.[120]

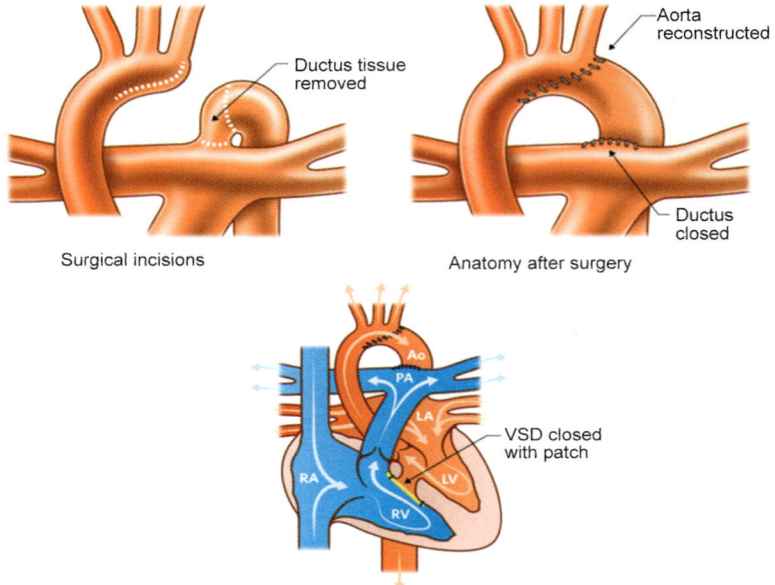

**Fig. 5.181:** Surgical repair of interrupted aortic arch. Patent ductus arteriosus is closed and the aorta is repaired by means of end-to-end anastomisis

### NURSING OBSERVATION

*Technique for surgical correction are similar to those of coarctation repair and include end-to-end anastomosis of the remaining segments with or without patch augmentation. However, IAA repair is commonly performed through a median sternotomy and cardiopulmonary bypass support with or without circulatory arrest. In case of severe hypoplasia of the aorta, a homograft, Gore-Tex™ graft or other patch material may be used to augment the aorta. In most cases regional cerebral perfusion may be employed. Aortic cannula is inserted in the innominate artery (which will perfuse the brain). A second aortic cannula is inserted in the main pulmonary artery (PA), (which is connected to a large PDA in IAA (Figs 5.179 and 5.182), and when left and right PAs are occluded, will perfuse the lower body through the PDA). A Y-adapter is placed in the arterial line of the pump, so that both aortic cannulae can be connected to the arterial pump line.* Except for very small infants for whom a single atrial cannula is employed, venous return is with bicaval cannulation, and avoiding the need for circulatory arrest. The head and neck vessels are encircled with snares, which are tightened during the period of regional cerebral perfusion.

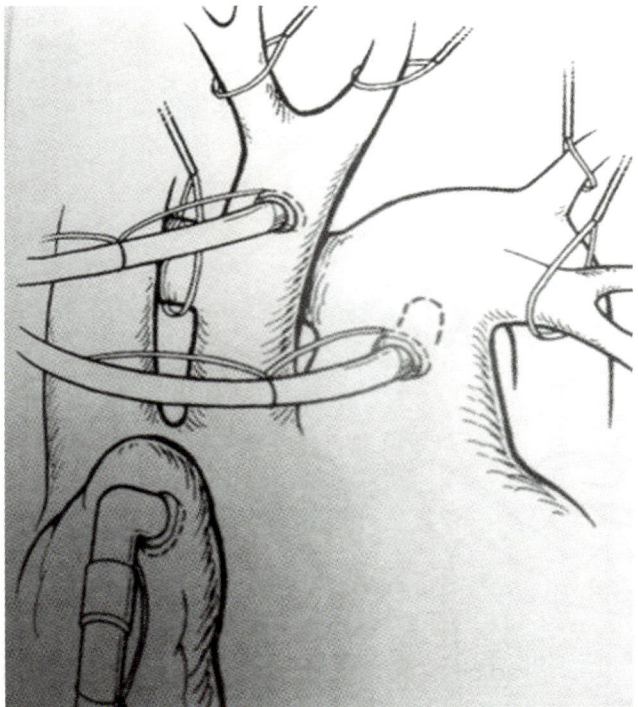

**Fig. 5.182:** A second aortic cannula is inserted in the main pulmonary artery (PA), (which is connected to a large PDA in IAA, and when left and right PAs are occluded, will perfuse the lower body through the PDA)

## AORTOPULMONARY WINDOW (APW)

### Introduction

Aortopulmonary window (APW) is a rare congenital anomaly in which there is a connection (window) between the ascending aorta and the main pulmonary artery (Fig. 5.183). It may occur just above the semilunar valves (pulmonary and aortic valve) or between the more distal ascending aorta and main pulmonary artery. The anomaly can occur as an isolated defect or is associated with other cardiac anomalies. More than half of children with aortopulmonary window have additional associated lesions of which patent ductus arteriosus, atrial septal defect, interrupted aortic arch and tetralogy of Fallot are the most common.[121]

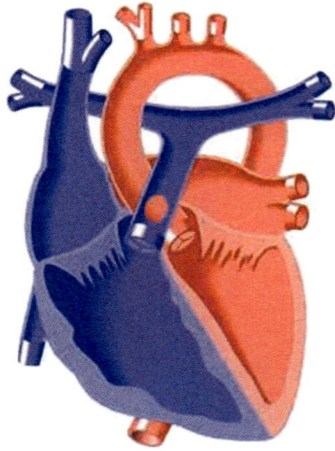

**Fig. 5.183:** Aortopulmonary window (APW). APW is a rare congenital anomaly in which there is a connection (window) between the ascending aorta and the main pulmonary artery

## What Causes an Aortopulmonary Window

APW occurs when the aorta and the pulmonary artery fail to divide completely during foetal development. It is separate from truncus arteriosus in that it is associated with essentially normal aortic and pulmonary valves. The defect usually begins just above the sinuses of Valsalva and then extends a variable distance distally into the arch.

## Prevalence

APW represents approximately 0.2% of all congenital cardiac lesions. It affects males equally as females.[122]

## Symptoms

The haemodynamic changes are similar to those seen with a large, unrestrictive ventricular septal defect. An aortopulmonary window allows oxygenated blood from the aorta to pass, or shunt (left-to-right shunt), into the pulmonary artery. Shunting of blood becomes progressively worse as pulmonary vascular resistance falls during the newborn period. Volume overload and pulmonary overcirculation lead to progressive left ventricular dysfunction and congestive heart failure. Shunting of blood into the pulmonary circulation occurs during both systole and diastole under high aortic pressures. These children may develop Eisenmenger syndrome at an early age if the defect is large, and unrestricted.

## Treatment

Initial intravenous prostaglandins may be required to maintain patency of the ductus arteriosus in infants with interrupted aortic arch in order to provide blood flow to the lower-half of the body. The presence of an APW is indicative for surgical repair. Spontaneous closure is not known in the medical literature. Early repair is necessary to prevent pulmonary hypertension and Eisenmenger syndrome. Most lesions are repaired by direct patch repair of the defect. Associated lesions are usually repaired during the same surgery.

## Aortopulmonary Window Repair—Technique

Cardiopulmonary bypass is used to perform the surgical repair.
1. Exposure is obtained through a median sternotomy.
2. The aorta is cannulated as distally as possible.
3. A single right atrial cannula is used. If an atrial septal defect or ventricular septal defect is present, bicaval cannulae must be used.
4. Cardiopulmonary bypass is initiated, and the procedure is performed using moderate hypothermia.
5. Deep hypothermic circulatory arrest may be necessary:
   - If the lesion is complex or extends distally into the arch of the aorta,
   - If the child requires repair of an interrupted aortic arch.
6. The right and left pulmonary arteries must be snared before the administration of cardioplegia
   - The snares should be tightened to ensure good coronary flow
   - To prevent run-off of cardioplegia into the pulmonary circulation.
7. The defect is entered from:
   - The anterior aspect of the aorta,
   - The main pulmonary artery, or
   - The aortopulmonary window itself.
8. The aortopulmonary window is then closed using patch material.
9. The child is warmed and weaned off cardiopulmonary bypass.

10. Protamine is administered to reverse the heparin, and the child is decannulated.
11. Chest drains are inserted and the chest is closed in a standard fashion.

---

**NURSING OBSERVATION**

*Technique for this procedure may vary from standard cardiopulmonary bypass using deep circulatory arrest. The perioperative nurse should be familiar and be prepared for whatever technique may be necessary.*

*The right and left pulmonary arteries must be snared before the administration of cardioplegia; be familiar, which technique the surgeon uses to occlude the left and right pulmonary artery; aneurysm clips, bulldogs or ties/tape with a tourniquet. Have patch material available for closing of the defect. Also tissue glue and other haemostatic material may be required.*

---

### Outcome of Surgical Repair

Outcomes continue to improve with better management during the perioperative period. The prognosis of aortopulmonary window is excellent if repaired in infancy and preferably before the onset of significant pulmonary hypertension. The mortality rate for simple aortopulmonary window without other associated anomalies should be near 0%.

## HYPOPLASTIC LEFT HEART SYNDROME

### Introduction

Hypoplastic left heart syndrome (HLHS) is a rare congenital heart defect. In this defect, the left ventricle and the ascending aorta are severely underdeveloped (Fig. 5.184). The aortic and mitral valves are atretic, hypoplastic, or stenotic. A patent foramen ovale, or an atrial septal defect is usually present to sustain life. The ventricular septum is usually intact and is not considered as part of the condition. The left ventricle is unable to support the systemic circulation, which is maintained by the right ventricle through a patent ductus arteriosus. Typically a large patent ductus arteriosus supplies blood to the systemic circulation. Coarctation of the aorta may be present[123, 124], but interrupted aortic arch is rare. The right side of the heart may be normal or markedly enlarged. Similar to other congenital heart defects, hypoplastic left heart syndrome has various types of severity.[125]

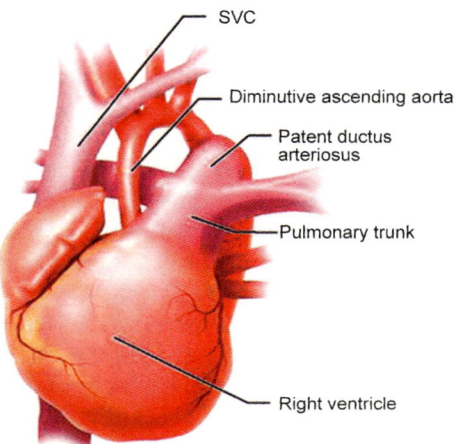

**Fig. 5.184:** Anatomic manifestations of hypoplastic left heart syndrome: mitral stenosis or atresia, hypoplasia of the left ventricle, aortic stenosis or atresia, hypoplastic aortic arch, and ductal dependent systemic cardiac output

## What Causes Hypoplastic Left Heart Syndrome (HLHS)?

The cause of HLHS is unknown. The medical literature suggests that severe underdevelopment of the left ventricular outflow tract (aortic valve stenosis, or atresia) results in abnormal blood flow to the aorta and causes subsequent underdevelopment of the ascending and aortic arch.

### Prevalence

HLHS accounts for approximately 1.5% of all congenital heart defects[126, 127], and was responsible for up to 25% of all deaths within the first week of life before treatment became available.[128] Without surgical palliation, 95% of children die within the first month of life. Prevalence of HLHS is for unknown reasons higher in males than in females.

### Symptoms

Severity of symptoms depends on: (1) adequacy of interatrial communication, (2) patency of the ductus arteriosus, and (3) level of pulmonary vascular resistance. Hypoplastic left heart syndrome typically presents within the first 24–48 hours of life. Symptoms occur as soon as the ductus arteriosus constricts, thereby decreasing systemic blood flow. At the same time, saturated pulmonary venous blood returning to the left atrium cannot flow into the left ventricle because of atresia, hypoplasia, or stenosis of the mitral valve. Therefore, pulmonary venous blood must cross the atrial septum. This blood mixes with desaturated systemic venous blood in the right atrium. The right ventricle then must pump this mixed blood to both the pulmonary and the systemic circulations that are connected in parallel, rather than in series, by the ductus arteriosus. Blood exiting the right ventricle may flow (1) to the lungs via the branch pulmonary arteries (left and right pulmonary arteries) or (2) to the body via the ductus arteriosus. The amount of blood that flows into each circulation is based on the resistance in each circuit. Following birth, pulmonary vascular resistance decreases, which allows a higher percentage of blood flow in the right ventricle to go to the lungs instead of the body. Although increased pulmonary blood flow results in higher oxygen saturation, systemic blood flow is decreased. Perfusion becomes poor and cyanosis results. Alternatively, if pulmonary vascular resistance is significantly higher than systemic vascular resistance, systemic blood flow is increased however at the expense of pulmonary blood flow. This may result in hypoxemia and the child may develop symptoms of shock (become pale, sweaty, heavy and/or rapid breathing, fast heart rate, cold hands and feet with diminished pulses). A delicate balance between pulmonary and systemic vascular resistances should be maintained to ensure adequate oxygenation and tissue perfusion.

### Treatment

Treatment for HLHS is ultimately surgical intervention; either staged reconstructive surgery or heart transplantation. The staged reconstructive surgery consists of the Norwood procedure, usually performed in the first week of life, the Glenn procedure, usually performed six months after the Norwood, and the final Fontan procedure, which is usually performed between two and four years of age.

In 1983, Norwood et al. reported the first successful surgical palliation of HLHS, which consisted of a Norwood procedure followed by the Fontan procedure.[129] In 1990, Bridges et al. described the bidirectional cavopulmonary anastomosis as an intermediate staging operation for the management of high-risk candidates for the Fontan procedure, such as infants with HLHS.[130] At present, this three stage surgical palliation remains the most common treatment for infants with HLHS.

## Norwood Procedure—Overview

The procedure has been technically refined since the initial procedure but the main principles of the norwood remain much the same:

1. Atrial septectomy, to establish unrestricted interatrial communication to provide mixing of blood and at the same time avoid overload of pulmonary blood flow,
2. Anastomosis of the proximal pulmonary artery to the aorta with homograft augmentation of the aortic arch, and
3. Systemic-to-pulmonary shunt by means of a Blalock-Taussig shunt or right ventricle-to-pulmonary artery conduit (Sano shunt) to provide pulmonary circulation (Figs 5.185–5.188).

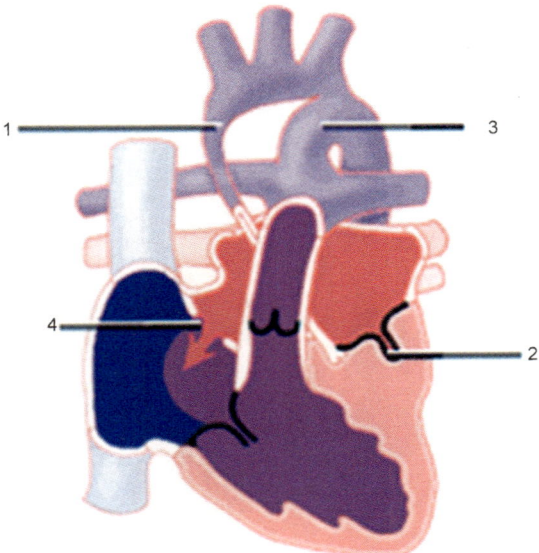

**Fig. 5.185:** Hypoplastic left heart syndrome (HLHS) consists of the following defects: Hypoplastic ascending aorta and aortic arch(1). Hypoplastic left ventricle (2). Large patent ductus arteriosus supplying the only source of blood flow to the body (3). Atrial septal defect allowing blood returning from lungs to reach the single ventricle (4)

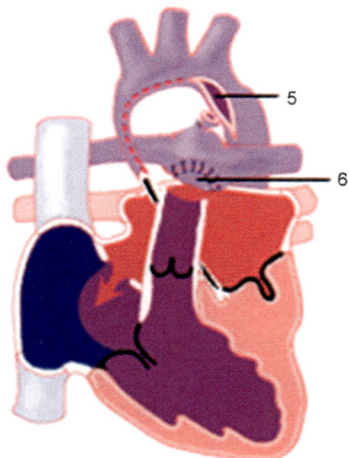

**Fig. 5.186:** The PDA has been ligated and the hypoplastic aorta is opened longitudinally from the descending aorta to near its origin at the heart (5). The main pulmonary artery has been divided and the distal end closed (6)

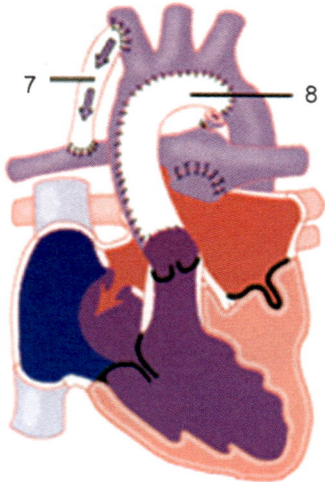

**Fig. 5.187:** A Gore-Tex™ modified Blalock–Taussig shunt from the innominate artery to the right pulmonary artery supplies blood flow to the lungs (7). The aorta has been reconstructed using the proximal main pulmonary artery, hypoplastic aortic arch, and a patch. Instead of a patch, a homograft can be used (8)

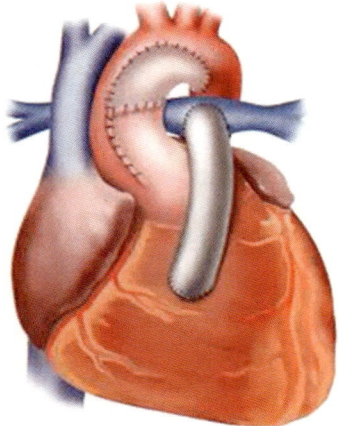

**Fig. 5.188:** Systemic-to-pulmonary shunt, by means of a right ventricle-to-pulmonary artery conduit (Sano shunt)

In 2003, Sano and colleagues reported a modification of the Norwood procedure by placing a larger Gore-Tex™ graft between the right ventricle and the pulmonary arteries.[131] This right ventricle to pulmonary arteries (RV to PA) conduit has been proposed as a better alternative to a modified BT shunt and preliminary data from one or two centres has suggested a better outcome (Fig. 5.189).[132, 133]

### Norwood Procedure—Technique

Individual surgeons may perform the Norwood procedure in different ways. The following operative technique for Norwood described here, is the one using the technique of deep hypothermic circulatory arrest:

1. A full midline sternotomy is performed.
2. The thymus is removed and pericardium opened and suspended with silk sutures.
3. The ascending and descending aorta, the head vessels, ductus arteriosus, and pulmonary arteries are extensively mobilized (Fig 5.190).
4. Purse string sutures are placed in the proximal main pulmonary artery and atrial appendage (Fig. 5.191). Some surgeons may prefer to also put a purse string in the superior vena cava (SVC).

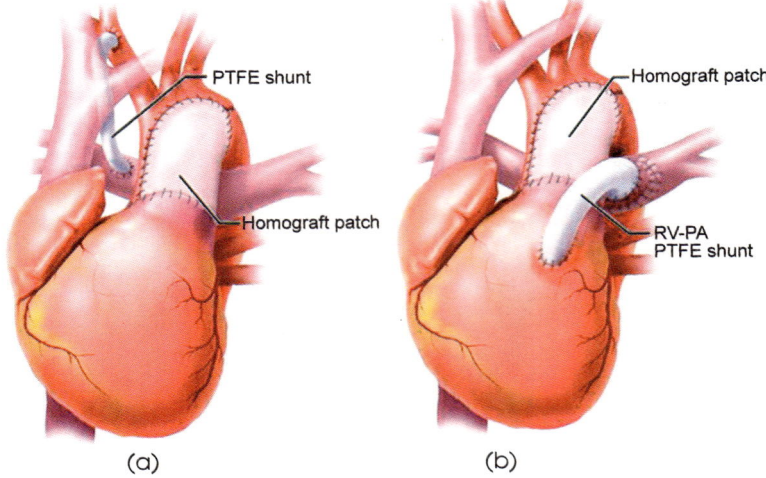

(a)                           (b)

**Fig. 5.189:** The final appearance of a completed Norwood operation (a) The ascending aorta and arch have been reconstructed with homograft patch augmentation. The shunt between the distal innominate artery and the central pulmonary arteries is demonstrated. The final appearance of a completed Sano modification using the RV-PA shunt. The ascending aorta and arch have been reconstructed with homograft patch augmentation. The shunt between the right ventricle and the central pulmonary arteries including an autologous pericardium cuff is demonstrated. PTFE indicates polytetrafluoroethylene (b)

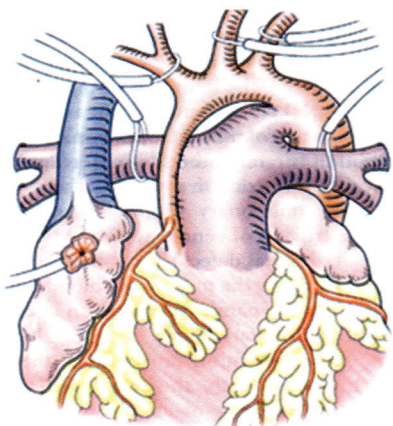

**Fig. 5.190:** The ascending and descending aorta, the head vessels, ductus arteriosus, and pulmonary arteries are extensively mobilized

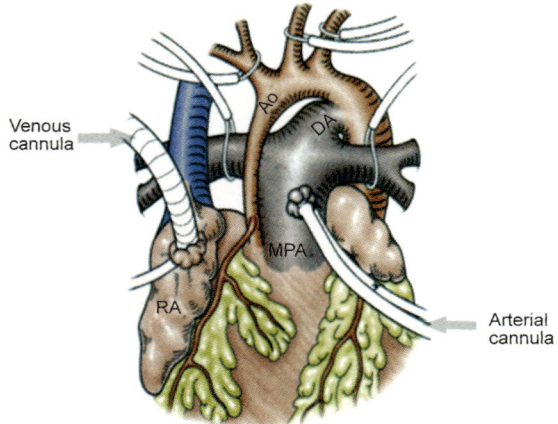

**Fig. 5.191:** Cannulation is achieved with the arterial cannula in the main pulmonary artery and a single venous cannula in the atrial appendage

5. Infant is cannulated with the arterial cannula in the main pulmonary artery and a single venous cannula in the atrial appendage—or two venous cannulae, first in the atrial appendage and the second in the SVC.

6. Cardiopulmonary bypass is initiated and tapes brought down around the left and right pulmonary arteries. Tapes are placed around the head vessels, which will be occluded during the first stage of repair. Instead of tapes, some surgeons may use silk tie and tourniquets, or aneurysm clips.

7. Infant is cooled to 18°C, during which time the surgeon may perform any further dissection.

8. Next, the proximal end of a Blalock-Taussig shunt is anastomosed to the innominate artery by placing a side-biting clamp on the innominate artery. Then a small incision is made into the innominate artery and the graft is sewn onto it in an end-to-side fashion with a 6-0 or 7-0 polypropylene suture (Fig. 5.192).

9. The surgeon removes the clamp to assess the blood flow, and may put a haemoclip to occlude the graft temporarily (Fig. 5.193).

10. When/If circulatory arrest is begun tapes are brought down around the head vessels and tightened with snuggers, (alternatively, the surgeon may use haemoclips or neuroclips

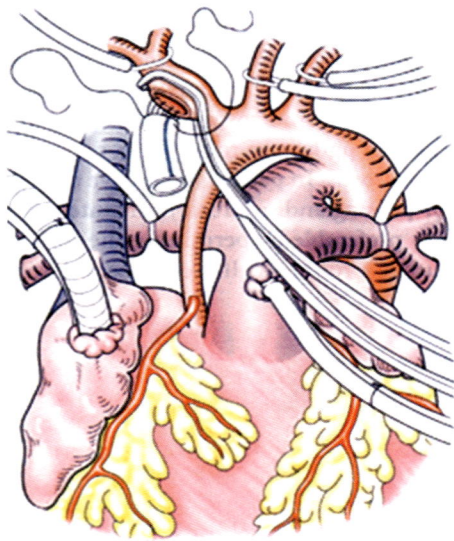

**Fig. 5.192:** The proximal end of a Blalock-Taussig shunt is anastomosed to the innominate artery by placing a side-biting clamp on the innominate artery. Then a small incision is made into the innominate artery and the graft is sewn onto it in an end-to-side fashion

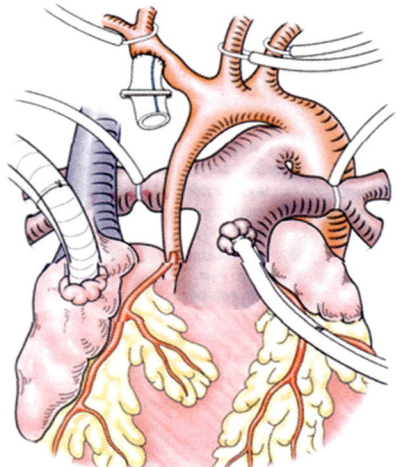

**Fig. 5.193:** The vascular clamp is removed to assess the blood flow, and a haemoclip is applied to occlude the graft temporarily

to occlude the head vessels). A vascular clamp is placed on the descending aorta distal to the patent ductus arteriosus (Fig. 5.194).

11. Cardioplegia is given through either a separate cardioplegia needle inserted into the main pulmonary artery (MPA) or via a side port on the arterial cannula.

12. After draining the heart, the arterial and venous cannulae are removed. The tapes around both left and right pulmonary arteries are removed.

13. Next, the ductus arteriosus is ligated close to the pulmonary artery and divided on the aortic side (Fig. 5.195).

14. First, an atrial septectomy is performed, through the atrial purse string (Fig. 5.196).

15. Second, the main pulmonary artery is divided near the confluence and the defect in the distal pulmonary artery is closed with a piece of homograft, or pericardial patch (Fig. 5.197).

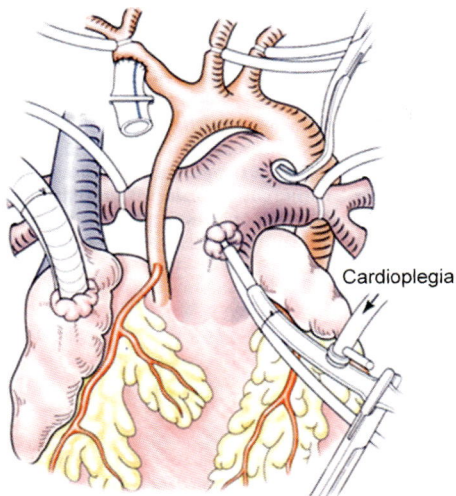

Cardioplegia

**Fig. 5.194:** At the time of circulatory arrest, tapes are brought down around the head vessels and tightened with snuggers, (alternatively, the surgeon may use haemoclips or neuroclips to occlude the head vessels). A vascular clamp is placed on the descending aorta distal to the patent ductus arteriosus. Cardioplegia is given through either a separate cardioplegia needle inserted into the MPA or via a side port on the arterial cannula

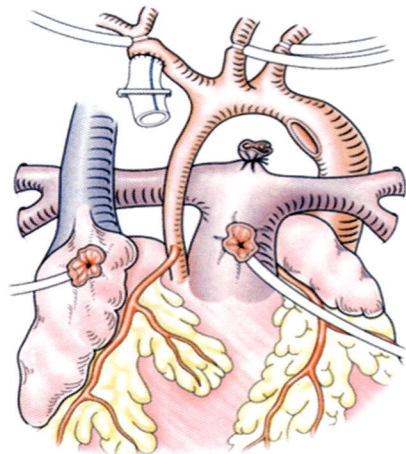

**Fig. 5.195:** After draining the heart, the arterial and venous cannulae are removed. The tapes around both left and right pulmonary arteries are removed. Next, the ductus arteriosus is ligated close to the pulmonary artery and divided on the aortic side

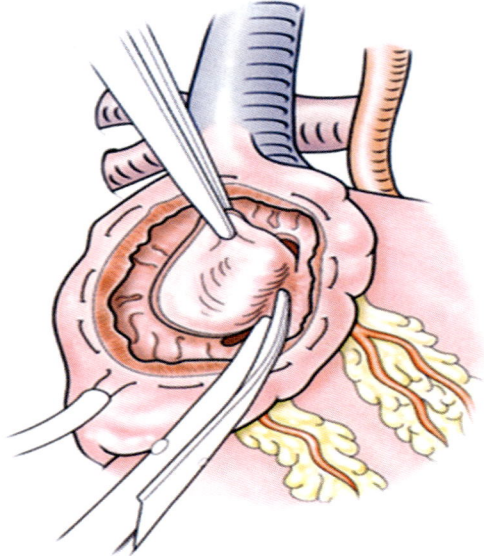

**Fig. 5.196:** An atrial septectomy is performed, through the atrial purse string

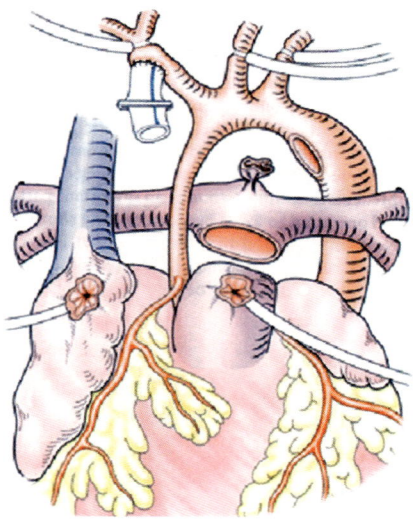

**Fig. 5.197:** Then, the main pulmonary artery is divided near the confluence and the defect in the distal pulmonary artery is closed with a piece of homograft, or pericardial patch

16. Third, the surgeon will perform the distal Blalock-Taussig-shunt-to-pulmonary artery anastomosis and the previous applied haemoclip is removed from the graft (Figs 5.198 and 5.199).
17. Last, an incision is made in the hypoplastic aorta and the proximal aortic-to-proximal pulmonary artery anastomosis is performed. The aortic arch is further augmented with a homograft (Figs 5.189 and 5.202).
18. Some surgeons may prefer not to use further material for the anastomosis of the pulmonary artery to the aorta (Fig. 5.200).
19. The arterial and venous cannulae are reinserted and cardio-pulmonary bypass is restarted.
20. The child is slowly rewarmed, during which stage the surgeon will rigorously check all anastomoses for obvious bleeding.
21. The child is then weaned off cardiopulmonary bypass, with pacing wires and chest drains routinely inserted.
22. If the child is haemodynamically stable, the chest will be closed. In some cases the surgeon may be cautious and the sternum is left open for 12 to 24 hours postsurgery.

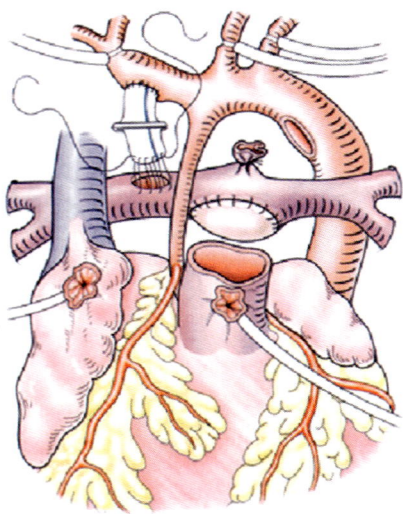

**Fig. 5.198:** The distal Blalock-Taussig-shunt-to-pulmonary artery anastomosis is performed next and the previous applied haemoclip is removed from the graft. Closure of the distal pulmonary artery can be seen

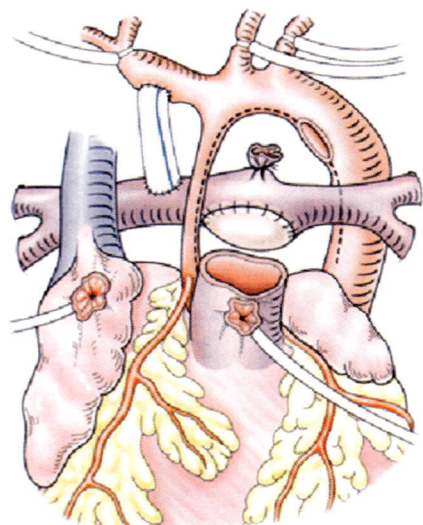

**Fig. 5.199:** Last, an incision is made in the hypoplastic aorta and the proximal aortic-to-proximal pulmonary artery anastomosis is performed

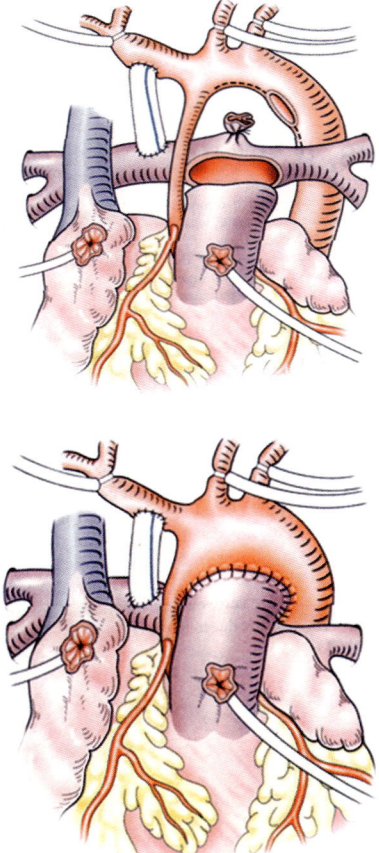

**Fig. 5.200:** Some surgeons may prefer not to use further material for the anastomosis of the pulmonary artery to the aorta, depending on the child's anatomy

Some surgeons may prefer not to use further material for the anastomosis of the pulmonary artery to the aorta.[134] However, most would prefer to use a homograft for augmentation and reconstruction of the aorta (Figs 5.189 and 5.202).

If regional cerebral perfusion is intended, the proximal anastomosis of the Gore-tex™ shunt is performed and the arterial cannula can be placed into the shunt. Perfusion is administered through the innominate artery (Fig. 5.201).

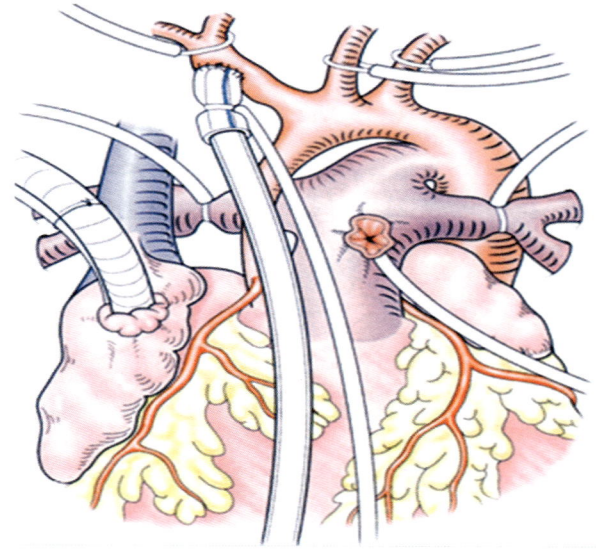

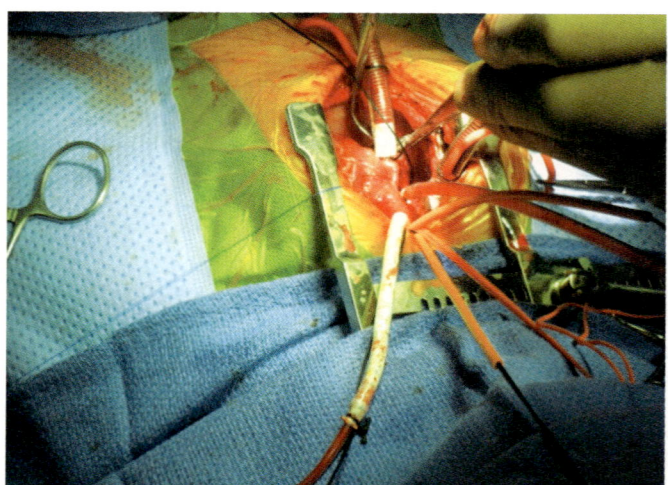

**Fig. 5.201:** If regional cerebral perfusion is intended, the proximal anastomosis of the Gore-Tex™ shunt is performed and the arterial cannula can be placed into the shunt. Perfusion is administered to the innominate artery. *(Photo by EDJ, courtesy of KAMC, National Guard Hospital, Riyadh, Saudi Arabia)*

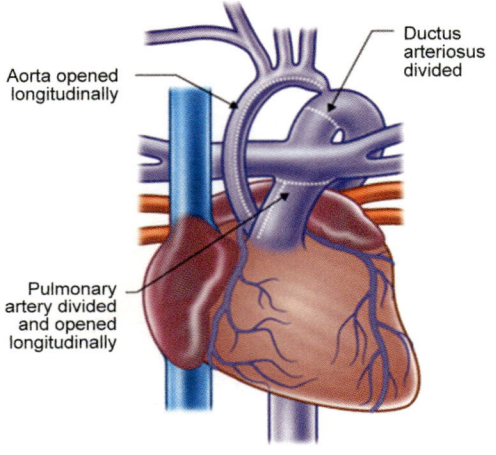

Ductus
arteriosus
divided

Aorta opened
longitudinally

Pulmonary
artery divided
and opened
longitudinally

Preoperative anatomy

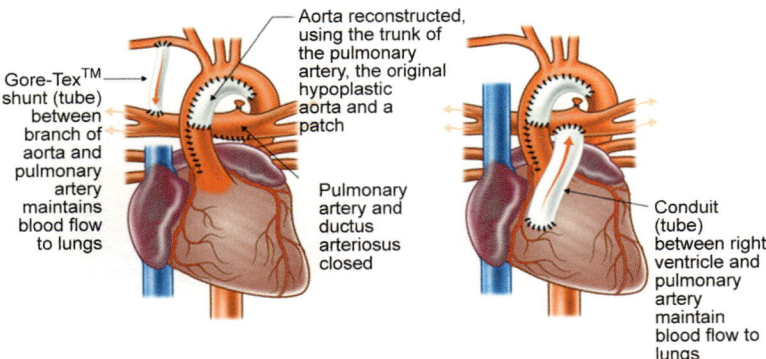

Aorta reconstructed,
using the trunk of
the pulmonary
artery, the original
hypoplastic
aorta and a
patch

Gore-Tex™
shunt (tube)
between
branch of
aorta and
pulmonary
artery
maintains
blood flow
to lungs

Pulmonary
artery and
ductus
arteriosus
closed

Conduit
(tube)
between right
ventricle and
pulmonary
artery
maintain
blood flow to
lungs

**Fig. 5.202:** The Norwood operation involves connecting the origin of the pulmonary artery to the aorta, to allow the right ventricle to pump blood to the main circulation and a shunt (BT shunt) operation, involving insertion of a tiny piece of artificial tube (made from Gore-Tex™) between the right subclavian or the innominate artery and the right pulmonary artery, to maintain blood flow to the lungs. Another option that is sometimes used, involves a Gore-Tex™ tube from the RV to the pulmonary artery (Sano shunt) instead of the BT shunt

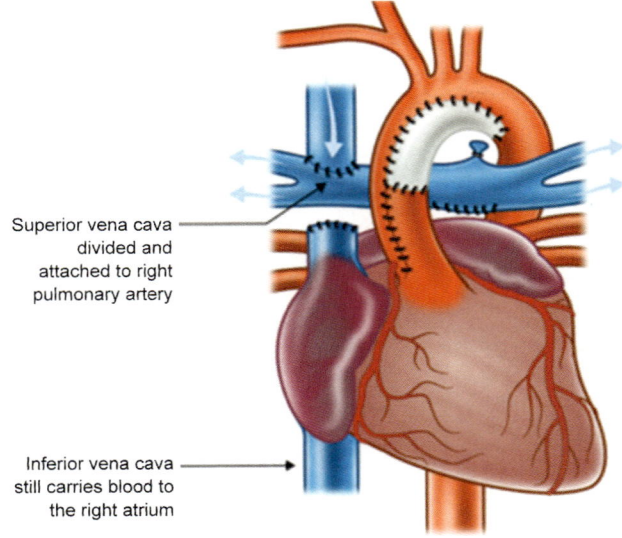

Superior vena cava divided and attached to right pulmonary artery

Inferior vena cava still carries blood to the right atrium

**Fig. 5.203:** A second operation, the Glenn Shunt, follows after about three months and is also called a cavo-pulmonary shunt

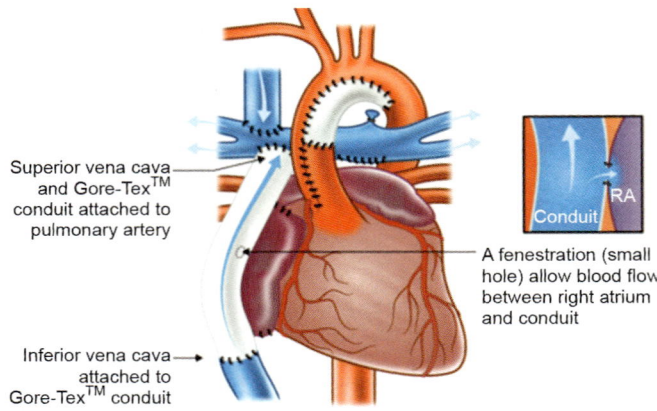

Superior vena cava and Gore-Tex™ conduit attached to pulmonary artery

A fenestration (small hole) allow blood flow between right atrium and conduit

Inferior vena cava attached to Gore-Tex™ conduit

Fontan operation with extracardiac conduit

**Fig. 5.204:** At a later stage (around three to four years old) a Fontan operation may be performed. This involves connecting the veins from the main circulation (SVC and IVC) directly to the pulmonary arteries. Blue blood is thus directed into the lungs rather than to the left atrium. A patch is placed to prevent blood passing from the RA to the LA—though sometimes a small hole (a Fenestration) is deliberately left

*It is important for the cardiac nurse to be prepared for whatever perfusion repair technique the surgeon may use, for example, deep hypothermic circulatory arrest, with or without selective antegrade continuous cerebral perfusion. Knowledge of these techniques and their requirements save valuable time in the operating theatre. Furthermore, surgical repair of HLHS may vary significantly depending on surgeon's philosophies and the various anatomical manifestations of HLHS. The perioperative scrub nurse should be familiar with the individual surgeon's technique for repair. During repair, most commonly, tapes are placed around the head vessels, which will be occluded during the first stage of repair. Instead of tapes, some surgeons may use silk tie and tourniquets, or aneurysm clips. Have various sizes of Gore-Tex™ shunts for the Blalock–Taussig shunt available. If regional cerebral perfusion is intended, the proximal anastomosis of the Gore-Tex™ shunt is performed and the arterial cannula can be placed into the shunt. Perfusion is administered to the innominate artery. Another option that is sometimes used, involves a Gore-Tex™ tube from the right ventricle to the pulmonary artery (Sano shunt) instead of the BT shunt. When the main pulmonary artery is divided near the confluence, the defect in the distal pulmonary artery is closed with either a piece of homograft, or pericardial patch, depending on surgeon's preference and child's anatomy. Have a homograft folder available in the room and discuss with the surgeon, which homograft he/she intends to use, if any. Also have other patch material available as well as haemostatic agents, such as gelfoam, surgical or tisseel glue. During the haemostasis phase, a good supply of irrigation fluid, irrigation syringes and fine sutures should be available.*

## *Outcome of Surgical Repair*

The variety of treatment approaches are based on different surgical philosophies and each approach has its unique advantages and disadvantages. Nonetheless, multiple experienced cardiac centres have reported improved outcomes in each one of those surgical varieties. Hypoplastic left heart syndrome is fatal, if left untreated. Outcome after surgical palliation for HLHS has been improved substantially. This has been attributed to these modifications in surgical technique. Perioperative medical care, together with a better understanding of postoperative physiology has also contributed to improved survival. Survival after the first stage is now more than 75%. The overall survival rate of the staged

Norwood procedure is 70% after 5 years. The risk factors for poor result are multiple and vary between health care centres.

Another approach to the treatment of HLHS is heart transplantation. The advantage of cardiac transplantation is replacement of an abnormal circulation with a normal 4-chambered heart in a single operation. However, disadvantages of this approach are the limited availability of donor hearts, rejection, infection and the requirement for lifelong immunosuppression.

A recently developed alternative procedure for the treatment of HLHS is the so-called hybrid procedure. In this procedure a stent is placed in the patent ductus arteriosus to keep it open. In addition, an atrial septostomy is performed and both the left and right pulmonary arteries are banded to control the blood flow to the lungs (Fig. 5.205). This procedure is carried out in the catheterization laboratory or cath lab. The ultimate goal is to avoid major surgery in the neonatal period (Norwood procedure) in the hope to improve long-term outcomes. The second stage of the surgery then combines elements of the Norwood procedure and the Glenn procedure. The third and final surgical repair is the Fontan procedure.

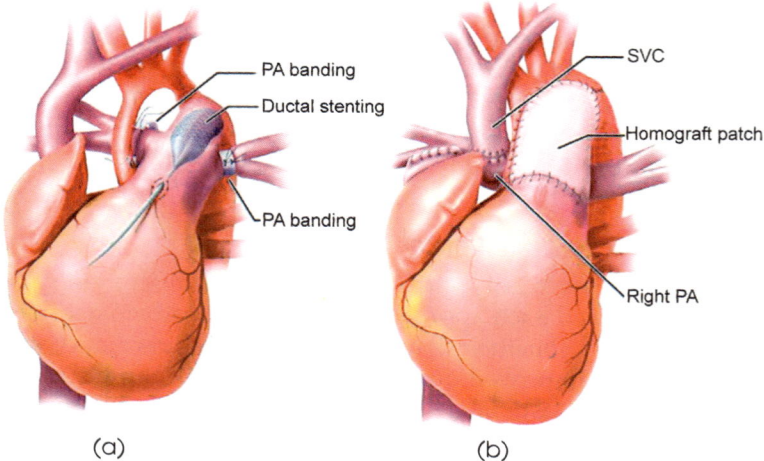

(a)        (b)

**Fig. 5.205:** First-stage hybrid pulmonary artery banding and ductal stenting (a). Second-stage reconstruction (b). The ascending aorta and arch have been reconstructed with homograft patch augmentation. BDCPA (Bidirectional cavopulmonary anastomosis) between the superior vena cava and the right pulmonary artery is demonstrated

## The Yasui Procedure—Overview

At the other end of the spectrum are milder forms of HLHS with aortic stenosis/severe left ventricular outflow tract obstruction (LVOTO), hypoplastic aortic arch or interrupted aortic arch, and mitral stenosis with a reasonable sized left ventricle. Often a ventricular septal defect is also present. Surgical management for this group of children is a biventricular repair depending on an adequate size mitral valve i.e. adequate blood flow into the left ventricle and the size or dimension of the left ventricle. The biventricular repair consists of a Stansel connection and arch augmentation (as in Norwood), ventricular septal defect baffle of left ventricle to pulmonary artery, and right ventricle to pulmonary artery valved conduit (Rastelli).[135]

This approach was first described by Yasui and is referred to as the **Yasui procedure** (Fig. 5.206). The Yasui procedure is also described as a Norwood arch reconstruction with a Rastelli connection establishing a biventricular repair in children born with

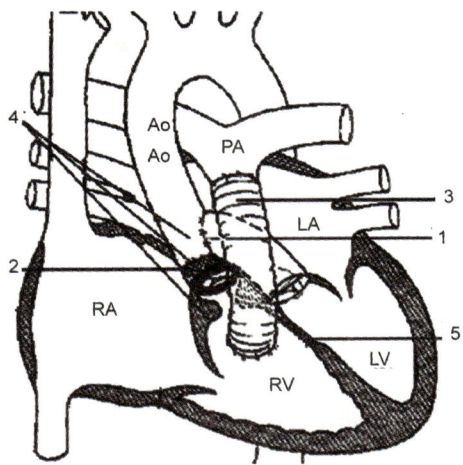

**Fig. 5.206:** Yasui procedure—Damus-Kaye-Stansel procedure with Rastelli Repair. Main pulmonary artery to ascending aorta (end-to-side) anastomosis (1). Patch closure of aortic orifice (2). Conduit interposition from right ventricle to distal pulmonary artery (3). Transposition of the great arteries with valvular and subvalvular aortic stenosis (4). Patch closure of ventricular septal defect (5). Postoperative: main pulmonary artery to ascending aorta (end-to-side) anastomosis with patch closure

interrupted aortic arch (IAA) and left ventricular outflow tract obstruction (LVOTO) or aortic atresia (AA), severe stenosis with ventricular septal defect (VSD) and two adequate sized ventricles. The term 'Norelli' procedure has been applied to this modification of the Yasui procedure, combining the essential elements of the Norwood procedure with the Rastelli procedure to establish a biventricular repair (Figs 5.206–5.209).[136]

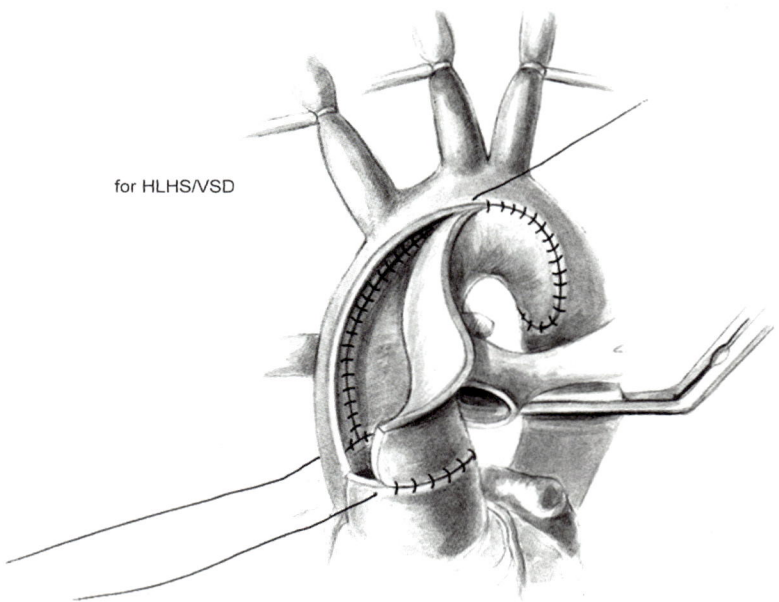

for HLHS/VSD

**Fig. 5.207:** For patients with aortic atresia and 2 good ventricles (HLHS/VSD), a typical Norwood arch reconstruction is performed. If there is a coarctation, a coarctectomy is performed (not shown); otherwise, just a patch is used to enlarge the undersurface of the hypoplastic arch from the descending aorta beyond the ductal insertion site down to the previously created junction of the hypoplastic ascending aorta and the proximal pulmonary trunk. HLHS, hypoplastic left heart syndrome; VSD, ventricular septal defect

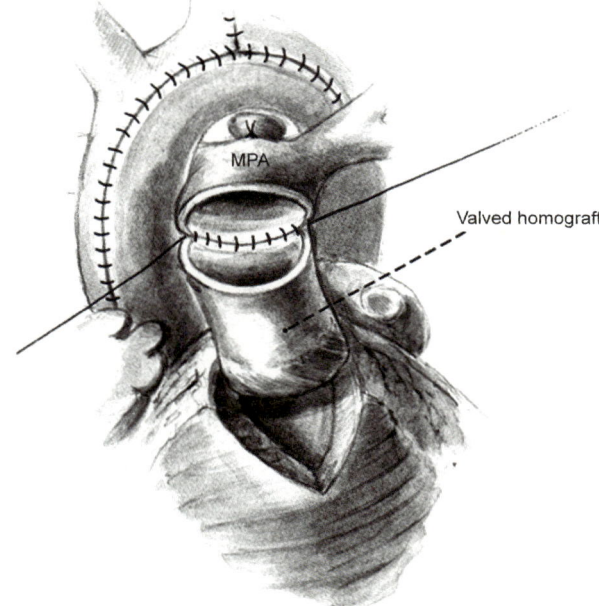

MPA

Valved homograft

**Fig. 5.208:** A valved homograft is used to establish right ventricular to pulmonary artery continuity (Rastelli). This can be achieved by placing a cryopreserved pulmonary homograft of 10 to 14 mm. If a pulmonary homograft is unavailable, then an aortic homograft is used. If no suitable homograft is available, then a Contegra bovine jugular vein valved conduit (Medtronic) is used. The graft first is trimmed and then an end-to-end anastomosis between the distal homograft and the pulmonary bifurcation is performed with a continuous 6-0 polypropylene suture. MPA, main pulmonary artery. Note the hypoplastic aortic arch repair (Norwood)

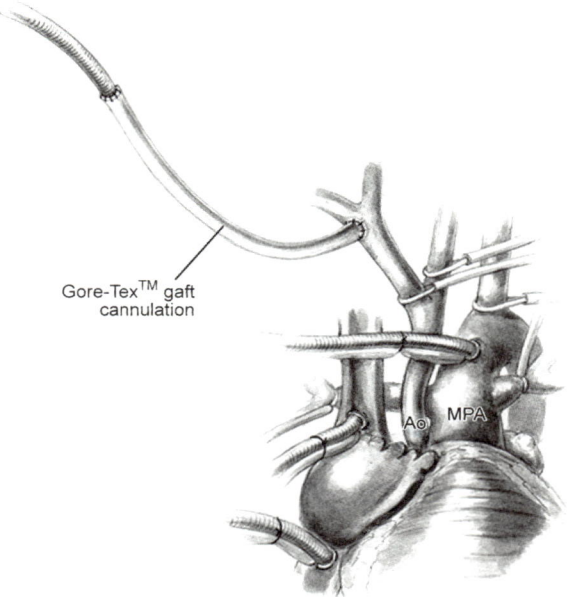

Gore-Tex™ gaft
cannulation

Ao MPA

**Fig. 5.209:** For the patient with IAA/LVOTO, arterial perfusion is established with a 3.5 mm PTFE graft anastomosed to the distal innominate artery. The graft is cannulated with an 8-French cannula. The descending aorta is cannulated directly through the proximal ductus arteriosus also with an 8-French cannula and the 2 cannulae are connected to the arterial perfusion line. For patients with HLHS/VSD, if there is a significant coarctation, 2 arterial cannulae may be used. If there is only a mild coarctation, just the PTFE graft to the innominate artery for arterial perfusion may suffice. Except for very small infants for whom a single atrial cannula is employed, venous return is with bicaval cannulation, thus avoiding the need for circulatory arrest. The head and neck vessels are encircled with snares, which are tightened during the period of regional perfusion. Alternatively, 'Yasargil' aneurysm clips can be used to control these vessels. Ao, aorta; MPA, main pulmonary artery

## *Outcome of Surgical Treatment*

The literature suggests that the Yasui operation is effective for patients with IAA/LVOTO and AA/VSD. Reoperation after biventricular repair seems inevitable, mostly for conduit replacement.

## Section 4.2: Anomalies of the Venous Connections
## Anomalies of Pulmonary Veins

Normally, pulmonary veins are those veins that carry blood from the lungs and to the left atrium (Fig. 5.210). The major pulmonary vein emerges from the lungs and branches out immediately into right and left pulmonary veins. The right pulmonary veins collect blood from the right lung and the left pulmonary veins collect blood from the left lung. One of the special characteristics of these veins is that pulmonary veins are the only veins that perform the function of transporting oxygenated blood.

Congenital anomalies of the systemic venous connection to the heart represent a extensive group of malformations, whose physiological consequences may vary from nil to the most severe form of systemic arterial desaturation. Such anomalies are reviewed in this section with particular respect to their surgical implications.

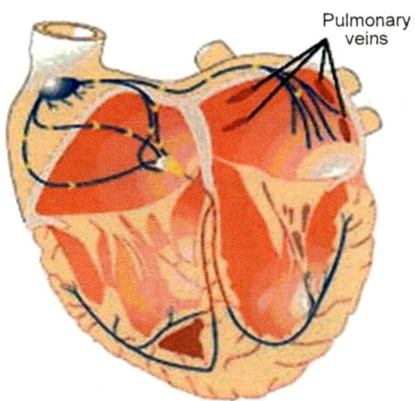

Pulmonary veins

**Fig. 5.210:** The pulmonary veins are those veins that carry blood from the lungs to the left atrium

## PARTIAL AND TOTAL ANOMALOUS PULMONARY VENOUS RETURN OR DRAINAGE (PAPVD, TAPVD)
### Introduction

Abnormal development of the pulmonary veins may result in either anomalous connection of at least one but not all four pulmonary veins into the right atrium (partial anomalous pulmonary venous return, PAPVR) or, anomalous connection of all four pulmonary veins into the right atrium (total anomalous pulmonary venous return, TAPVR). Normally, the pulmonary veins carrying oxygenated blood from the lungs connect to the left atrium. Thus, in PAPVR and TAPVR, one or more, or all four pulmonary veins, carry oxygenated blood from the lungs to the right atrium instead of the left atrium, as in a normal heart. The anomalous pulmonary vein or veins may be connected directly to the right atrium. They may also be connected to the inferior vena cava or the superior vena cava. There are many variations of this anomaly. The most common form of PAPVR is one in which the right upper pulmonary vein connects to the right atrium or the superior vena cava. This is the supracardiac type (Fig. 5.211). This type is almost always associated with an atrial septal defect. An interatrial communication, such as a patent foramen ovale or an atrial septal defect is also commonly present in TAPVR and considered part of the complex. These lesions are essential for shunting (mixing) of blood to the left heart. Both TAPVR and PAPVR are frequently isolated lesions, however, TAPVR has been

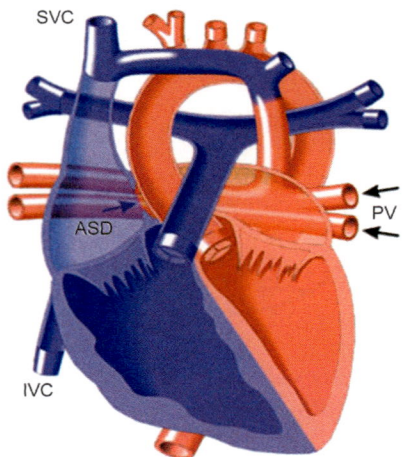

**Fig. 5.211:** Total anomalous pulmonary venous connection, (showing pulmonary veins connected to the left innominate vein. This is the supracardiac type. Oxygenated blood returning from the lungs is routed back into the superior vena cava, rather than the left atrium. The presence of an atrial septal defect is necessary to allow partially oxygenated blood to reach the left side of the heart

diagnosed with valvular stenosis or atresia, ventricular septal defect, transposition of the great arteries, tetralogy of Fallot, double outlet right ventricle and atrioventricular canal.

## Prevalence

Total and partial anomalous pulmonary venous return is relatively uncommon and occurs in about one out of every 10,000 live births.[137]

TAPVR is classified in three types to describe the various routes of pulmonary venous drainage (Fig. 5.212).

## Types of Total Anomalous Pulmonary Venous Return (TAPVR)

These are classfied into the following types:

1. **Supracardiac TAPVR:** In supracardiac TAPVR, all four pulmonary veins drain via a common vertical pulmonary vein into the innominate vein. The innominate vein is connected to the superior vena cava and blood then drains into the right atrium. This is the most common type, and occurs in approximately 45% of patients (Fig. 5.213).
2. **Cardiac TAPVR:** In cardiac TAPVR, the common pulmonary vein drains into the coronary sinus or in rare cases, the pulmonary veins are connected individually to the right atrium (Fig. 5.212).
3. **Infracardiac TAPVR:** In infracardiac TAPVR, the common pulmonary vein drains through the diaphragm into the portal vein or ductus venosus, which carries blood to the inferior vena cava and back to the right atrium (Fig. 5.214).

## Symptoms

Both congestive heart failure and pulmonary hypertension may develop soon after birth and is dependent on the severity of the lesion. The severity of symptoms is largely determined by the presence and the degree of obstruction to pulmonary venous return and the presence of an interatrial communication (patent foramen ovale or an atrial septal defect). Neonates with unobstructed TAPVR have few or no symptoms and present with signs and symptoms similar to that of an atrial septal defect. In neonates with obstructed TAPVR, however, venous drainage is obstructed leading to pulmonary venous hypertension, eventually leading to pulmonary arterial hypertension. These neonates present early, after birth, with profound cyanosis from pulmonary hypertension and oedema.

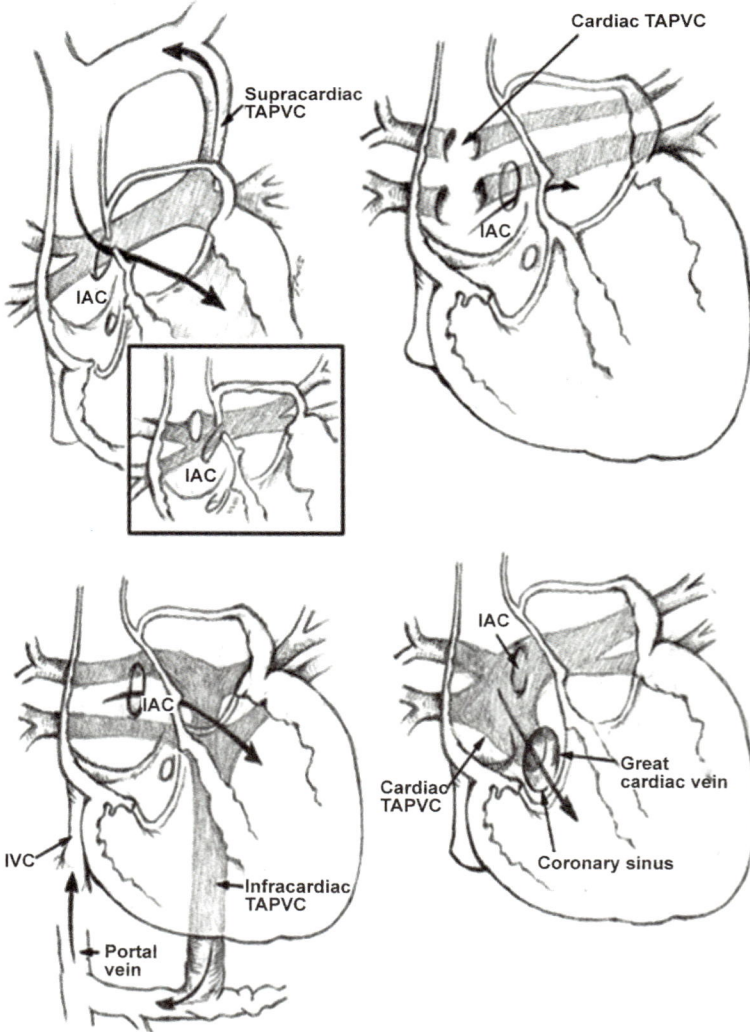

**Fig. 5.212:** Types of total anomalous pulmonary venous connection

The infradiaphragmatic or infracardiac drainage type is invariably severely obstructed, leading to dramatic pulmonary oedema and cyanosis unresponsive to supplemental oxygen

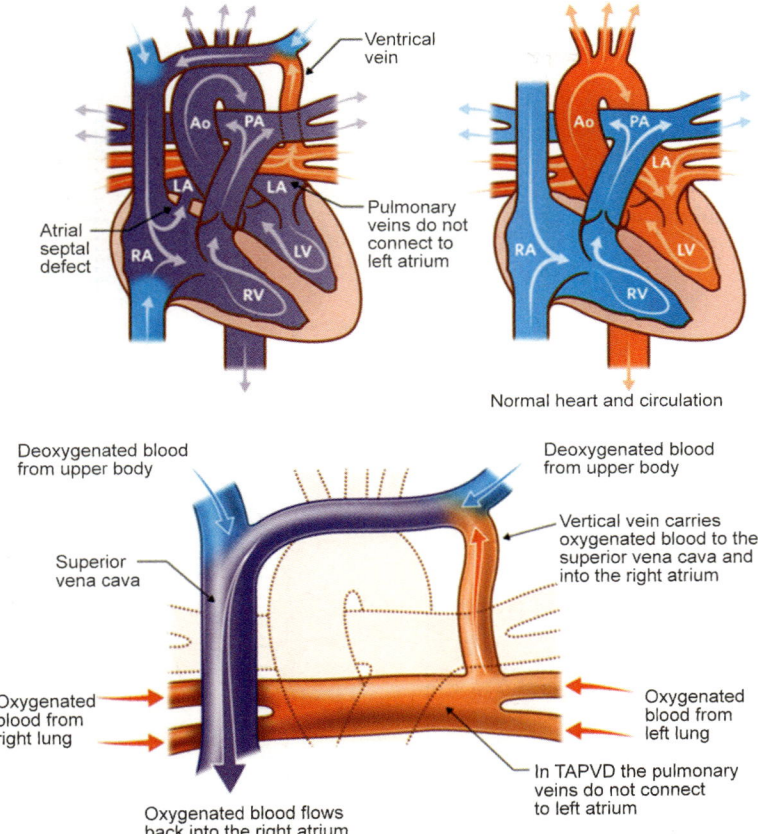

Ventrical vein

Atrial septal defect

Pulmonary veins do not connect to left atrium

Ao  PA
LA  LA
RA  LV
RV

Normal heart and circulation

Ao  PA
LA
RA  LV
RV

Deoxygenated blood from upper body

Deoxygenated blood from upper body

Superior vena cava

Vertical vein carries oxygenated blood to the superior vena cava and into the right atrium

Oxygenated blood from right lung

Oxygenated blood from left lung

In TAPVD the pulmonary veins do not connect to left atrium

Oxygenated blood flows back into the right atrium

**Fig. 5.213:** Supracardiac TAPVR: The pulmonary veins, which carry blood back to the heart after it has circulated through the lungs, are not connected to the left atrium. Instead they are connected to one of the veins from the main circulation so that the blood returning from the lungs drains back to the right side of the heart. The affected babies may be blue or show signs of heart failure. Most of them require surgical repair in the newborn period

therapy. The other two types do not typically involve obstruction and lead to mild signs of heart failure and mild cyanosis in the first month of life.

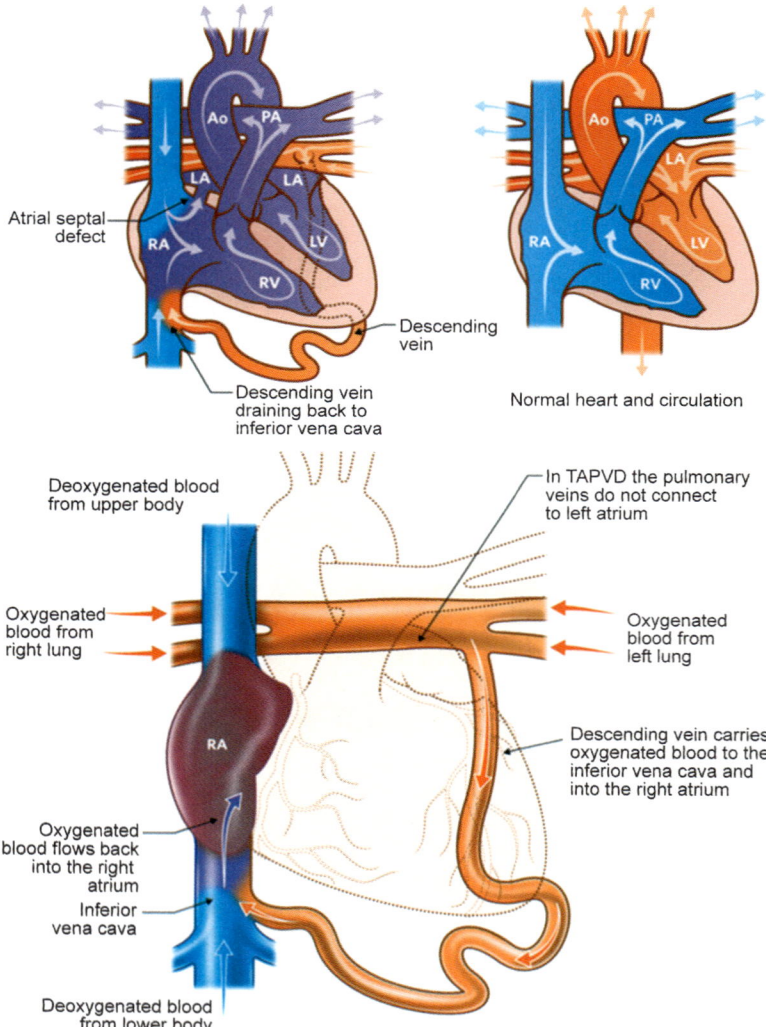

Atrial septal defect

Descending vein

Descending vein draining back to inferior vena cava

Normal heart and circulation

Deoxygenated blood from upper body

In TAPVD the pulmonary veins do not connect to left atrium

Oxygenated blood from right lung

Oxygenated blood from left lung

Descending vein carries oxygenated blood to the inferior vena cava and into the right atrium

Oxygenated blood flows back into the right atrium

Inferior vena cava

Deoxygenated blood from lower body

**Fig. 5.214:** Infracardiac TAPVR: The common pulmonary vein drains through the diaphragm into the portal vein or ductus venosus, which carries blood to the inferior vena cava and back to the right atrium

## Treatment

The treatment of PAPVD and TAPVD is surgical correction. The abnormal pulmonary venous connection to the right side of the heart is obliterated and the pulmonary venous blood is redirected to the left atrium. The main aim of the surgical correction is to ensure that there is no kinking or obstruction in the new connection between pulmonary veins and the left atrium. With the above aim of surgery, there are some differences in the surgical technique of correction depending upon the type of the venous abnormality.

## PAPVD Repair—Technique

1. A full midline sternotomy is performed.
2. The pericardium is opened and the abnormal connection of the pulmonary veins is identified. The most common form of defect involves abnormal connection of right upper pulmonary veins to the superior vena cava near its junction with right atrium. This is associated with the presence of a sinus venosus type atrial septal defect, which is present in the superior part of the interatrial septum. This abnormal connection is exposed with dissection.
3. Ascending aorta and inferior vena cava are cannulated in the usual manner. However, the superior vena caval cannula is inserted above the level of the attachment of abnormal pulmonary vein or into the innominate vein. In this way, the cannula stays away from the area of surgery.
4. Usual cardiopulmonary bypass is commenced and ascending aorta is clamped. Cardioplegia is given into the aortic root as usual.
5. Tapes are then passed around the superior and inferior caval cannulae to control systemic venous return. The abnormal openings of the right upper pulmonary veins and the sinus venosus atrial septal defect are then exposed. Some surgeons open the right atrium for repair while others make an incision on the side of the superior vena cava right atrium junction.
6. A generous patch of autologous pericardium is then fashioned and sutured to the edges of the pulmonary vein ostea and the sinus venosus atrial septal defect (ASD) to direct the blood from these veins through ASD towards the left atrium. It is important to ensure that the superior vena cava does not become narrow as a result of the above repair. If there is any doubt, a part of the autologous pericardial patch is used to augment the superior vena cava.

7. Air is removed from the left heart and aortic cross clamp is removed. Patient is rewarmed if required.

8. Weaning from the cardiopulmonary bypass is carried out usually without any problems.

9. After completion of the repair, the child is weaned from cardiopulmonary bypass. Pacing wires and chest drains are inserted in a standard fashion. The sternum is closed if the child is stable.

## TAPVD (Supracardiac and Infracardiac) Repair—Technique

1. A full midline sternotomy is performed.

2. Ascending aortic and bicaval cannulation is done in the usual manner and cardiopulmonary bypass is commenced.

3. Some surgeons carryout the procedure under hypothermic circulatory arrest and thus deep hypothermia is induced. This avoids constant flow of blood from pulmonary veins during repair and pulmonary veins do not require to be clamped. Other surgeons carryout repair without circulatory arrest but they have to dissect all pulmonary veins and put clamps on them to avoid flooding of operating field.

4. In cases of supracardiac and infracardiac type of TAPVD, all the pulmonary veins join together to form a confluence behind the left atrium which then drains through a vertical vein upwards (supracardiac) or downwards (infracardiac) to the systemic veins.

5. The vertical vein is dissected, doubly ligated and then divided. The right atrium is opened and atrial septal defect is enlarged to achieve good access to the left atrium. An opening is made in the posterior wall of the left atrium and the pulmonary venous confluence lying behind the left atrium is identified.

6. If circulatory arrest is not carried out, all the pulmonary veins draining into the confluence are dissected and controlled with fine clips.

7. The pulmonary confluence is then opened by an incision parallel to the incision in the back wall of the left atrium. A wide anastomosis is then made between the left atrium and the pulmonary confluence, ensuring no kinking at the anastomosis. A patch of autologous pericardium is then used

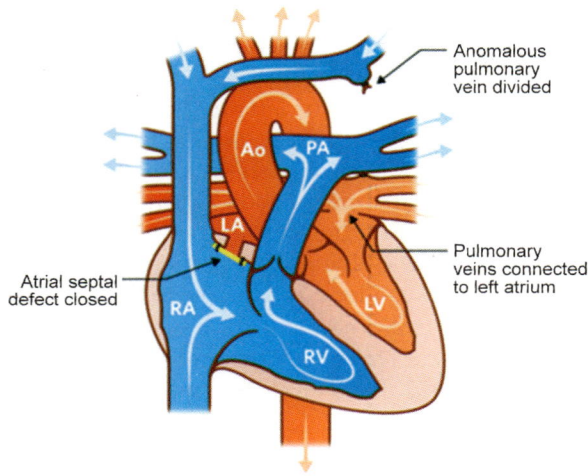

Anomalous
pulmonary
vein divided

Pulmonary
veins connected
to left atrium

Atrial septal
defect closed

**Fig. 5.215:** Surgical repair for supracardiac TAPVD consists of creating a wide anastomosis between the pulmonary venous confluence and the posterior wall of the left atrium, along with ligation of the vertical vein

to close the atrial septal defect and air is removed from the left heart. If circulation was stopped, it is started again at this stage and rewarming is commenced (Fig. 5.215).

8. Aortic cross clamp is removed and right atrium is closed.
9. Patient is weaned from cardiopulmonary bypass and cannulae are removed. Pacing wires and chest drains are inserted in a standard fashion.
10. Chest is closed when patient is stable.

### TAPVD (cardiac) Repair—Technique

1. A full midline sternotomy is performed.
2. Ascending aortic and bicaval venous cannulation is done in the usual manner and cardiopulmonary bypass is commenced. Moderate hypothermia is observed.
3. Ascending aorta is clamped and cardioplegia is given.
4. In cardiac type of TAPVD, the pulmonary veins drain directly to the right atrium or more commonly join the coronary sinus which, opens into the right atrium.

5. Superior and inferior vena cavae are snared and right atrium is opened. The atrial septal defect and an enlarged ostium of the coronary sinus are prominently seen. The roof of the coronary sinus separates it from the left atrial cavity. An incision is made into the roof of the coronary sinus to make a direct communication from the sinus to the left atrium. Then a wide patch of autologous pericardium is used in the form of a baffle covering the atrial septal defect and the osteum of the coronary sinus. Thus, all the blood in the coronary sinus including the pulmonary venous blood is directed to the left atrium.

6. The venous blood from the heart draining into the coronary sinus also gets directed to the left atrium creating a small right-to-left shunt but it is of no clinical significance and is well-tolerated by the patient.

7. In cases where the pulmonary veins open directly into the right atrium, a patch of autologous pericardium is used to form a baffle in the right atrium directing the blood from the pulmonary veins through ASD to left atrium.

8. Air is removed from the left heart and aortic clamp is removed.

9. Patient is weaned from the bypass circuit and cannulae are removed. Pacing wires and chest drains are inserted in a standard fashion.

10. Closure of chest is performed when patient is stable.

### SURGEON'S COMMENT

*Standard routines of paediatric cannulation should be observed. The choice of cannulae should be checked with the surgeon and may vary depending upon the congenital defect.*

*The scrub nurse should be familiar with surgeon's preference for preservation of autologous pericardial patch.*

*A generous supply of fine clips and clamps used by the surgeon should be available. During the haeostasis phase, a good supply of irrigation fluid, irrigation syringes and fine sutures should be available.*

## SCIMITAR SYNDROME

### Introduction

Scimitar syndrome is a rare congenital heart anomaly in which, usually a part of the pulmonary venous blood return, typically, from the right lung, returns to the inferior vena cava and drains into the right atrium instead of the left atrium. When seen in an X-ray, the anomalous vein resembles the shape of a scimitar (Turkish sword, Fig. 5.216), hence the name Scimitar syndrome (Fig 5.217).[138]

Associated anomalies are right lung hypoplasia, with dextro-position of the heart, and pulmonary artery hypoplasia.

About 50% of patients with Scimitar syndrome are asymptomatic, despite varying degrees of pulmonary hypoplasia and pulmonary artery hypertension. Neonates display worst symptoms of pulmonary hypertension, while older children or adults may only be diagnosed after complaints of recurrent respiratory infections caused by pulmonary venous hypertension and oedema of the lungs.

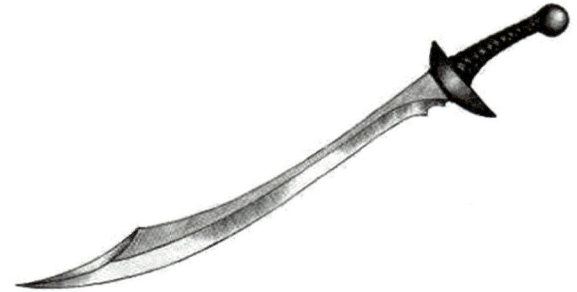

**Fig. 5.216:** The anomalous pulmonary vein resembles the shape of a Turkish sword (Scimitar)

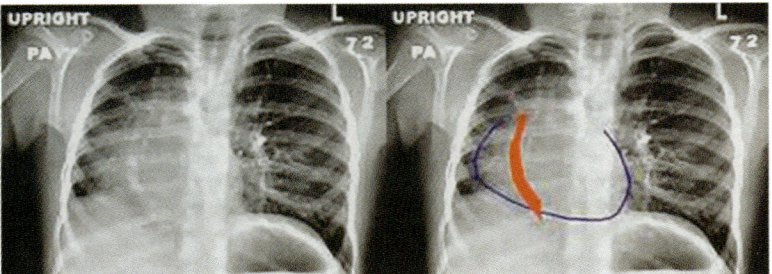

**Fig. 5.217:** Chest X-ray of a five-year-old girl with Scimitar syndrome. The heart (blue outline) is shifted to the right (dextro-position), and the anomalous pulmonary vein (red) has the shape of a Scimitar

Surgery involves the creation of an interatrial baffle (atrial septal defect) to redirect the anomalous pulmonary venous return into the left atrium. Alternatively, the anomalous vein can be reimplanted directly into the left atrium.

## Repair of Scimitar Anomaly—Technique

1. A standard median sternotomy is carried out.
2. Inferior vena cava is dissected and the Scimitar venous connection is exposed.
3. The dissection may be extended into the lower part of the right pleural cavity to identify the course of Scimitar vein.
4. Cannulation of the aorta and superior vena cava is carried out in the usual manner.
5. Inferior vena caval cannulation is done as low as possible so that the opening of the Scimitar vein into the inferior vena cava may be approached.
6. Aorta is clamped and cardioplegia is given.
7. Both cavae are snared and the lower part of the right atrium is opened.
8. An ASD is usually present but if the atrial septum is intact, an opening is made in the lower part of the septum.
9. If the ostium of the Scimitar vein is easily accessible, a patch of autologous pericardium is used to form a baffle between the ostium of the vein and the atrial septal defect. In this way, the drainage from the Scimitar vein is directed towards the left atrial cavity.
10. In some instances, the Scimitar vein may be inserted so low in the inferior vena cava that an intra-atrial baffle construction is not possible. In this case, the Scimitar vein is disconnected from the inferior vena cava and is directly anastomosed to the left atrium by a wide anastomosis. A small patch of autologous pericardium may be used to augment the anastomosis.
11. Air is removed from the left heart and aortic clamp is removed.
12. Right atrium is closed and patient is rewarmed.
13. Patient is weaned from cardiopulmonary bypass and cannulae are removed.
14. Chest is closed when patient is stable.

Section 5

## OTHER CARDIAC ANOMALIES

## COR TRIATRIATUM

### Introduction

Cor triatriatum is a heart with three atria. It is a congenital cardiac anomaly in which the left atrium, or in rare cases, the right atrium, is divided into two parts by a fold of tissue or a membrane. Most common, the left atrium is divided into an upper chamber, that receives blood from all four, or from one or two pulmonary veins, and a lower chamber that communicates with the left atrial appendage and the mitral valve (Fig. 5.218).

### Prevalence

Cor triatriatum has a prevalence of 0.1% and may be associated with other cardiac anomalies such as, atrial septal defect, partial anomalous pulmonary venous connection, ventricular septal defect, tetralogy of Fallot, atrioventricular defect, and double outlet right ventricle.[139]

### Symptoms

Thus, the symptoms depend on the communication between the upper and lower chamber and the number of pulmonary veins draining into the upper chamber. If the opening between the upper and lower chamber is small, less oxygenated blood will be able to pass through the mitral valve into the left ventricle and rest of the body. The obstruction will cause congestive heart failure and pulmonary oedema and a neonate diagnosed with this lesion may be critically ill. If the opening between the two chambers is large, children may present in childhood or later in life with symptoms similar to mitral valve stenosis, including pulmonary hypertension and heart failure.

### Treatment

Surgical resection of the accessory membrane has been successful in symptomatic children with cor triatriatum. Complete resection of the membrane and closure of the atrial septum with a pericardial patch is a common approach. Associated congenital defects need to be corrected at the same time.

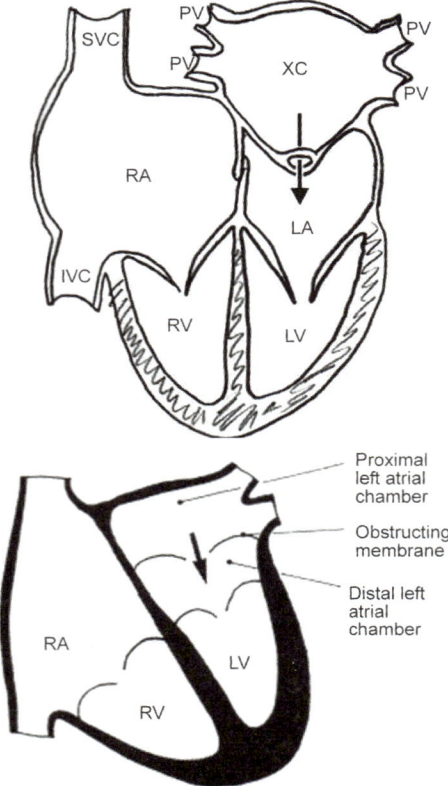

**Fig. 5.218:** Cor triatriatum—the left atrium, or in rare cases, the right atrium, is divided into two parts by a fold of tissue or a membrane

## VASCULAR RINGS/SLINGS

### Introduction

A vascular ring or sling is a vascular structure, usually the aortic arch and/or associated blood vessels, which during early development of the embryo encircles partial (vascular sling) or completely (vascular ring) the oesophagus and the trachea.[140] Most common is double aortic arch (Figs 5.219 and 5.220). In this anomaly, the aorta is divided into two arches, which encircle the trachea and oesophagus. In about 30% of these cases, one of the aortic arches is small, but still in continuation with the descending aorta and thus forming a complete vascular ring, compressing both the trachea and the oesophagus. Double arch typically produces the most severe airway compression in infants as a result of a tight ring around the trachea and oesophagus. Liquids (breastfeeding or mik) are usually well-tolerated. However, when infants start on solid foods, this may not be tolerated so well and vomiting may occur. In 20% of these cases the defect is associated with other cardiac anomalies, with ventricular septal defect and tetralolgy of Fallot being the most common.[141]

## Prevalence

Vascular rings and slings are rare congenital anomalies and account for less than 1% of congenital cardiac anomalies. Most common is double aortic arch and right aortic arch (85–90%).[142, 143]

## Symptoms

Double aortic arch typically produces the most severe airway compression in infants as a result of a tight ring around the trachea and oesophagus. Liquids (breastfeeding or milk) is usually well-tolerated. However, when infants start on solid foods, this may not be tolerated so well and vomiting may occur.

Typically, all vascular rings/slings cause compression on the airway and/or oesophagus in various degrees depending on the severity of the defect. Infants may present with cyanosis, wheezing, respiratory distress and difficulty feeding if oesophagus is

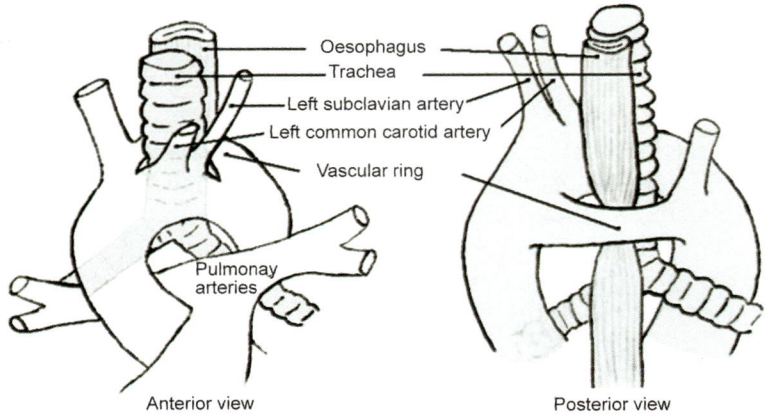

Anterior view          Posterior view

**Fig. 5.219:** Double aortic arch

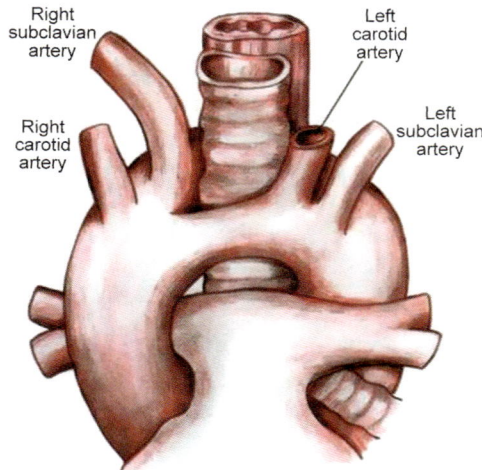

Right subclavian artery

Right carotid artery

Left carotid artery

Left subclavian artery

**Fig. 5.220:** Double aortic arch—in this anomaly, the aorta is divided into two arches, which encircle the trachea and oesophagus

involved. In some cases the anomaly may not present till adulthood.[144] One of the first reported cases of vascular slings was in the 18th century of a woman, who had suffered dysphagia for years and eventually died of starvation.

Another type of vascular ring is the anomalous left pulmonary artery or pulmonary artery sling. In this defect the left pulmonary artery arises from the right pulmonary artery and slings between the trachea and oesophagus to the left lung (Fig. 5.221). This lesion is often associated with abnormalities of the trachea and/or bronchus. Also, in 20% of these cases, other intracardiac defects are seen.

## Treatment

Surgical intervention is indicated in all symptomatic children and usually consists of dividing the ring/sling.[145] A left thoracotomy approach can be used to repair most vascular ring anomalies.

Many surgeons approach a pulmonary artery sling with a median sternotomy and perform cardiopulmonary bypass. Aortic and single atrial cannulation is used. The usual tracheal anomaly associated with a pulmonary artery sling is tracheal stenosis. The choice of repair of tracheal stenosis depends on the length of the trachea involved. Resection with end-to-end anastomosis is used for short segments, whereas tracheoplasty is used for long-segment anomalies.[146]

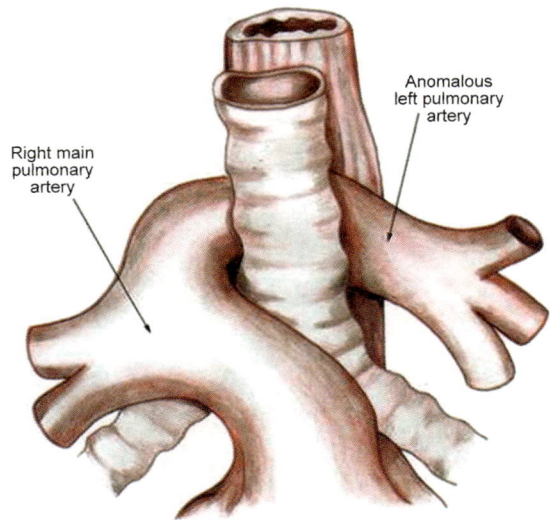

**Fig. 5.221:** Aberrant left pulmonary artery or pulmonary artery sling. In this defect the left pulmonary artery arises from the right pulmonary artery and slings between the trachea and oesophagus to the left lung.

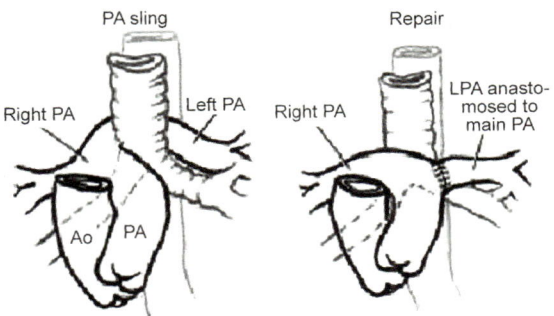

**Fig. 5.222:** Repair of pulmonary artery sling

## *Outcome of Surgical Repair*

Approximately 95% of children undergoing operative correction of an isolated vascular ring anomaly have a normal lifespan and is asymptomatic. Children with less-than-optimal long-term results are those with anomalous left pulmonary artery with and without complete tracheal rings and those with severe associated intracardiac defects.[147]

## ECTOPIA CORDIS

### Introduction

Ectopia cordis (Latin word **Ectopia** means *outside/away* and **cardis** means *heart*) is a congenital malformation in which the heart is abnormally located either partially or totally outside of the thorax. The ectopic heart can be found along a spectrum of anatomical locations, including the neck, chest, or abdomen (Fig. 5.223). In most cases, the heart protrudes outside the chest through a split sternum.[148]

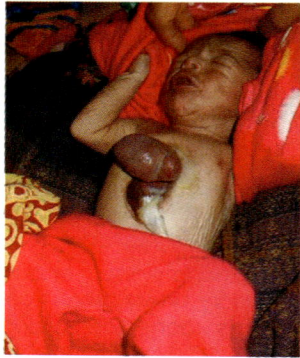

**Fig. 5.223:** Ectopia cordis—the ectopic heart can be found along a spectrum of anatomical locations, including the neck, chest, or abdomen

### Prevalence

The occurrence of ectopic cordis is 8 per 1 million births.[149]

### Treatment

As ectopia cordis is so rare and most children die soon after birth, limited treatment options have been developed. Successful surgeries have been performed, but the mortality rate remains high. However, with the advances in all aspects of medicine, the number of infants who undergo successful repair and survive is steadily increasing.[150]

# References

1. American Heart Association. Congenital Heart Disease.
2. British Heart Foundation. Congenital Heart Disease.
3. Perioperative Standards and Recommended Practices for Inpatient and Ambulatory Settings. AORN. 2011. AORN: Association of perioperative Registered Nurses.
4. Hoffman J, Kaplan S. The incidence of congenital heart disease. *J Am Coll Cardiol.* 2002; **39**(12): 1890–1900.
5. Freeman SB, Taft LF, Dooley KJ, et al. Population-based study of congenital heart defects in Down syndrome. *Am J Med Genet.* 1988; **80**(3): 213–7.
6. Kaemmerer H, Oechslin E, Seidel H, et al. Marfan syndrome: What internists and pediatric or adult cardiologists need to know? *Expert Rev Cardiovasc Ther.* 2005; 3: 891–909.
7. Nora JJ, Nora HH. Maternal transmission of congenital heart diseases: New recurrence risk figures and the questions of cytoplasmic inheritance and vulnerability to teratogens. *Am J Cardiol.* 1987; **59**(5): 5459–63.
8. Becker S M, Al Halees Z, Molina C, et al. Consanguinity and congenital heart disease in Saudi Arabia. *Am J Med Genet.* 2001; **99**(1): 8–13
9. Barnes–Powell LL. Infants of diabetic mothers: The effects of hyperglycemia on the fetus and neonate. *Neonat Netw.* 2007; **26**(5): 283–90.
10. Nielsen GL, Norgard B, Puho E, et al. Risk of specific congenital abnormalities in offspring of women with diabetes. *Diabet Med.* 2005; 22: 693–96.
11. Campbell M. Place of maternal rubella in the aetiology of congenital heart disease. *BMJ.* 1961; 1: 691–96.
12. McIntosh ED, Menser ME. A fifty-year follow-up of congenital rubella. *Lancet* 1992: 340–414.
13. Tikkanen J, Heinonen OP. Risk factors for atrial septal defect. *Eur J Epidemiol.* 1992; 8: 509–15.
14. Cohen LS, Friedman JM, Jefferson JW, et al. A re-evaluation of risk of *in utero* exposure to lithium. *JAMA.* 1994; 271: 146–150.
15. American pregnancy association. Last updated February 2014.
16. Malik S, Cleves MA, Honein MA, et al. National Birth Defects Study. *Pediatrics.* 2008: **121**(4): e810–16.

17. Kallen K. Maternal smoking and congenital heart defects. *Eur J Epidemiol*. 1999; 15: 731–37.
18. American Heart Association. Infective endocarditis. Updated 1214.
19. Diller GP, Gatzoulis MA. Pulmonary vascular disease in adults with congenital heart disease. Circulation. 2007; **115**(8): 1039–50.
20. Rashkind WJ, Miller WW. Creation of an atrial septal defect without thoracotomy: A palliative approach to complete transposition of the great arteries. *JAMA*. 1966; **196**(11): 991–92.
21. Perloff JK, Warnes CA. Challenges posed by adults with repaired congenital heart disease. Circulation. 2001; 103: 2637–43.
22. Nieminen HP, Jokinen EV, Sairanen HI. Late results of pediatric surgery in Finland: a population-based study with 96% follow-up. Circulation 2001; **104**(5): 570–75.
23. Van Praagh R. The segmental approach to diagnosis in congenital heart disease. In: Bergsma D, editor. Birth Defects (Original Article Series). 1972; 8:4–23.
24. Higgins CB. Essentials of cardiac radiology and imaging. Philadelphia, Pa: JB Lippincott Co; 1992: 283–331.
25. Wilhelm A. Situs inversus imaging. Medscape. 2013.
26. Maldjian PD, Saric M. Approach to dextro-cardia in adults: review. *AJR Am J Roentgenol*. 2007; **188**(6): 39–49.
27. Gindes L, Hegesh J, Barkai G, Jacobson JM, Achiron R. Isolated levocardia: Prenatal diagnosis, clinical importance, and literature review. *J Ultrasound Med*. 2007; **26**(3): 361–65.
28. Fung TY, Chan DL, Leung TN, et al. Dextro-cardia in pregnancy: 20 years' experience. *J Reprod Med*. 2006; **51**(7): 573–77.
29. Anderson RH, Shinebourne EA, Gerlis LH. Criss-cross atrioventricular relationships producing paradoxical atrioventricular concordance or discordance: their significance to nomenclature of congenital heart disease. *Circulation*. 1974; 50: 176–80.
30. LeRoy S, Elixson E M, O'Brien P, et al. AHA scientific statement. Recommendations for preparing children and adolescents for invasive cardiac procedures. A statement from the american heart association pediatric nursing subcommittee of the council on cardiovascular nursing in collaboration With the council on cardiovascular diseases of the young. *Circulation,* 2003; 108: 2550–64.
31. Perioperative standards and recommended practices. AORN. 2011.
32. Cohn LH, Fifty years of open-heart surgery. *Circulation*. 2003; 107: 2168–70.
33. Cooley DA. C. Walton Lillehei. the "Father of open heart surgery". *Circulation*. 1999; 100: 1364–65.
34. Schure AY. Cardiopulmonary bypass in infants and children: what's new? *S Afr J Anaesthesiol Analg*. 2010; **16**(1).

35. Eisenmenger V. Die angeborenen Defecte der Kammerscheidewand des Herzens. *Z Klin Med.* 1897; 32: 1–28.

36. Burke RP. Patent ductus arteriosus. Mastery of cardiothoracic surgery, 2nd ed. 2007; 73: 716–21.

37. Hillman ND, Mavroudis C, Backer CL. Patent ductus arteriosus. In: Mavroudis C, Backer CL, editors. *Pediat Cardiac Surg.* Philadelphia: Mosby; 2003: 223–33.

38. Koch J, Hensley G, Roy L, et al. Prevalence of spontaneous closure of the ductus arteriosus in neonates at a birth weight of 1000 grams or less. Pediatrics. 2006; **117**(4): 1113–21.

39. Victor Alzamora–Castro, Guido Battilana, Ricardo Abugattas, et al. Patent ductus arteriosus and high altitude. Am J Cardiol. 1960; 5(6): 761–63. University of San Marcos Medical School and the Hospital Dos de Mayo, Lima, Peru.

40. Hoffman JIE, Kaplan S. The incidence of congenital heart disease. *J Am Coll Cardiol.* 2002; 39: 1890–1900.

41. Tavera MC, Bassareo PP, Biddau R, et al. Role of echocardiography on the evaluation of patent ductus arteriosus in newborns. *J Matern Fetal Neonat Med.* 2009;1–4.

42. Hamrick SEG, Hansmann G, Patent Ductus Arteriosus of the Preterm Infant. Pediatrics. 2010; **125**(5).

43. Valentík P, Omeje IC, and Nosál M. Surgical closure of patent ductus arteriosus in pre-term babies. Images Paediatr. *Cardiol.* 2007; **9**(2): 27–36.

44. Kaemmerer H, Meisner H, Hess J, et al. Surgical treatment of patent ductus arteriosus: A new historical perspective. *Am J Cardiol.* 2004; **94**(9): 1153–54.

45. Shah SN. Patent Foramen Ovale. Medscape. Updated: 2014.

46. Hanna JP, Ping Sun J, Furlan AJ, et al. Patent foramen ovale and brain infarct: echocardiographic predictors, recurrence, and prevention. Stroke. 1994; 25: 782–86.

47. Movsowitz C, Podolsky LA, Meyerowitz CB, Jacobs LE, Kotler MN. Patent foramen ovale: A non-functional embryological remmant or a potential cause of significant pathology? *J Am Soc Echocardiogr.* 1992; 5: 259–70.

48. De Castro S, Cartoni D, Conti G, et al. Continuous monitoring by biplane transesophageal echocardiography of pulmonary and paradoxical embolism. *J Am Soc Echocardiogr.* 1995; 8: 217–20.

49. Hagen PT, Scholz DG, Edwards WD. Incidence and size of patent foramen ovale during the first 10 decades of life: An autopsy study of 965 normal hearts. *Mayo Clin Proc.* 1984; 59: 17–20.

50. Mainwaring RD, Lamberti JJ. Atrial septal defects. Mastery of cardiothoracic surgery, 2nd ed. 2007. 739–49.

51. Reller MD, Strickland MJ, Riehle-Colarusso T, et al. Prevalence of Congenital heart Defects in Metropolitan Atlanta, 1998–2005. J Pediatr. 2008; 153: 807–13.

52. Markham LW. Atrial septal defect. Medscape. Updated: 2014.

53. Hufnagel C, Gillespie J. Closure of interaurical septal defects. Bull Georgetown. *Univ Med Cent.* 1951; 4: 137–39.

54. Roos-Hesselink JW, Meijboom FJ, Spitaels SE, et al. Excellent survival and low incidence of arrhythmias, stroke and heart failure long-term after surgical ASD closure at young age. A prospective follow-up study of 21–33 years. *Eur Heart J.* 2003; 24: 190–97.

55. Botto LD, Correa A, Erickson D. Racial and temporal variations in the prevalence of heart defects. *Pediatrics.* 2001; **107**(3): e32.

56. Bjornard K, Riehle-Colarusso T, Gilboa SM, et al. Patterns in the prevalence of congenital heart defects, metropolitan Atlanta, 1978 to 2005. Birth defects. *Res Part A Clin Mol Teratol.* 2013; **97**(2): 87–94.

57. Ramaswamy P. Ventricular Septal Defects. Medscape. 2013.

58. Baslaim G. Modification of Trusler's formula for pulmonary artery banding. *Heart Lung Circ.* 2009; **18**(5): 353–7.

59. Meijboom F, Szatmari A, Utens E, et al. Long-term follow-up after surgical closure of ventricular septal defect in infancy and childhood. *J Am Coll Cardiol.* 1994; 24: 1358–64.

60. Hoffman JIE. Incidence of congenital heart disease: Postnatal incidence. *Pediatr Cardiol.* 1995; 16: 103–113.

61. Rosenthal GL, Wilson PD, Permutt T, et al. Birth weight and cardiovascular malformations: A population-based study. The Baltimore–Washington Infant Study. *Am J Epidemiol.* 1991; **133**(12): 1273–81.

62. Webb G, Gatzoulis MA. Atrial septal defects in the adult. Recent progress and overview. *Circulation.* 2006; 114: 1645–53.

63. Najm HK, Coles JG, Endo M, et al. Complete atrioventricualr septal defects: Results of repair, risk factors, and freedom from reoperation. Circulation 1997; **96**(9 Suppl): II-3 11–5.

64. Pettersen MD. Pediatric complete atrioventricular septal defects treatment and management. *Medscape* 2013.

65. Atz AM, Hawkins JA, Lu M, et al. Surgical management of complete atrioventricular septal defect: Associations with surgical technique, age, and trisomy 21. *J Thorac Cardiovasc Surg.* 2011; **141**(6): 1371–79.

66. Blalock A, Taussig HB. The surgical treatment of malformations of the heart. *JAMA* 1945; **128**(3): 189–202.

67. Von Bernuth G, Ritter DG, Frye RL, et al. Evaluation of patients with tetralogy of Fallot and Potts anastomosis. *Am J Cardiol.* 1971; **27**(3): 259–63.

68. Glenn WW. Circulatory bypass of the right side of the heart. Shunt between superiorvena cava and distal right pulmonary artery; report of clinical application. *N Engl J Med.* 1958; **259**(3): 117–20.

69. Kawashima Y, Kitamura S, Matsuda H, et al. Total cavo-pulmonary shunt operation in complex cardiac anomalies. A new operation. *J Thorac Cardiovasc Surg* 1984; 87: 74–81.

70. Fontan F, Baudet E. Surgical repair of tricuspid atresia. Thorax. 1971; **26**(3): 240–8.

71. Kreutzer G, Galindez E, Bono H, et al. An operation for the correction of tricuspid atresia. *J Thorac Cardiovasc Surg.* 1973; **66**(4): 613–21.

72. Weber HS, Gleason MM, Myers JL, et al. The fontan operation in infants less than 2 years of age. *J Am Coll Cardiol.* 1992; **19**(4): 828–33.

73. Baslaim G, Hussain A, Kouatli A, et al. Bovine valved xenograft conduits in the extracardiac Fontan procedure. *J Thorac Cardiovasc Surg.* 2003: 126: 586–88.

74. Baslaim G. Bovine valved xenograft (Contegra) conduit in the extracardiac fontan procedure: The preliminary experience. *J Card. Surg.* 2008: 23: 146–9.

75. Tandon R, Edwards JE. Tricuspid atresia. A re-evaluation and classification. *J Thorac Cardiovasc Surg.* 1974; **67**(4): 530–42.

76. Weinberg PM. Anatomy of tricuspid atresia and its relevance to current forms of surgical therapy. *Ann Thorac Surg.* 1980; **29**(4): 306–11.

77. Nadas AS, Fyler DC. Tricuspid Atresia. Pediatric Cardiology. 3rd ed. Philadelphia, PA: WB Saunders; 1972.

78. Mann RJ, Lie JT. The life story of Wilhelm Ebstein (1836–1912) and his almost overlooked description of a congenital heart disease. *Mayo Clin Proc.* 1979; 54: 197–204.

79. Riaz K. Ebstein anomaly. *Medscape.* Updated 2014.

80. Attenhofer Jost CH, Connolly HM, Dearani JA, et al. Congenital heart disease for the adult cardiologist. Ebstein's anomaly. *Circulation.* 2007; 115: 277–85.

81. Pettersen MD. Tetralogy of Fallot with pulmonary atresia. *Medscape.* Udated 2014.

82. Schneider DJ. Pediatric subvalvular aortic stenosis. *Medscape.* Updated: Oct 2013.

83. Parry AJ, Kovalchin JP, Suda K, et al. Hanley FL. Resection of subaortic stenosis: Can a more aggressive approach be justified? *Eur J Cardiothorac.* 1999; 15: 631–8.

84. Ross DN. Replacement of aortic and mitral valves with a pulmonary autigraft. *Lancet.* 1967; **2**(7523): 956–8.

85. Alsoufi B, Al Halees Z, Manlhiot C, et al. Superior results following the Ross procedure in patients with congenital heart disease. *J Heart Valve Dis.* 2010; **19**(3): 269–77.

86. Bentall HH, DeBonno A. A technique for complete replacement of the ascending aorta. *Thorax.* 1968; 23: 338–39.

87. Cook AC, Anderson RH. The anatomy of hearts with double inlet ventricle. *Cardiol Young.* 2006; **16**(suppl 1): 22–6.

88. Vyas H, Hagler DJ. Double inlet left ventricle. Current treatment options in cardiovascular medicine. 2007; **9**(5): 391–98.
89. Baas AS. Congenitally corrected transposition. *Medscape.* 2014.
90. Sloth AD, Jensen JK, Steffensen FH, et al. Congenitally corrected transposition of the great arteries newly diagnosed in a 76-year-old woman. *Ugeskr Laeger.* 2009; **171**(5): 319–21.
91. Al Habib HF, Jacobs JP, Mavroudis C, et al. Contemporary patterns of management of tetralogy of Fallot: data from the society of thoracic surgeons database. *Ann Thorac Surg.* 2010; **90**(3): 813–19.
92. Alghamdi AA. Double outlet right ventricle. *Medscape.* Updated: 2012.
93. Demir MT, Amasyall Y, Kopuz C, et al. The double outlet right ventricle with additional cardiac malformations: An anatomic and echocardiographic study. *Folia Morphol (Warsz).* 2009; **68**(2): 104–8.
94. Tchervenkov CI, Walters HL, Chu VF. Congenital heart surgery nomenclature and database Project: Double outlet left ventricle. *Ann Thorac Surg.* 2000; 69: 264–69.
95. McElhinney DB.Truncus Arteriosus. *Medscape. Updated:* 2012.
96. Collett RW, Edwards JE. Persistent truncus arteriosus: A classification according to anatomic types. *Surg Clin North Am.* 1949; 29: 1245–70.
97. Van Praagh R, Van Praagh S. The anatomy of common aortopulmonary trunk (truncus arteriosus communis) and its embryologic implications. A study of 57 necropsy cases. *Am J Cardiol.* 1965; **16**(3): 406–25.
98. Russell HM, Pasquali SK, Jacobs JP, et al. Outcomes of repair of common arterial trunk with truncal valve surgery: A review of the society of thoracic surgeons congenital heart surgery database. *Ann Thorac Surg.* 2012; 93:164.
99. Rajasinghe HA, McElhinney DB, Reddy VM, et al. Long-term follow-up of truncus arteriosus repaired in infancy: A twenty-year experience. *J Thorac Cardiovasc Surg.* 1997; 113: 869.
100. Senning A. Surgical correction of transposition of the great vessels. *Surgery.* 1959; **45**(6): 966–80.
101. Mustard WT. Successful two-stage correction of transposition of the great arteries. Surgery. 1964; 55: 469.
102. Jatene AD, Fontes VF, Paulista PP, et al. Successful anatomic correction of transposition of the great vessels. A preliminary report. *Arq Bras Cardiol.* 1975; (4): 461–64.
103. Jatene AD, Fontes VF, Paulista PP, et al. Anatomic correction of transposition of the great vessels. *J Thorac Cardiovasc Surg.* 1976; **72**(3): 364–70.
104. Rastelli GC. A new approach to anatomic repair of transposition of the great arteries. *Mayo Clin Proc.* 1969; 44: 1.
105. Alsoufi B, Awan A, Al-Omrani A, et al. The rastelli procedure for transposition of the great arteries: Resection of the infundibular septum diminishes recurrent left ventricular outflow tract obstruction risk. *Ann Thorac Surg.* 2009; (88): 137–43.

106. Nikaidoh H. Aortic translocation and biventricular outflow tract reconstruction: A new surgical repair for transposition of the great arteries associated with a ventricular septal defect and pulmonary stenosis. *J Thorac Cardiovasc Surg.* 1984; 88: 365–72.

107. Morrell VO, Jacobs JP, Quintessenza JA. Aortic translocation and biventricular outflow tract reconstruction in the management of complex transposition of the great arteries with ventricular septal defect and pulmonary stenosis: Results and follow-up. *Ann Thorac Surg.* 2005; 79: 2089–93.

108. Kreutzer C, De Vive J, Oppido G, et al. Twenty-five-year experience with rastelli repair for transposition of the great arteries. *J Thorac Cardiovasc Surg.* 2000; (120): 211–23.

109. Damus PS. Correspondence. *Ann Thorac Surg.* 1975; (20): 724–25.

110. Kaye MP. Anatomical correction of transposition of the great arteries. *Mayo Clin Proc.* 1975; (50): 638–40.

111. Stansel HC Jr. A new operation for d-loop transposition of the great arteries. *Ann Thorac Surg.* 1975; (19): 565–67.

112. Bland EF. Congenital anomalies of the coronary arteries: Report of an unusual case associated with cardiac hypertrophy. 1933; (8): 787–801.

113. Mancini MC. Surgical approach to anomalous left coronary artery from the pulmonary artery. *Medscape.* 2012.

114. Mancini MC. Anomalous left coronary artery from the pulmonary artery. *Medscape.* Updated: 2014.

115. Takeuchi S, Imamura H, Katsumoto K, et al. New surgical method for repair of anomalous left coronary artery from pulmonary artery. *J Thorac Cardiovasc Surg.* 1979; **78**(1): 7–11.

116. Jonas RA, Quaegebeur JM, Kirklin JW, et al. Outcomes in patients with interrupted aortic arch and ventricular septal defect: a multi-institutional study. *J Thorac Cardiovasc Surg.* 1994; (107): 1099.

117. Freedom RM, Bain HH, Esplugas E, et al. Ventricular septal defect in interruption of aortic arch. *Am J Cardiol.* 1977; (39): 572–82.

118. Koutlas TC. Surgical approach to coarctation of the aorta and interrupted aortic arch. *Medscape.* Updated: 2014.

119. Schreiber C, Matzzitelli D, Haehnel JC, et al. The interrupted aortic arch: an overview after 20 years of surgical treatment. *Eur J Cardiothorac Surg.* 1997; **12**(3): 466–69.

120. Serraf A, Lacour-Gayet F, Robotin M, et al. Repair of interrupted aortic arch: A ten-year experience. *J Thorac Cardiovasc Surg.* 1996; **112**(5); 1150–60.

121. Barnes ME, Mitchell ME, Tweddell JS. Aortopulmonary window. *Semin Thorac Cardiovasc Surg Pediatr Card Surg Annu.* 2011; **14**(1): 67–74.

122. Backer CL, Mavroudis C. Surgical management of aortopulmonary window: A 40-year experience. *Eur J Cardiothorac Surg.* 2002; **21**(5): 773–9.

123. Norwood WI, Kirklin JK, Sanders SP, Hypoplastic left heart syndrome: Experience with palliative surgery. *Am J Cardiol.* 1980; **45**(1): 87–91.

124. Bharati S, Lev M. The surgical anatomy of hypoplasia of aortic tract complex. *J Thorac Cardiovasc Surg.* 1984; **88**(1): 97–101.

125. Rao PS, Striepe V, Merrill WH. Hypoplastic left heart syndrome. In: Kambam J, editor. Cardiac anesthesia for infants and children. St. Louis, MO: Mosby-Year Book; 1994: 296–309.

126. Freedom RM. Aortic atresia. In: Keith JD, Rowe RD, Vlad P, editors Heart disease in infants and children. 3rd ed. New York: McMillian; 1978.

127. Fyler DC. Prevalence trends. In: Fyler DC, editor. Nadas' Pediatric Cardiology Hanley & Belfus. Philadelphia: 1992.

128. Norwood WI Jr. Hypoplastic left heart syndrome. *Ann Thorac Surg.* 1991; **52**(3): 688–95.

129. Norwood WI, Lang P, Hansen DD. Physiologic repair of aortic atresia-hypoplastic left heart syndrome. *N Engl J Med.* 6 1983; **308**(1): 23–6.

130. Bridges ND, Lock JE, Castaneda AR. Baffle fenestration with subsequent transcatheter closure. Modification of the Fontan operation for patients at increased risk. *Circulation.* 1990; **82**(5): 1681–89.

131. Sano S, Ishino K, Kawada M, et al. Right ventricle-pulmonary artery shunt in first stage palliation of hypoplastic left heart syndrome. *J Thorac Cardiovasc Surg.* 2003.

132. Malec E, Januszewska K, Kolcz J, et al. Right ventricle-to-pulmonary artery shunt versus modified Blalock–Taussig shunt in the Norwood procedure for hypoplastic left heart syndrome–influence on early and late haemodynamic status. *Eur J Cardiothorac Surg.* 2003.

133. Pizarro C, Norwood W I. Right ventricle to pulmonary artery conduit has a favourable impact on postoperative physiology after stage I Norwood: preliminary results. *Eur J Cardiothoarac Surg.* 2003.

134. Alsoufi B, Bennetts J, Verma S, et al. New developments in the treatment of hypoplastic left heart syndrome. Pediatrics 2007; **119**(1): 109–17.

135. Kanter, KR. The Yasui operation. *Operat Tech Thorac Cardiovasc Surg.* 2010; 15: 206–22.

136. Kanter KR, Kirshbom PM, Kogon BE. Biventricular repair with the Yasui operation (Norwood/Rastelli) for systemic outflow tract obstruction with two adequate ventricles. The *Annals of Thoracic Surgery.* 2012; **93**(6): 1999–2006.

137. Bjornard K, Riehle-Colarusso T, Gilboa SM, Correa A. Patterns in the prevalence of congenital heart defects, metropolitan Atlanta, 1978 to 2005. *Birth Defects Res Part A: Clin Mol Teratol.* 2013; 97: 87–94.

138. Vanderheyden M, Goethals M, Van Hoe L. Partial anomalous pulmonary venous connection or scimitar syndrome. Heart. 2003; **89**(7): 761.

139. Thakrar A, Shapiro MD, Jassal DS, et al. Cor triatriatum: the utility of cardiovascular imaging. *Can J Cardiol.* 2007; **23**(2): 143–45.

140. Mancini MC. Vascular ring and sling surgery. *Medscape.* Updated: 2013.

141. Yamamoto LG. Difficulty breathing throughout infancy. In: Yamamoto LG, Inaba AS, DiMauro R editors. Radiology cases in pediatric emergency medicine, 1999, volume 6.

142. Humphry C, Duncan K, Fletcher S. Decade of experience with vascular rings at a single institution. *Pediatrics.* 2006; **117**(5): e903–8.

143. Greiner A, Perkmann R, Rieger M, et al. Vascular ring causing tracheal *compression in an adult patient. Ann Thorac Surg.* 2003; **75**(6): 1959–60.

144. Yildirim A, Karabulut N, Dogan S, Herek D. Congenital thoracic arterial anomalies in adults: A CT overview. *Diagn Interv Radiol.* 2011; **17**(4): 352–62.

145. Backer CL, Mavroudis C. Surgical approach to vascular rings. *Adv Card Surg.* 1997; 9: 29–64.

146. Bai S, Li XF, Liu CX, et al. Surgical treatment for vascular anomalies and tracheoesophageal compression. *Chin Med J (Engl).* 2012; **125**(8): 1504–07.

147. Humphrey C, Duncan K, Fletcher S. Decade of experience with vascular rings at a single institution. *Pediatrics.* 2006; **117**(5): e903–8.

148. Kumar B, Sharma C, Sinha DD, et al. Ectopia cordis associated with Cantrell's pentalogy. *Ann Thorac Med.* 2008; 3(4): 152–53.

149. Hornberger LK, Colan SD, Lock JF, et al. Outcome of patients with ectopia cordis and significant intracardiac defects. *Circulation.* 1996; 94: 32–7.

150. Kabbani MS, Rasheed K, Mallick MS, et al. Thoraco-abdominal ectopia cordis: Case report. *Annals of Saudi Medicine.* 2002; vol. 22: 5–6.

## FURTHER READING

1. Alexander's Nursing Practice. Margaret F. Alexander, Maggie Nicol, Christine Brooker. Elsevier, Health Science Division, 2011.

2. Cardiopulmonary bypass: Principles and practice, 2nd ed. Edited by Glenn P. Gravlee, M.D. Richard F. Davis, M.D., (Mark Kursz, C.C.P. and Joe R. Utley, M.D.2000 by Lippincott Williams & Wilkins.

3. Mastery of cardiothoracic surgery. 2nd ed. Larry R. Kaiser, Irving L Kron, Thomas L. Spray. 2007 by Lippincott Williams & Wilkins.

4. Perioperative standards and recommended practices for inpatient and ambulatory settings. AORN. 2011. AORN: Association of perioperative registered nurses.

# Index

## A

Adib Domingos Jatene 282
Adolescent 51
Alfred Blalock 117
Antegrade paediatric aortic root
    cannula (DLP) 86
Aortic cannulation 91
Atresia and hypoplastic 40
Atrial septostomy 24
Atrioventricular 42
Autologous pericardium 146

## B

Balanced 165
Balloon 24
Bentall 231
Blalock-Taussig shunt 193

## C

Canal type VSD 154
Cardiac catheterization (cath) 19
Cardiac chambers and ventricular
    loop 43
Cardiac positions 32
Cardiac registry 29
Cardiac TAPVR 357
Cardioplegia 93, 105
Cardiopulmonary bypass 65
Chest X-ray 17, 19
Chylothorax 60
Circulation 10
Clubbing 119
Complete atrioventricular septal
    defect 164

Computed tomography (CT) 17
Computed tomography (CT) scan
    19
Concordant and discordant 40
Congenital 1
Congestive heart failure (CHF) 22
Consanguineous 4
Consanguinity 4
Coronary sinus 140
Crisscross heart 45
Cryoprecipitate or cryo 102
Cyanosis 7

## D

Deep hypothermic circulatory
    arrest (DHCA) 105
Defibrillation paddles 106
Dextro 34
Dextrocardia 34
Diaphragmatic plication 59
DiGeorge syndrome 251
Donald Ross 219
Double outlet right ventricle with
    a doubly committed VSD 261
Double outlet right ventricle with
    noncommitted VSD 261
Double outlet right ventricle with
    subaortic VSD 260
Double outlet right ventricle with
    subpulmonary VSD 260
Doubly committed 42
Down's syndrome 3, 163
Dr Hisashi Nikaidoh 293
Dr Mustard 281
Dr Senning 281

## E

Echocardiogram (echo) 19
Eisenmenger syndrome 119
Electrocardiogram 17
Electrocardiogram (ECG or
  EKG) 19
Embolism 21
Endocarditis 19
Extracorporeal membrane
  oxygenation (ECMO) 112

## F

Foetal and newborn 10
Fontan procedure 193
Fresh frozen plasma (FFP) 102

## G

Giancarlo Rastelli 290, 291
Glenn shunt 193

## H

Haemodilution 98
Heart murmur 7
Helen Taussig 117
Heparin 73
Hippocratic fingers 121
Hypothermia 105

## I

Infants 48
Inflammatory response 99
Infracardiac TAPVR 357
Infracristal 152
Inlet 42
Interventional cardiac
  catheterization 26
Intracardiac anatomy 38

## J

Jatene 281
John gibbon 65

## K

Kawashima procedure 182
Konno procedure 229

## L

LeCompte manoeuvre 286
Levo 34
Levocardia 34

## M

Magnetic resonance imaging
  (MRI) 17
Magnetic resonance imaging
  (MRI) 19
Major aortopulmonary collateral
  arteries or MAPCAs 203
Marfan syndrome 3, 229
Mesocardia 37
Muscular VSD 154
Mustard operation 250

## N

Newborns 48
Normally committed 42

## O

Oscillating or vibrating sternal
  saw 70
Ostium primum 139
Ostium secundum 137
Outlet 42

## P

Packed red blood cells (PRBCs)
  103
Partial or incomplete atrioventri-
  cular septal defect 164
Patent 121
Perfusionist 66
Peritoneal dialysis catheter 104
Phrenic nerve 57
Platelets or thrombocytes 102
Postoperative bleeding 100

Potts shunt  173
Premedication  52
Preschool age  50
Pulmonary hypertension  22, 101

**R**

Rashkind and Miller  24
Recessive  4
Reciprocating sternal saw  68
Recurrent laryngeal nerve  57
Retrograde cardioplegia  82
Richard Van Praagh  29

**S**

Sano  337
School age  50
Senning  250, 279
Septa  42
Sequential segmental
    classification  30
Sinus venosus  140
Stella Van Praagh  29
Supracardiac TAPVR  357
Supracristal  153

**T**

Taussig-Bing anomaly  264
Temporary pacing wires  89, 108
Thebesianvii veins  83
Thoracic duct  57

Three types of cardiac position 34
Toddlers  49
Toronto general  236
Transcatheter device occlusion
    125
Transitional or intermediate
    atrioventricular septal defect
    165

**U**

Ultrafiltration and modified
    ultrafiltration  104
Unbalanced atrioventricular
    septal defects  165

**V**

Venous cannulation  92
Vent  94
Ventriculo-arterial connections 42
Viscero-atrial situs  31
Vivien Thomas  117

**W**

Walton Lillehei  65
Waterston/Cooley shunt  173

**Y**

Yasui procedure  351